T0260894

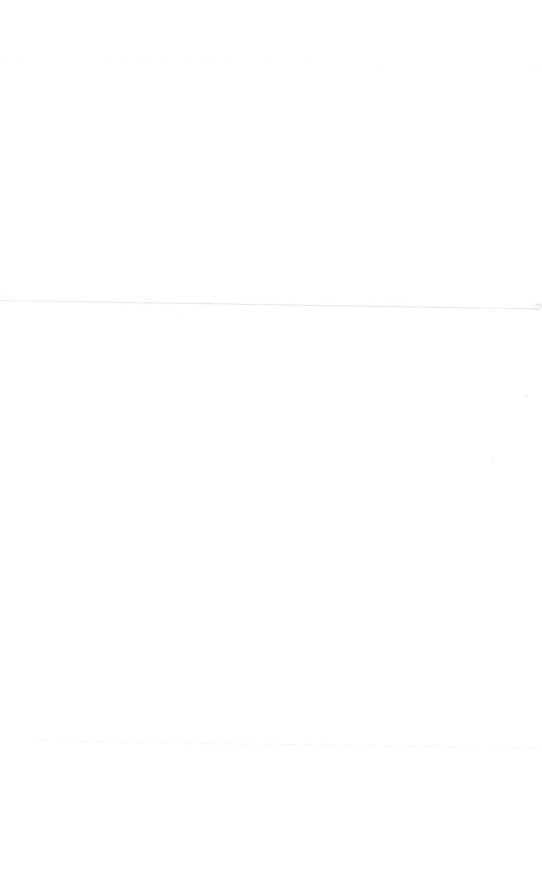

Rotten Bodies

Rotten Bodies

*Class and Contagion in
Eighteenth-Century Britain*

Kevin Siena

Yale

UNIVERSITY PRESS

NEW HAVEN AND LONDON

Published with assistance from the foundation established in memory of James Wesley Cooper of the Class of 1865, Yale College.

Published with assistance from the Annie Burr Lewis Fund.

Yale University Press books may be purchased in quantity for educational, business, or promotional use. For information, please e-mail sales.press@yale.edu (U.S. office) or sales@yaleup.co.uk (U.K. office).

Set in Fournier MT type by IDS Infotech Ltd.
Printed in the United States of America.

Library of Congress Control Number: 2018940908
ISBN 978-0-300-23352-0 (hardcover : alk. paper)

A catalogue record for this book is available from the British Library.

This paper meets the requirements of ANSI/NISO Z39.48-1992 (Permanence of Paper).

10 9 8 7 6 5 4 3 2 1

For Kate

Contents

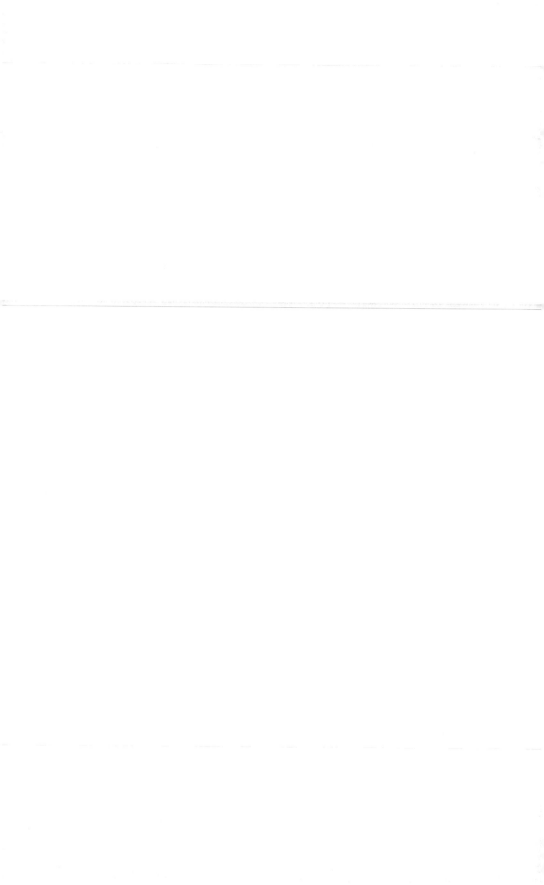

Acknowledgments

I have incurred many debts while writing this book. Indeed, it has taken so long to complete that I am certain to forget some of the many kind people who took the time to share their expertise, alert me to sources, correct grievous errors, read drafts, or act as sounding boards. To them I apologize. I honed the logic of this book on such willing and patient sharpening stones as Tim Hitchcock, Robert Shoemaker, Simon Devereaux, Mary Fissell, Donna Andrew, Jeremy Boulton, Olivia Weisser, Matthew Newsom Kerr, Susannah Ottaway, Mark Harrison, Erica Charters, Graham Mooney, Jonathan Reinarz, Paul Slack, Margaret Pelling, and Joanna Innes. The anonymous readers also offered much valued advice in their reports. Naturally, none of them bears responsibility for any blunders that I have persisted in making despite their sage advice. Considerable good fortune came my way when I was welcomed as a visiting fellow by the History Department of Oxford Brookes University in 2011. The entire department deserves my thanks, but especially Alysa Levene and Jane Stevens Crawshaw, who not only made my visit intellectually thrilling but acted as such gracious hosts. Several chapters simply could not have been written without the research conducted on that trip. It was also there, in seminar presentations at Oxford Brookes and at Oxford University's Wellcome Unit for the History of Medicine, that I first began to shape and articulate the core ideas found in this book. Audiences at too many conferences to name similarly have my gratitude for their many insights, but special mention is owed to the community of the Institute for the History of Medicine at Johns Hopkins, which thoroughly workshopped Chapter 1. I benefited from the hard work and care of many librarians and archivists, including those at the British Library, Bodleian Library, Wellcome Library, London Metropolitan Archives, Royal Free Archive Centre, Westminster Abbey Library and Muniments Room, Guildhall Library, Senate House Library, and the Bata Library at Trent University. I am grateful for the keen editorial eye of Dan Heaton at Yale University Press. Preliminary research was supported by the Social Science and Humanities Research Council of Canada.

My children, Simon and Isabelle, have lived with this book for their entire lives. I thank them for sharing their dad when he has had to travel, for schlepping to England for reasons they cannot possibly have understood at the time, and for making me smile when I come home each evening. And now we come to the point where these acknowledgments must fail, for I am just not a good enough writer to convey my thanks to Kate. While I was in the middle of writing this book life handed our family a terrifying shock. She steered us through it. She encouraged me to continue with my work when doing so was the last thing on my mind. In a very real sense this could not have been written without her. Compared with all that she gives me, dedicating this book to her is a paltry gift, but one I offer with all my love.

Rotten Bodies

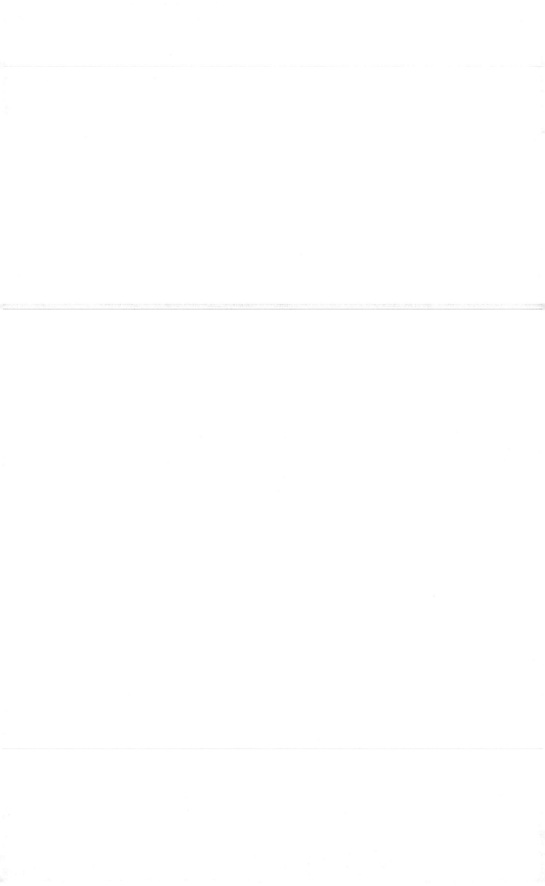

Introduction

Poore People, (by reason of their great want) living sluttishly, feeding nastily
on offals, or the worst & unholsomest meates; and many times too long
lacking food altogether; have bothe their bodies much corrupted, and
their Sprits exceedingly weakened: whereby they become (of all
others) most subject to this Sicknesse. And therefore we see the
Plague sweeps up such people in greatest heapes.
—Steven Bradwell, 1625

Predisponent Causes [of Plague]: Whatever increases the putrescency
of the system, want of exercise and usual labour, especially in the lower
class, who are accustomed to it, and, in consequence of this to perspire
copiously; living on putrid animal food; want of fresh vegetables,
good bread, sugar, wine and other antisceptics; foul air, in consequence
of nastiness, and the want of free ventilation, which is seldom found
in the houses of the lower class of people, among whom this disease
is most frequent and fatal.
—John Gregory, 1788

The British frequently pinned their epidemics on the poor. We have known
this for a long time about seventeenth-century plague and for an equally
long time about nineteenth-century scourges like cholera.[1] They did so as
well during the period that fell between these bookends, but this remains to
be shown.

Steven Bradwell, an early-seventeenth-century London physician, and
John Gregory, a late-eighteenth-century professor of medicine at Edinburgh,
spoke a surprisingly similar language. They shouldn't have. A vast intellectual gulf comprising a scientific revolution and subsequent Enlightenment

separated them. Yet near the end of the eighteenth century Gregory still imparted to his students as doctrine the same idea that Bradwell had advanced in the 1620s: The poor were uniquely prone to diseases like plague because their bodies were corrupt. The poor had rotten bodies, and as a result they were dangerous.

In this book I argue that the plebeian body was the subject of constant concern in medical discussions of epidemic disease throughout the period of roughly 1650–1800. By charting this concern from its inception in the early seventeenth century through the dawn of the nineteenth century, I hope not just to fill a gap in the history of long-eighteenth-century medicine but to demonstrate how a focus on the plebeian body may offer a new way to move in a direct line from the age of plague to the age of cholera.

It turns out that plague cast an enormous shadow over eighteenth-century culture. As places like London became ever more crowded, respectable eighteenth-century Britons remained frightened of catching diseases from the lower orders long after plague's last attack in 1666. Lacking the benefit of our historical hindsight, they had no idea that plague would not return. Indeed, they feared few things more. For too long, however, body counts have driven where historians of epidemics have focused. Eighteenth-century Britain was gripped by a powerful fear of epidemics, one for which greater scrutiny is overdue. As Enlightenment Britons prepared for the epidemic they felt sure could alight at any moment, they relied on history as a medical tool, looking back to plague times for lessons that might protect them. One of those lessons—that epidemics usually started among the poor—rang especially true.

As the eighteenth century unfolded Britons applied these lessons to diseases other than plague. We will see that Britain had quite a scare when plague struck Marseilles in the 1720s. But it was spared then and for the rest of the century. In the absence of actual plague, a form of fever took center stage.[2] A contagious ailment frequently called "pestilential" or "putrid" fever became the primary disease associated with the poor. Intimately linked to plague—many thought it merely a weaker version of the disease—it came to have many names. One of the most common was "jail fever," a designation that highlights a context that, for a period, came to dominate discussions of domestic epidemics involving the poor. If a plague was going to strike, many thought it was more likely to start in a prison than anywhere else because here was a dense concentration of plebeian bodies in a filthy, tight

space. Debates about prisons provide one of the clearest venues for charting
the influence of medical ideas about poor bodies beyond the realm of medical
treatises. Prison reformers worked closely with physicians, and as prison
reform became a national issue in the 1770s, debates about the plebeian body
made their way into the national political conversation. Moreover, concerns
expressed by citizens in newspapers about jails reveal just how strongly class-
based contagion anxieties influenced the general public.

I contend that such anxieties need to be registered as a more important
eighteenth-century cultural force than has been allowed, producing episodes
like what I call the Jail Fever Panic of the 1770s and 1780s, which itself
needs to be acknowledged as a significant development in British history. For
example, it played a much greater role animating the prison reform movement
than is usually allowed, as propertied Britons moved to protect themselves
from a significant health menace, creating heroes out of men like John Howard
who risked their lives inspecting the toxic spaces within prisons in the name of
national safety. While the era of Howard represents the moment when contagion anxieties about prisoners reached their zenith, we will see that such
concerns were much older. Hence a series of chapters on prisons in earlier
periods must precede our reevaluation of Howard's era in order to spotlight
how indebted late-eighteenth-century developments were to earlier ideas and
practices. We will see that a particular 1750 epidemic in London with profound
class dynamics (explored in Chapters 4 and 5) provided a touchstone event
stirring medical concerns about prisons to new levels. Moreover, a recurrence
of this episode in 1772—the same disease, killing the same kinds of people in
the very same room, and blamed on prisoners from the same jail—provided
the immediate spark that ignited the Howardian golden age of British prison
reform. It is also important that many discussions of disease in prisons focused
on the peculiar plight of debtors. In Chapter 3 I explore a revealing conun-
drum. While debtors were officially impoverished (in the sense that they
lacked the resources to pay their debts), they often hailed from the propertied
classes and thus complicated eighteenth-century opinions about "the poor."
Calls to cordon off such respectable prisoners from threatening poor ones
nicely demonstrate the eighteenth-century tendency to respond to contagion
through mechanisms of class segregation.

However, although we will explore prisons for several chapters, we
will see that they represented but one forum of danger. If prisons bred
disease by crowding putrid bodies in filth, then slums were dangerous by the

same logic. Indeed, it was the poor neighborhood that had formed the crux of worry in plague times, and this fear never dissipated. Whether in London in 1665 or 1720, or in new industrial towns at the end of the eighteenth century, beliefs about the dangers of plebeian bodies powerfully informed anxieties about the health hazards associated with slums. In Chapter 7 I thus look primarily to 1790s Manchester, where concerns about poor neighborhoods and epidemics in early cotton mills demonstrate how, even at the dawn of the nineteenth century, ideas rooted in early modern plague still represented cutting-edge science—ideas that continued to inform medical thinking well into the choleric age of the Victorians.

Although we will chart the history of an idea, it is important to make the point that the idea itself should not be seen as the catalyst of events. Quite the opposite. Events often drive the story, for we will see that contagion anxieties were episodic, flaring up at particular moments because of developments on the ground: the great epidemic of 1665/6, the Marseilles plague scare of the 1720s, or outbreaks of fever in London courtrooms in 1750 and 1772. It may well be that an institutional disease—so-called jail fever—became such a prominent worry precisely because urban Britons saw their cities changing, with institutions for the poor mushrooming all around them in the form of hospitals, orphanages, and, perhaps most important, workhouses, drawing together hundreds of paupers at a time under a single roof. Social tensions informed doctors' and reformers' claims about the poor and what should be done about them. Roy Porter, with his characteristically good ear for medical metaphors, paraphrased respectable eighteenth-century complaints that "the miasmatic plebs were threatening to pollute everything."[3]

Scholarship on the eighteenth-century poor has largely explored their interactions with one of two administrative systems: the criminal justice system and the poor law. When eighteenth-century medical historians, myself included, have worked on the poor, we have tended to do so through the prism of charity, usually in the form of the history of hospitals. The best work weaves that story into the wider picture of eighteenth-century social conflict and urbanization, and thus has explored medical institutionalization as a way of enhancing our understanding of the contested processes by which a place like London became modern. Intellectual history related to eighteenth-century poverty has similarly tended to focus on debates about the poor within discourses on crime, institutionalization, morality, or social welfare. Science, however, has been largely omitted from these discussions.

For although historians have explored how some of the emerging *social* sciences informed eighteenth-century programs connected to the poor, we as yet lack a history of eighteenth-century ideas about the poor drawn from the biological sciences.[4]

This is a shame because we know how vital Enlightenment-era medicine was to the larger project of the history of the body. Cultural historians have demonstrated that the eighteenth century was a crucial moment in the development of both gender and race, as medical science inscribed these identity categories onto bodily structures, whether skin, hair, nerves, genitals, or skeletons. As research matured scholars like Dror Wahrman, Kathleen Wilson, Londa Schiebinger, and Felicity Nussbaum highlighted the dynamic interplay among these categories, which were not formed in isolation but were mutually constituted.[5] Doctors' theories about the biology of the poor offer an opportunity to bring class more fully into this conversation. To put a fine point on it, class was, at least in certain respects, physiological in the eighteenth century. I will have my hands full making this case for class and so can address gender and race only sparingly in the body of the book. However, my Conclusion takes the form of a lengthy thought-experiment suggesting how I believe we can situate the medical construction of class dynamically alongside a category like race. This research may be especially timely, as developments in the field of epigenetics have recently called attention to the possible impact of poverty at the genetic level, signaling a potential renaissance of the idea that class may have a physiological component.[6]

Of course, the applicability of the category class for the period before the nineteenth century has been the subject of considerable debate. Challenges have argued that the premodern social order did not neatly conform to Marx's description of it, that the term *class* is anachronistic before industrialization, and that contemporaries lacked class consciousness because they identified themselves according to factors other than their relationship to production. The linguistic turn had a multivalent impact on this scholarship, at once leading to important work on the discursive construction of class, but also calling the utility of the concept further into question and fueling heated debates on the so-called death of social history.[7] Certainly, for the premodern period this development had the effect of encouraging many young early modern scholars to focus much more attention on categories like gender. It was hardly a secret for my generation of early modernists (those of us working on doctorates in the mid-1990s) that a dissertation on class had become a risky proposition for one staring down the barrel of the academic job market.[8] To be clear, this book is a cultural history of ideas, not an economic analysis of the social order. I seek to contribute to scholarship that has explored how identity categories in the seventeenth and eighteenth century were discursively constructed, relational, and contingent. I hope to add to the study of class a new body of texts—seventeenth- and eighteenth-century medical treatises about contagion—that have yet to be mined in the exploration of how social rank was embodied.

Given the debates, it is important to establish that the term *class* was indeed employed in the period under study. John Gregory, whose words appear at the start of this Introduction, has already provided evidence. Penelope Corfield's important exploration of the issue has shown that the term was used as a specific referent of the socioeconomic order as early as the 1650s. Her somewhat passing insight about class's importance within science—specifically as a category in taxonomies alongside terms like *genus, family,* and *species*—offers a tantalizing clue about the potential of looking to scientific texts on this issue. Indeed, one of Corfield's primary examples of early attempts to sketch Britain's class structure was the 1753 five-class schema offered not by an economic or political thinker but by a medical man, London apothecary James Nelson, who opined: "Every nation has its Custom of dividing the People into Classes." Of course, there was little agreement on what those classes might be. Daniel Defoe suggested that there were seven, seventeenth-century statistician Gregory King eight. Keith Wrightson has noted that although the language of class can certainly be detected by 1700, many formulations of the social order in the early modern period tended to opt for terms like *rank, order,* or *sorts.* His work demonstrates beyond doubt that by the eighteenth century there was considerable attention to social rank, even if the ideas and nomenclature remained in flux, and even though economic status was only one of many means by which eighteenth-century Britons forged identities.[9] As heated as the debates have been, historians generally agree that whatever class might be, it took form during the eighteenth century. This position is held both by those who tether class to industrialization, and who thus point for its similar origins sometime after 1750, and by cultural historians like Wahrman, who, studying political discourse, sees the emergence of the modern language of class in the era of the French Revolution.[10]

Concerning these debates, I share Wahrman's assessment that, despite the attacks on his position, E. P. Thompson's formulation has held up rather well. We will see that it certainly has much to recommend for medical historians. Thompson described class functioning in the eighteenth century as what he called a "field of force," not unlike competing magnets that drew people toward bipolar positions of the patrician elite or plebeian poor. This is not to suggest that interim levels between these poles were nonexistent or without influence. But Corfield's study goes some way to confirm Thompson's picture, showing that many eighteenth-century descriptions of the social order avoided the messy issue of sorting out fine medial gradations and opted instead for simplistic formulations that described society as devised of the rich and the poor, a tendency she calls "rich/poor dualism." Wrightson similarly found that early formulations of the social order were frequently expressed through a binary language of "sorts," with the "richer" or "better" sorts distinguished from the "poorer" or "meaner" ones. Speaking about the seventeenth century, Craig Muldrew concurs and comments on the moral rather than strictly economic assumptions that drove these characterizations, noting, "In this sense there is an element of what I think we could term class formation occurring here with group generalisations being made in moral terms, based on wealth, between the better and poorer in society." An early form of class consciousness—or perhaps more precisely consciousness *about* class—was the wide agreement on the rather obvious fact that there were considerable distinctions between the wealthy and needy.[11]

Important to our study, doctors discussing contagion endorsed precisely this view. Coming chapters will show that throughout the long eighteenth century physicians tended to speak in binary terms. Of course, we know that this was a vast oversimplification of the social hierarchy. Leaving aside the complex middle orders, the poor were themselves frequently compartmentalized: the working and nonworking poor, the urban as compared with rural poor, skilled artisans and unskilled laborers, the respectable poor versus criminals, worthy objects of charity or immoral beggars.[12] However, when doctors discussed class in treatises about epidemic disease, they were remarkably inexact. They usually made no such distinctions and instead spoke in vague formulations. In the quotations opening this chapter Bradwell simply identified "Poore People," while Gregory never bothered specifying whom he meant by "the lower class." Physicians' laziness in defining their categories turns out to be a key element of our story. When they wrote in these ways they did not break from tradition but rather employed the pervasive parlance of morally tinged rich/poor dualism. In practice there were many Britons with the means to stake out positions between the patricians and the plebs. Physicians were among them. But as early ideas about class took form, they were often expressed in terms of stark simplicity.

Wahrman has commented on the subtle power of this eighteenth-century vagueness. Perhaps what made medical proclamations about the poor so effective was this very simplicity. By avoiding the more complex middling orders, and by deftly failing to clarify whom they meant, physicians discussing epidemics were able to make powerful claims about social rank that were unlikely to be challenged or analyzed too closely. Moreover, because these claims were expressed outside of political or economic genres there was little encouragement for readers encountering them to dwell on socioeconomic or political details. The point of the discussions in which these claims were advanced—what philosopher John L. Austin called their illocutionary force—always addressed a different, and at that moment much more pressing concern: deadly disease. In other words, the purpose of reading a treatise on plague or fever was not to ascertain England's social structure but to learn how to prevent or treat contagion. Thus medical treatises provided an effective medium for advancing claims about class that were unlikely to be challenged on finicky details. Yet because doctors were medical experts, their words carried the weighty epistemic authority of Enlightenment science, despite conveniently lacking much of its alleged penchant for specificity. We will see that physicians' proclamations about poverty were so sweeping that, although they may have had in mind specific groups like the urban poor or shiftless beggars, their words read as universal claims about the poor generally. Such formulations would certainly frustrate social historians hoping to identify precise economic gradations or looking for expressions of working-class consciousness. But for the cultural historian of the body these unreflective assertions offer quite rich material. Thus, in the context of eighteenth-century medicine, economic rank—poorly defined—was deployed as a legitimate scientific category. Although the physiological elements of class in the eighteenth century have received little attention, the recent work of Timothy McInerney on notions of blood and the nobility may suggest that that is changing. Moreover, Roy Porter and George Rousseau's study of eighteenth-century gout, a disease that they called "the most visible insignia of the upper-class," offers at least one example of how doctors in the period wrote about classed physiologies specifically within discussions of susceptibility to a particular disease.[13]

Yet we still may face an issue of terminology. Some may contend that, given the period under study, I should simply employ a safer term such as *order* or *sort* and be done with it. Allow me to address that point by way of a thought-experiment. Imagine for a moment that early modern historians were inhibited from using the term *gender* to explore ideas about maleness and femaleness, or that scholars exploring Europeans' early ideas about the distant peoples they were colonizing were similarly inhibited from employing the term *race*. In both cases arguments similar to those that contest the use of *class* in early modernity can be easily imagined. First, neither *gender* nor *race* was a primary term used by the historical actors. Commentators had numerous terms for speaking about sexual difference, but *gender,* though in use, was hardly their only choice, sharing time with a panoply of terms (for example, "the stronger/weaker sex"), while contemporaries referring to non-Europeans were just as likely to use terms like *nations, peoples,* or *savages* as they were to use *race*. Second, just as traditional ideas about the social order differed markedly from later ones (moving, for example, from vertical conceptions of the Great Chain of Being to horizontal conceptions of class), early modern ideas about race and gender were vastly different—many would say incommensurate—with the nineteenth- and twentieth-century notions that replaced them. In the case of gender, in the early modern period a one-sex model dominated, under which men and women shared the same biological structures, while the scholarly definition of gender, which distinguishes it from biological sex, was still centuries off. For race, the dominant theory was monogenism, the notion that all humans were part of a single family, descended from Adam and Eve, and that physiological difference resulted primarily from climate. Early moderns thought and spoke quite differently about the things we call race and gender.[14] Yet we do not inhibit early modern scholars from using those terms, and we are undoubtedly correct not to do so. Our understanding of the generation of these concepts over the *longue durée* would be much obfuscated if we create an unbridgeable gulf between early and later modernity.

Andy Wood comments on this very point for class. In addition to providing compelling evidence for class consciousness in the seventeenth and even sixteenth centuries, Wood highlights the cleaving impact of the decision to bind class to industrialization and nineteenth-century developments like the nation-state: "Social historians have failed to communicate across the historiographical and conceptual divide of the Industrial Revolution. Early modern social historians have long been hesitant in using the term 'class' as an analytical category, convinced that it was a product of nineteenth-century modernity."[15] One of the unintended consequences of setting early and later modernity on opposite sides of industrialization has been to discourage analyses that might cross this great divide. However, if instead of privileging modes of production we allow ourselves think in terms of the history of ideas, then a different event than industrialization can take center stage: namely, the Enlightenment. That development, of course, is viewed not as a sharp divide between early modernity and the modern world but rather— because it dates to the later seventeenth century and is often seen as birthing modernity itself—as a kind of connective tissue between eras. This is certainly how the period looks within the scholarship on ideas about human variety as evidenced by the work on gender and race; it therefore seems a worthwhile exercise to explore ideas about the related category of class in this period through the prism of such quintessentially enlightened actors as doctors.[16] I contend that since contemporaries were using the term *class* to refer to the social hierarchy as early as 1650, and since even cautious historians agree that the term is useful by the 1780s (at the very least as a shorthand), it makes little sense to try to shift within this book from *rank* or *sort* in the early chapters to *class* in the later ones—if only because the point at which such a shift might make sense would be hopelessly difficult to pin down and inevitably contested. Is it 1700? 1750? 1780? (Moreover, if anyone should decide such timing, it should hardly be a medical historian!) The point is, seventeenth- and early-eighteenth-century commentary about economic strata clearly influenced and developed into late-eighteenth- and early-nineteenth-century ideas about what we call class. This is especially true if we look at medical discussions because, as the opening quotations suggested, doctors' claims about the plebeian body were remarkably durable over a very long time. Put simply, when we consider physiological claims about the poor, it makes far more sense to connect the seventeenth and nineteenth centuries than to divide them.

It is also important to clarify that unlike scholars like Wood, I am not attempting to demonstrate working-class consciousness. To do so one would need to explore entirely different records from those I have examined, records that would shed light on how poor and working people thought and acted.[17] Indeed, one of the most important developments of the past twenty years regarding the British poor has been the flourishing of an approach that seeks to do just that, sometimes termed a "New History from Below."[18] Historians have interrogated sources like institutional and criminal justice records, reading them against the grain to recapture the outlooks, experiences, and survival strategies of the early modern and eighteenth-century poor. My first monograph employed this very methodology, highlighting the agency of the London poor as they negotiated their way through various institutions seeking medical care for syphilis. For this book, however, I have moved in a decidedly different direction. By and large it is a history of ideas *about* the poor. Whenever possible I strive to reflect on how the discourses under exploration may have affected the lives of common Britons. However, it is primarily an exploration of how the propertied conceptualized the needy. In this way it is a book meant to raise questions for further research. For example, whether and how the British poor internalized the images that eighteenth-century doctors conveyed about them must for now remain open to speculation. It is likely that they understood well the contagion anxieties that so animated their social betters. Following on Tim Hitchcock's research on London beggars, I think it entirely possible that some paupers strategized to play on these fears at opportune moments. However, more often they probably had to work oppositely, to convince landlords, employers, or other authorities that they were healthy, clean, and thus not dangerously contagious. This was probably a particularly sensitive issue for that huge class of workers who resided in the very homes of their polite employers, namely domestic servants. Moreover, we must never forget—even though it is something that my sources allowed me to analyze only occasionally—that plebeian men and women must have been themselves struck by the fears that the discourses under study did so much to fan. After all, they inhabited the spaces and lived the lifestyles that the experts claimed were treacherous. Impassioned pleas in court not to be imprisoned in filthy jails and daring prison breaks at the height of jail epidemics offer a few tantalizing clues about how the poor reacted to episodes like the Jail Fever Panic.

In terms of ideas about the poor, those found within plague and fever treatises unsurprisingly reflect those encountered throughout wider British culture. We are told that opinions about poverty shifted during our period, thanks largely to the tumult that remade the British social and economic landscape over that time. When our study begins, the impact of the Price Revolution was already making itself felt. Population boom and inflation drove structural changes characterized by the consolidation of land in fewer hands, enriching the gentry and above but rendering a huge swath of the underclass poorer. A new kind of poverty can be detected by the early seventeenth century, one affecting a larger portion of the population than ever before and not confined as was previously typical primarily to the aged or infirm. As poverty deepened and expanded, opinions toward it toughened, exemplified by the criminalization of behaviors like begging and vagrancy.[19] Although real wages rebounded some by the eighteenth century, the pressures of urbanization resulted in the institutionalization of poor relief in workhouses and considerable concern about poverty and disorder expressed through worried commentary on issues from crime and drinking to irreligion and sexuality.[20]

Feelings remained mixed, however. When caricatured by Hogarth, the eighteenth-century poor could be menacing and riotous but also sympathetic and worthy. Lynn Hollen Lees and Alysa Levene confirm that ambiguous attitudes toward the poor characterize much of the eighteenth century. Vestiges of the *noblesse oblige* survived alongside the newly hardening opinions so that many among the downtrodden remained eligible for sympathy and care, whether through voluntary charity or the poor law. David Hitchcock's recent study of vagrancy similarly conveys a variegated set of representations in the century after 1650, though with complaints about immorality seeming to have greater impact as time went on. Lees then suggests, with support from scholars like Gertrude Himmelfarb, that by the end of the eighteenth century a further shift can be detected whereby the darker attitudes toward *some* of the poor increasingly came to apply to all of them. Poor law debates show that by the 1790s Victorian-style complaints about so-called pauperism were emerging to craft the poor as a separate group, one "pushed outside the world of the respectable" and characterized by moral failure. Perhaps tellingly for our purposes, Lees explains that by this point the poor were often represented as physiologically distinct in graphic depictions, and that enmity frequently expressed itself through commentary on filth and disease: "Perhaps, many thought, urban pollution and disease came not from economic ill health but from moral failure. In the conception of the pauper, we can see the English wrestling with multiple anxieties. They transferred their hostility to the dirt, disease, and decay of early industrial society onto the figures of the dependent poor."[21]

This fusion of the medical and the moral can be detected even earlier, however. Even in the seventeenth century we already find doctors medicalizing the emerging resentment toward paupers, as when they advanced theories about the physiological dangers of such cardinal sins as "idleness." At various points we will encounter physicians offering medical support to policing discourses by presenting the poor as predisposed to disease because of intemperate habits, sexual license, or proclivity to drink. In Chapter 1 I begin to unpack what I call the moral biology of the British poor, whereby transgressive actions were inscribed physiologically with considerable relevance for medicine. However, the issue is hardly clear-cut, because even into the age of the New Poor Law, with its heavily moralized lens, illness remained a widely accepted excuse for poverty, the sick often spared the harsh rhetoric thrown at beggars or vagrants. Thus medical presentations of the sick poor were just as frequently sympathetic or morally neutral as they were condemning. For example, we will see that the relatively mundane issue of diet occurs as a much more common feature in theories of plebeian fever than did such morally loaded issues as alcohol or sex. Doctors' treatises thus reflect a somewhat ambiguous eighteenth century, with some overtly condemning the poor but many others resisting that urge. In terms of contagion, the poor were undoubtedly dangerous, but not everyone held that this was their fault.

Such varied constructions of diseases like "jail fever" thus reveal that commentators often made of them what they wished. But that does not mitigate the fact that the epidemics that caused so much consternation killed. A disease of many names—we will see it variously termed pestilential, putrid, malignant, or violent fever, spotted or petechial fever (because of its skin eruptions), or jail, hospital, ship, or camp fever (because of where doctors believed it struck)—it took on a modern title as the eighteenth century closed: typhus. The disease of that name is a lethal bacterial infection spread by the human louse, one which indeed can prey on the poor and dispossessed, as grim experiences of refugee camps attest. Anne Frank in Bergen-Belsen concentration camp may be its most famous victim. It is also a disease with a rich history. Harvard bacteriologist Hans Zinsser's groundbreaking 1935 biography of the disease paved the way for an approach to medical history that is still practiced today. Charles Creighton explored numerous typhus epidemics in his even earlier and equally foundational *History of Epidemics in Britain* (1891). However, I resist treating the disease as modern typhus to avoid the problems associated with retrodiagnosis.[22] Given the state of early modern records and the worldviews of those who recorded them, it is often impossible to know what people actually suffered from. In Chapter 6, for example, I show that coroners' reports on prison deaths were often vague to the point of being diagnostically useless.

Even if for a moment we were to take at face value that "fever" was frequently typhus, it remains difficult to correlate medical and popular discourses with what may have been occurring on the ground. For example, historical demographers have long pointed to a vital shift in the eighteenth century when mortality began to fall steadily. Life expectancy improved during the last decades of the century, and whereas scholars like McKeown once attributed this to better nutrition, it now appears to have resulted primarily from declining mortality due to disease, with typhus playing a prominent role (alongside smallpox) in this improving regime.[23] For example, all of the eleven severe mortality crises identified by Wrigley and Schofield (when mortality spiked 30 percent higher than the norm) occurred before 1750, and the last second-order crisis (mortality elevated 20 percent) occurred in the early 1760s. Fever deaths recorded in London's *Bills of Mortality* increased steadily to a peak in the 1740s before starting a clear, steady fall that continued well into the nineteenth century. Scholars thus suggest that mortality from typhus in places like London was probably worse in the early and middle parts of the century than it was after about 1770.[24] The problem for us is that it was in these later decades of the century that public concerns about typhus spiked to their highest levels. In other words, the Jail Fever Panic may have coincided with an ebb rather than a flow in actual mortality rates from typhus (to the extent to which these can even be estimated). Such a disconnect supports my reading that to understand the contours of eighteenth-century debates about poverty and fever it may be most fruitful to look to particular noteworthy epidemics that captured the public imagination. We will see that it was often the issues of who died and where, rather than how many died, that mattered most.

That said, there is no reason to doubt that the poor suffered terrible rates of infection and mortality. Commentary linking poverty to diseases like plague and fever hardly arose from thin air. We know that factors like malnutrition led the British poor to be physically shorter than the eighteenth-century peerage, though the impact of such factors on disease remains debated.[25] Plague was famous for ravaging poor neighborhoods in the seventeenth century, and demographers studying the eighteenth century correlate areas of poverty with higher rates of fever burials thanks to factors like poor housing and crowding, with periodic spikes associated with local economic crises, especially following wars. Certainly after 1750 a shift seems under way that produced the clear social gradient in mortality statistics apparent by the nineteenth century.[26] It can be fascinating to think about how premodern and current understandings of the disease could at times be so close and yet so very far apart. In cases when episodes of fever were caused by the bacteria *Rickettsia prowazekii,* doctors who presented poor hygiene and crowding as contributing factors made claims that hold up nicely today. Indeed, scholars like Landers, Chambers, Riley, and Razzell have all suggested that some of the hygiene polices that we will see doctors advancing—such as boiling clothing, which would have helped eradicate lice and which became more feasible at the end of our period with the increased availability of cotton cloth—probably contributed to the improving epidemiological regime.[27] Yet when doctors based their advice on suggestions that the disease was airborne and caused by the foul breath of paupers whose blood was putrid, they made assertions that belong to a different world, one that modern bacteriology can do little to help us decode.

Indeed, among historical diseases "fever" is notorious as one of the most amorphous, mercurial, and complicated disease concepts of the premodern age. What will become for us just a symptom was for centuries a disease unto itself, one with a dizzying variety of forms—a point that complicates attempts to generate epidemiological information from burial data. I should stress at the outset that mine is not a comprehensive history of eighteenth-century fever; many ideas related to many different forms of fever receive no coverage.[28] Thankfully, Christopher Hamlin's recent biography of fever tackles the disease head-on with excellent results. One of his many contributions is to spotlight how certain fever discourses framed the eighteenth-century poor as "biological land mines," a term that nicely captures the sense of looming danger underpinning much of what we will explore. Only Candace Ward's excellent chapter on jail fever in her literary analysis of fever in the novel goes as far to highlight the question of class in eighteenth-century fever texts. However, much of the best work on fever remains focused on the nineteenth century.[29]

Although my work concerns the earlier period, I will try to converse with this scholarship. That said, I break with one of its traditions. Inspired by the groundbreaking work of Erwin Ackerknect, considerable effort has sorted through Victorian debates between contagionists and miasmatic theorists, often to plot this divide politically. I am able to move beyond this question in part because Margaret DeLacy's recent companion volumes on the genesis of contagion theory have done much of the heavy lifting for the long eighteenth century. DeLacy's earlier work already showed that the divide between contagionists and miasmatic theorists was far from clear-cut.[30] To the contrary, attempts to categorize physicians in this way often reveal how blurred the lines were. Doctors could be contagionists for some diseases and miasmatists for others, and many used *contagion* and *miasm* interchangeably. Margaret Pelling showed that even in the early nineteenth century a muddy middle ground characterized by the phrase "contingent contagionism" frequently prevailed.[31] However, through painstaking research DeLacy has now picked through the complex structures of seventeenth- and eighteenth-century disease theory to chart the gradual emergence of more clearly defined contagionism, especially after 1750. Her intellectual prosopography demonstrates that the most committed contagionists tended to share characteristics and backgrounds, especially as religious dissenters educated outside Oxford and Cambridge.[32] For our purposes, this question matters surprisingly little, because when it came to the issue of the poor and their role in epidemics there was virtually no debate at all. The stances of many of the leading contagionists identified by DeLacy—doctors like Richard Mead, John Pringle, and John Ferriar—will be explored as the book unfolds. But even when clear opponents can be identified, one often finds quite standard thinking about paupers' infectiousness.[33] Throughout the following chapters we will see that assumptions about plebeian putridity lay quite deep, and that doctors who debated other issues or held competing theoretical frameworks never bothered to fight about whether the poor were predisposed to epidemic disease. Seventeenth-century plague treatises had established that point as doctrine, and it found no opposition in the eighteenth century.

Moving beyond such debates can allow for new perspectives. One such is an ability to showcase continuity, in this case between Victorian approaches to public health and those of the preceding two centuries. Historians of fever and public health often see origins of nineteenth-century features in the ideas and practices of the very late eighteenth century, with John Pickstone's work on 1790s Manchester particularly important regarding strategies that would target the urban poor, especially the establishment of fever hospitals and intervention in plebeian homes via inspection and fumigation.[34] Indeed, DeLacy's task—charting how the precursors to germ theory gained traction over time—leads her to frame the coming of fever hospitals rather as novel harbingers of modernity.[35] Here our visions differ, for in Chapter 7 I will demonstrate that these developments were themselves still firmly rooted in much older thinking about poverty, disease, and the body. My application of the term *public health* to the eighteenth century follows that of Roy Porter, who challenged reductionist caricatures of the period as one with no public health movement because it lacked statutory initiatives on the scope of Chadwick's.[36] Pickstone's useful insights about continuities between 1790 and 1840 can thus be supported but considerably expanded on the earlier flank. Debates about fever in early factory towns had clear implications for modernity (in the form of industrialization), so it is understandable that historians would look forward from them, to good effect. However, we will see that building *to* the 1790s, rather than starting from them, can be equally valuable, if only because medical thought and action near the end of the century remained so powerfully influenced by plague. The focus on the poor, the centrality of putridity, the reliance on isolation hospitals—institutions that we will see openly compared to pesthouses—the regimens of hygiene and fumigation, the popularity of vinegar sniffing for personal protection, and the eagerness with which reformers looked to continental plague lazarettos as models for domestic institutions: these will all demonstrate how thoroughly steeped in early modern plague was a place like 1790s Manchester, an example that is so commonly framed as a seedbed of public health modernity. The final chapter thus concludes with a Coda that argues for acknowledging just how deep and old were the traditions that the Victorians maintained. When the sanitarians pointed to filth as a cause of fever (specifically identifying putrefaction as the key pathogenic process), identified the poor as the primary target of health initiatives, stressed technologies of hygiene, and colored these efforts with a hearty dose of moral condemnation, they took part in a conversation that had been going on for two centuries. The scholarly focus on separating contagionists from anticontagionists and the drive to stress what was new about Chadwick's program has had the effect of obscuring just how deeply indebted the sanitarians were to ideas that date back to plague times—ideas rooted in theories of the plebeian body that physicians can be found espousing at every point from 1625 forward. Even beyond the sanitarians, the legacy of plague may have echoed farther still in the work of British eugenicists, who were hardly the first to speculate on the degenerate—and heritable—physical constitutions of the British poor.

The nineteenth century, of course, lies far beyond the realm of this book. In *Rotten Bodies* I aspire merely to enhance our understanding of epidemic disease in the late seventeenth and eighteenth century. I argue that a focus on the history of the body as it relates to class holds the key for understanding the most worrying medical fears of the period. If my findings have value for scholars of modernity, all the better.

1. Plague, Putrefaction, and the Poor

This book concentrates on the perceived threat of plebeian bodies in the eighteenth century. One goal is to demonstrate that the ideas fueling those anxieties were quite old. Enlightened Britons inherited a set of ideas about impoverished bodies. In this chapter I explore what they inherited. By the time of the last great English plague epidemic of 1665–1666, medical constructions of the impoverished body demonstrate all of the features that commentators would recycle, reformat, and redeploy for the next century and a half. The formulation of this class-specific physiology centered on theories about plague.

Because it did, the origins of the pathogenic plebeian body may lie even earlier. However, because this book will progress to the dawn of the nineteenth century, we must satisfy ourselves with picking up the tail end of plague's story in Britain, with apologies to readers interested in medieval plague. Unlike most studies on plague in England, this one is oriented forward from 1666, beginning where most narratives end.[1] It makes the case that plague continued to exert enormous influence on British culture. We know that the British never again witnessed another domestic plague epidemic, but eighteenth-century Britons can be forgiven for not resting assured. We will see that they thought and wrote about plague constantly, time and again looking to past epidemics for useful knowledge. Therefore, for a chapter, we must also turn our minds to the seventeenth century. Early modern plague discourses bequeathed many legacies to Enlightenment culture, none more important than the belief that the bodies of the poor were different and dangerous.

At times, plague discourses pointed a moralizing finger at the rich, attributing epidemics to divine punishment for the elite's luxury or castigating civic leaders who fled. Such works tended to cast the urban poor as victims. It is difficult to determine precisely when attitudes shifted, but there seems little doubt that as the sixteenth century wore on, plague discourses increasingly portrayed the poor as a source of disorder and danger. We know that attitudes toward the poor moved in this direction, whether due to the influence of the Reformation, of urbanization, or of the Price Revolution. Samuel Cohn has recently argued from Italian material that by 1575 prevailing opinion held that plague was a disease of the urban poor; John Henderson locates the same shift a few decades earlier. Brian Pullan has proclaimed that by 1577 it was "axiomatic for many observers that plague . . . flourished chiefly among the poor." The leading historian of plague in England, Paul Slack, concurs that the link between poverty and plague "was already a cliché" by 1603.[2]

Historians have analyzed the connection between poverty and plague in numerous ways. Scholars like Slack, Cohn, Pullan, and Ann Carmichael have explored how plague policies reveal social tensions, especially those initiatives that targeted paupers, prostitutes, and immigrants. Historians of the state have pointed to the importance of these elements in plague orders to processes of state formation. No one analyzing burial data denies that the urban poor were struck especially hard. Contemporaries noted the high mortality rates in underprivileged parishes, crystallized in the *Bills of Mortality*, which presented plague deaths in the staggering cold facts of numerical tabulation. By the early seventeenth century writers like Thomas Dekker were calling it the "beggars plague," while Londoners frequently termed it simply the "poore's plague."[3]

Attention to the relationship between plague and poverty has thus tended to focus on social policy. Despite the depth of this scholarship, there remains an issue that rewards closer inspection: physicians' theories about *why* plague ravaged the poor. When plague historians address medical theory, they tend to focus on debates between adherents of two theories, of contagion and miasma. In this case, ideas about class were not matters of debate: the belief that epidemics began and raged most fiercely among the poor was a mainstay of both contagionist and miasmatic articulations of plague. Scholars also often embed discussions of the poor within larger analyses of issues like religion or social policing, analyzing medical theories about the poor only to make larger points about how plague discourses voiced concerns about disorder.[4] Of course, doctors certainly did that. Yet there is value in pursuing medical theories about the poor in their own right, if only because in the rest of this book I will demonstrate that these ideas had remarkably long lives.

Rotten Bodies: Putridity and Predisposition

Andrew Wear notes that plague forced doctors to reflect on the bodies of the poor more than ever before. Never had physicians had such a pressing reason to theorize about the physiological implications of status. Wear is correct that despite seeming singular in history, plague was not treated as unique but was situated within the traditional medical framework that explained all sickness.[5] Two elements of traditional medical thinking were vital to understanding how doctors attributed plague to the poor: putrefaction and predisposition. Let us address each in turn.

Putrefaction was central to sixteenth- and early-seventeenth-century pathology, a key element of Galenic thought, which would remain influential even as new paradigms arose. Disease was not merely an imbalance in one's humours, as is so frequently noted about classical medicine. It was often construed as rot. Blockages that caused fluids to stagnate or putrid matter that entered the body and spread corruption provided common explanations for many early modern diseases. "Health consisted in clearing and cleansing the body," writes Wear, and a wide range of purging therapies aimed to rid the body of foul matter lest it initiate the hazardous process of putrefaction. The suppression of menstruation, to take an example explored by historians of the female body, was one of many worrying situations in which the body found itself full of dangerous matter that might rot. The utility of putridity in explaining disease probably resulted from links between physical corruption and death that daily experience suggested. Rotting food, infected wounds, and festering corpses all suggested a connection. Those links were strengthened by Christian teachings that the Second Coming would reverse the corruption that followed death, and by Aristotelean philosophy that presented putrefaction both as a cause of death and a source of new life. Maggots growing out of rotting flesh offered a common example to make this last point, one perhaps most famously expressed by Carlo Ginzburg's doomed miller forced by the Inquisition to explain his cosmology that "the world had its origin in putrefaction."[6]

Hamlin shows that putrefaction was prominent in theories of fever dating back to Galen, and it was clearly central in explanations of plague from at least the fourteenth century. The bad air often thought responsible for epidemics was frequently said to stem from sources of rotting filth: refuse pits, dung heaps, marshes, and the like. Vanessa Harding and Mark Jenner have each pointed to the epidemic concerns embedded in municipal efforts to keep streets clean or monitor burial practices. Of course, moral and spiritual connotations of corruption mattered, so claims about the spiritual causes of plague rooted in sin should be understood as intertwined with medical claims about putrefaction: spiritual corruption and physical corruption went hand in hand.[7] That said, it is sometimes this linking of medical discourses to spiritual ones that has tended to draw scholarly attention away from deeper pursuit of medical claims in their own right.

Miasmatic theorists identified sources of filth and putridity to explain the evil vapors that caused plague, usually following their noses to identify foul-smelling situations. Health concerns about foul smells both predate and antedate the era of the current study and warrant invoking the influential ideas of Mary Douglas about pollution and Alain Corbin on odor. However, the connections between putrefaction and plague were also accepted by contagionists. The external source of the bodily corruption that plague brought on was equally easy to envisage as a particle or as a vapor. Cohn's analysis of Italian physicians' theories illustrates that while some believed filthy water contained putrid "atoms," others warned that it emitted "putrefied fumes." Frederick Gibbs demonstrates how the concept of poison bridged the gap between contagionist and miasmatic paradigms and that its connection to putrefaction was especially influential in early formulations of plague, points that Wear supports. Moreover, DeLacy's history of contagionism and my own research on the pox (syphilis) bear out that many doctors trying to explain communicable disease in the age before germ theory latched on to the explanatory convenience provided by the notion of poison and thus stressed putrefaction. Whether encountered via the bite of a mad dog or a venomous snake, during sex with a poxed partner, or in breathing in the "effluvia" exhaled by a plague victim, minuscule particles of a poison, doctors throughout the sixteenth, seventeenth, and, we will see, the eighteenth century believed, were essentially corrupt and carried the power to turn healthy matter to their own putrid quality. Like a single bruised apple in a basket, contagious effluvia could corrupt the entire system. If the metaphor of rotting fruit seems hackneyed, it is worth pointing out that William Austin's 1666 poem *Epiloimia epe; or, The anatomy of the pestilence* depicted contagion in the crowded city thus: "Fruit hoarded up, rots others by the touch."[8]

Throughout their discussions of plague's causes, treatments, symptoms, or preventatives, early modern doctors advanced the almost unanimous position that plague was putrid. For example, Paul Barbette argued that plague carbuncles arose from corrupted blood that was "apt to putrifye." Preventative strategies like burning fires and perfuming the air went hand in hand with advice for general cleanliness. Thomas Brasbridge's 1572 plague treatise gives a representative list of commonly held sources of plague. Corrupt air arose,

> particularly, in a fewe houses, or streetes, through the stinche of chanels, of filthie dung, of carion, of standing pudles, and stincking waters, of seeges, or stinking privies: of sheding of mans bloude, and of deade bodies, not deeply buried, (which happeneth among Souldiors:) of common pissing places, and such like. Finally a gret company dwelling or lying in a smal roome, (especially if those roomes be not very clenly kept, & perfumed,) do ingender a corrupt aire, apt to infect those that are in it: whiche infected persons and their infectious clothes, may infect a whole Citie.

Plague was generated in corruption and it corrupted in turn. Readers curious to know whether they or others were infected were told to look for symptoms that signaled internal corruption; those that stank threatened. Brasbridge followed classical theorists in seeing malodorous breath, fetid sweat, or foul-smelling urine as the clearest symptoms of internal rot. He recommended a diet that limited the possibility of generating corrupt humours.[9]

Brasbridge's treatise is telling in another way because it expressed a second crucial component of early modern thinking on epidemic danger. He listed four causes of the disease: 1) divine wrath, 2) astrological influences, 3) corruption of the air, and 4) "the aptnesse of mans body, through evill humors to receive ye effecte of a venomous aire, putrifying and corrupting the bodie." Some bodies were more apt than others to sicken during an epidemic. The common term for this quality was *predisposition*. This point offers the opportunity to raise a name that any discussion of early modern contagion must address, that of Gioralomo Fracastoro. While scholars question the novelty of the Italian physician's *De Contagione* (1546), he is often understood as the paramount architect of contagion theory. The antiquity of contagion theory is not immediately pertinent. However, Fracastoro makes two important claims that are. First, he placed corruption squarely at the heart of his theory: "Without some sort of putrefaction, there can be no contagion."[10] Moreover, like Brasbridge, he claimed that some bodies were predisposed to contagious illnesses. And he made the important direct link between predisposition and class.

Carmichael concludes her study of plague by examining a key passage from *De Contagione* that addressed a question that had vexed physicians for centuries, namely, why epidemics did not strike indiscriminately. As Nutton has shown, Galen had long ago suggested that contagious diseases struck only bodies "disposed" to receive infection. Both Galen and Fracastoro used the term *seeds* or *semina* to describe epidemic agents; keeping with that horticultural metaphor, predisposed bodies provided fertile soil for invading particles to take root, while other bodies were less welcoming. This idea accorded with a medical worldview that emphasized individual constitutional differences. It made little sense to a sixteenth- or seventeenth-century doctor to suggest that bodies would react uniformly to any foreign matter, force, or stimulus. Thousands of bodies were exposed to contagious effluvia or foul miasma in an urban epidemic, yet not all of them sickened. When Fracastoro addressed this issue, he pointed unmistakably to physiological class distinctions.

> Now the nobility, on account of their wealth and other conveniences which the populace lacks, can take greater precautions against the sort of contagion that is transmitted from one person to another; but they can defend themselves less well than the populace from the contagion that depends on the air, since that sort of contagion, though common to all, is more prone to attack those who are rather delicate and less robust, and those who are more full-blooded and of a less dry temperament, and the nobility have these characteristics because of their luxury and life of ease. The populace, on the other hand, are more robust and of a drier temperament, because they exert themselves strenuously, and their diet is more frugal.[11]

Numerous elements of this passage are important. First, it is clear that a body's reaction to epidemic disease hinged on its condition before the epidemic hit. As the prefix of *predisposed* suggests, a body's situation *prior* to an epidemic was a crucial variable. Brasbridge went so far as to consider it one of plague's "causes." Thus predisposition to disease must be understood as an essential quality that bodies possessed at all times. One had a level of predisposition to plague whether or not plague visited. Second, predisposition depended on many factors. Fracastoro here cites diet and work; hard-working commoners consuming a simple diet faced less risk than sedentary elites who ate rich food. This claim accorded with the age-old doctrine of the six nonnaturals, one of the longest surviving elements of Galenic medicine. Even after the decline of true humoural medicine—that is, the belief that health and disease hinge on balancing the four humours—it remained a point of doctrine that that health relied on the quality of one's 1) breathing, 2) eating and drinking, 3) sleeping, 4) activity, 5) emotions, and 6) evacuations.[12] This system allowed countless factors to explain sickness or health, and it provided the variability necessary for a medical paradigm based on individual, nonuniform bodies. However, one can see tension between the individual's constitution and the constitutional qualities being ascribed to large groups. Notwithstanding his commitment to individual constitutions elsewhere in his work, Fracastoro was here clearly generalizing about entire social ranks. Bodies internalized their class's lifestyle. Luxury or want, work or idleness, these factors inscribed deep changes in a body with profound implications for disease risk. Embedded in Fracastoro's assertion therefore is the claim that social distinctions were physiologically vital—vital, literally, for it was on these distinctions that life or death might hinge.

Two other elements of Fracastoro's claim warrant attention. First, this particular passage came from a discussion not of plague but of a closely related disease called pestilential fever (*Pestilentibus Febribus*).[13] Scholars often translate this as typhus, though as I suggested in the Introduction, such retrospective diagnosis is not always helpful. Pestilential fever has a long pedigree. Nutton shows that Galenic texts often discussed so-called "pestilent" fevers. Pestilential fever, we will see, was an important disease in the early modern schema. It would be nicknamed jail fever in the eighteenth century, and I devote a good deal of the rest of this book to exploring it. For now, it is important to note that many doctors, dating to classical times, regarded plague as simply the highest form of fever. By the seventeenth century it was a common belief that plague frequently grew out of pestilential fevers. In his treatise on plague Oxford physiologist Thomas Willis warned that improper treatment of patients could "kindle a Fever, which . . . soon turns to the Plague."[14]

This idea received its most important endorsement from Thomas Sydenham, who would be quoted on the topic for more than a century. Sydenham studied the Bills of Mortality and noted elevated rates of fever deaths both before and after epidemics, interpreting them to signal the coming and eventual waning of plague. Sydenham concluded that there must be a class of fever related to plague, which, he deduced, had the same causes and spread in the same way. Drawing on the tradition of Fracastoro and others, he termed this preplague fever "pestilential" or "malignant." For Sydenham, pestilential fever acted just like plague, but was less strong. It was lethal but not as lethal. It spread easily but not as far or rapidly. He then made a key claim, calling pestilential fever "truly of the same Species with the Plague, only 'tis a degree below it." One might be tempted to call it plague light. Sydenham demonstrated how the one disease became the other, describing pestilential fevers intensifying until they simply warranted the new name of plague. Analyzing the winter that preceded the 1665 epidemic, he stated: "[At] the beginning of March . . . a Pestilential Fever, soon after the Plague began to rage." Here his very syntax suggests that one disease mutated seamlessly into the other. It is entirely unclear where pestilential fever stops and plague begins. This suggested two important and worrying conclusions. First, plague had its origins in fever, and second, it was probably never going to be clear whether or not a pestilential fever might intensify into the even more deadly plague.[15] Pestilential fever thus forever contained within it the frightening *possibility* for plague, a quality that we will see terrified Britons into the nineteenth century. Thus when Fracastoro made his claim about elite bodies facing danger from "*pestilentibus febribus*," he addressed an issue of enormous import.

Fracastoro's claim about classed bodies made one further pertinent point. He warned elite readers that they faced the greatest risks in epidemics, while their social inferiors were relatively safe. He did not ascribe responsibility for plague to the poor. This stance is fitting considering that he wrote several decades before the period when Cohn suggests Italian plague theorists shifted to blaming the "plebs." In 1564 English physicians like William Bullein still emphasized the sins of the luxurious rich. His contemporary Brasbridge presented the rich and poor as facing roughly equal risks, though in a way that pointed toward corporeal distinctions between them: "Those things . . . must be avoyded, which ingender evyll humours, or otherwise make the bodie unable to expel evill aire. The firste of these, is the taking of

meate, and drinke out of measure, and too much lacke of it. Of the former
the riche are in daunger: by the latter the poore are pinched."[16] His point
nonetheless conveys the essence of Fracastoro's: social rank, via lifestyle,
had significant implications for disease risk. However, by the seventeenth
century, English readers of *De Contagione* surely would have thought that
Fracastoro had it backward. For by then prevailing opinion clearly held the
poor to be both a main cause of plague and the most highly susceptible to it.

Plague and the Physiology of Poverty

Steven Bradwell's *A Watch-Man for the Pest* (1625), cited in the Introduction,
shows how much opinion had changed by the early seventeenth century.
Medically, Bradwell was a traditionalist. His treatise is broadly Galenic
and emphasizes putrefaction along the lines we have seen. He warned of
vapors arising from such corrupt sources as "filthy sincks, stincking sewers,
channells, gutters, privies, sluttish corners, dunghils, and uncast ditches."
His description of symptoms similarly emphasized corruption: "Urine, and
Sweat, have an abhominable savour; the Breath is vile and noysome; evill
coloured Spots, Pustles, Blisters, Swellings; and Ulcers full of filthy matter
arise in the outward parts of the body." Moreover, he warned that plague
could evolve from fevers. Do not catch colds, he cautioned, "for there upon
follow putrid Feavors: and all of them are friends to the Plague."[17]

Bradwell was also a traditionalist on predisposition. When he came to
that vital question—"what bodies are most, or least apt to be Infected"—he
cited several groups at risk, including children and pregnant women, the
latter because "their bodies are full of excrementitious juices, & much heat."
Then, in the passage that appears as an epigraph to the Introduction, he identified the most susceptible bodies of all. Here it is once more: "*Poore People,*
(by reason of their great want) living sluttishly, feeding nastily on offals, or
the worst & unholsomest meates; and many times too long lacking food altogether; have bothe their bodies much corrupted, and their Sprits exceedingly
weakened: whereby they become (of all others) most subject to this Sicknesse. And therefore we see the *Plague* sweeps up such people in greatest
heapes." Here Bradwell likened paupers' innards to those other sources of
putrid filth that he and others itemized repeatedly. Like dunghills, marshes,
or sewers, paupers' bodies were to be understood as foul sources of corruption, rendering them most susceptible to deadly plague.[18]

Bradwell is especially instructive because he stressed that those factors did not simply make poor bodies disposed to catching the disease. Rather, he emphasized that their putrid humours enabled the poor to *produce* plague. He discussed two kinds of predisposed bodies: those "apt to receive infection from without" and others "from within." Echoing Fracastoro, he suggested that delicate bodies, like those of children, imbibed plague more easily from without. However, Bradwell categorized the poor in the second group, those who caught the disease from within. It may confuse modern readers to envision catching a disease from within oneself. To put it differently, the poor generated it. "From Within, they are most apt, whose veins and vessels are full of grose humours and corrupt juices, the evil matter (being thicke, and therefore cannot breath out through the pores) increasth her putrefaction (by the heat within) unto the greater malignity, and so becometh Pestilent." We cannot doubt that Bradwell implicated the poor here, for we saw just a moment ago that he held their bodies to be full of precisely this kind of corruption. Three further factors are important to note. First, the poor were considered actively pathogenic *before* plague struck. Their lifestyle, in this case their diet and hygiene, rendered their fluids corrupt, suggesting that this corrupt tendency was a quality found in impoverished bodies independent of epidemics. Second, it followed that if plague's effect was to render the blood putrid, and if paupers' blood was *already* putrid, then plebeian blood effectively shared a quality with plague-infested blood. There was an essential affinity between a pauper's blood and a plague victim's blood. Nathaniel Hodges made this point expressly describing predisposed blood as having "so great a Similitude to the pestilential poison, as greatly to encourage its Admission."[19] Finally, impoverished bodies had the dangerous capacity to intensify the malignity of disease agents that entered them. Now we can understand how doctors like Sydenham believed that lesser diseases could morph into plague. Bradwell claimed that when "evil matter" enters a corrupt body, it "increasth her putrefaction . . . and so *becometh* Pestilent." I emphasize "becometh" to stress that the matter was not pestilent when it entered the body. However, when it encountered the corruption therein, its malignancy intensified and it *became* pestilent. A disease that was not plague when it entered a pauper's body had become plague by the time it left. Paupers' blood could manufacture plague. The bodies of the poor were thus pathogenically powerful, capable of turning mundane fevers into the most deadly of all diseases. This concept wielded influence for almost two centuries.

Bradwell implicates the poor in other ways. These are less explicit but so numerous as to warrant attention. Read together, they would have made it impossible for readers to avoid concluding that the poor were dangerous. Take his advice on clothing. Plague's alleged "lurking qualitie" rendered it capable of lying dormant in furniture, walls, or cloth, sometimes for years. His instructions to purchase clothing unlikely to hold infection emphasized such expensive fabrics as silk. Moreover, safety required a large wardrobe to allow frequent shifting and airing. Aware that economic realities limited who could heed this advice, Bradwell recommending buying such a wardrobe "if your purse will serve." It would have been just as difficult to imagine poor Londoners heeding his advice about food, which ran for many pages and instructed readers to purchase only select meats and vegetables that reduced levels of predisposition. And how could a seventeenth-century Londoner not think of poorer citizens' homes and neighborhoods when reading of the dangerous places that safety-conscious citizens should avoid? "At all times avoyd all close alleys and lanes (especially to lodge in them) or neare common sewers, ditches, or such like noysome places. And keepe out of crowds and assemblies of people as much as you may." Bradwell's dictum—"Dwell not in an house that is pestred with much company in little roome"—could hardly have been heeded by those to whom it actually applied. Moreover, idleness, a common moral failing attributed to the poor in the period, was listed as a cause of plague, and the idle were discussed alongside drunks and whore-mongers as those especially prone. Attention to idleness is important because considerable scholarship has demonstrated that assumptions of laziness and unwillingness to work underscored the powerful charge of "idleness" that David Hitchcock tells us became a central defining feature in depictions of the destitute in the period. It was thus no accident that Bradwell cited it. The best regimen therefore included moderate exercise in a closed and perfumed room, even though the many herbs and medicines needed for such perfuming were "costly." Indeed, he included one basic recipe—water, vinegar, and rue—specifically for the poor who he acknowledged could not afford his perfuming concoctions. Finally, working Londoners could not have realisti-cally followed Bradwell's most prominent advice, namely to flee London.[20] Read in its entirety then, *A Watch-Man for the Pest* generated a powerful impression that poor Londoners were precisely the kind of people whom polite Londoners should keep at a distance, if not avoid altogether. Their diet, housing, clothing, work habits, moral failings, and general hygiene, their inability to avoid places with foul air or to preserve themselves from it by way of costly medicines, all contributed to Bradwell's conclusion that the poor had putrid blood coursing through their veins and were thus highly susceptible to plague.

Bradwell appears to offer the earliest English iteration of this idea. It is likely that he was channeling sixteenth-century Italian physicians like Francesco Tommasi, who in 1597 attributed plague to "filthy plebs" and Jews, "whose activities give rise to putrefied blood." For little about Bradwell suggests that he was a particularly innovative thinker. A licentiate of the College of Physicians and son-in-law to distinguished surgeon John Banister, he was admitted to the college without an M.D., in part for his courageous service treating plague in 1593. Michelle DiMeo connects him to the Hartlib circle, and Michael MacDonald suggests that he may have been influenced by Paracelsianism. However, Jonathan Gil Harris is correct to describe his medical thought as a hodgepodge of Galenic humouralism, Hippocratic miasma theory, and Fracastoran contagionism, noting that his explanation of the latter was "too vague to be in any way groundbreaking." Bradwell is best known for his publication of a medical self-help book for the poor and for his role in the notorious Mary Glover demonic possession trial, a case that exemplifies the role of social tensions in such cases. (He helped convict an elderly woman he notably charged with "importune begging.") These details afford us a few hints that he may have had an interest in issues related to the social order.[21] However, we have seen that English plague doctors like Brasbridge and Bullein were already discussing class, if somewhat more ambiguously, in the sixteenth century.

A wider look demonstrates that Bradwell's arguments were typical of seventeenth-century English opinion. Physicians Gideon Harvey and Nathaniel Hodges each witnessed the 1665 outbreak firsthand. Writing during the epidemic, Harvey answered that same perennial question—"Why are some Bodies more exposed to the Contagion than others?"—in traditional fashion, emphasizing predisposition and putrefaction especially among commoners, a point he signals with his reference to alehouses. "Because of their passive disposition of Body and Humours to receive the Infection, and of being vitiated [corrupted] by it; to wit, by foulness of their bodies, abundance of bloud, oppression of the Spirits, aperture of their pores, thinness of texture of body, intemperance, promiscuous converse with all sorts of people, whence the contagion oft lights in Taverns, Ale-houses, &c." Hodges painted a similar picture. He emphasized the dietary origins of putrescence, identifying "common people" whose intemperate diet "very much contribute[s] to that Disposition of Body as made the pestilential Taint more easily take Place. . . . Such a Way of Living may raise the Humours to a Degree of Putrefaction as brings Fevers, very malignant and causes epidemical Diseases." If there were any doubt who Hodges meant, comments in a different text, one written in the midst of the epidemic, offered clarification. Promising more on the topic in his next book he apologized: "I have intentionally omitted very much which may seem pertinent to this business, as to assign the reason why the poor were mostly infected which I might have ascribed to the rotten mutton they fed on the preceding Autume preparing their bodies for the Contagion, their being crowded in little roomes and close alleys, as also their unrestrainable mixing and converse with the infected, and their great want and poverty notwithstanding the Magistrates industrious provision for them." Like Bradwell, then, both Harvey and Hodges pointed to a quality in poor bodies that predated plague, and both used the term *disposition* to describe it. Each emphasized corruption and conveyed it in similar language: "putrefaction," "vitiate," "foulness." Hodges chastised paupers who ate immoderately when food was cheap and thus he, too, colored his picture with a moralizing tone about intemperance that accords in its own way with Bradwell's warning about idleness and Harvey's critique of taverns.[22]

While concerns about alehouses seemed to target the immoral or disorderly poor, claims about diet and living conditions, which were much more prominent in plague treatises, cast a much wider net. Such claims implicated the underclass generally rather than the immoral poor specifically. These assertions allowed discussions of the pathogenic plebeian body to cut across, even to resist, those categories into which early modern commentators often situated the poor. Reformers often set the idle, unruly, or immoral poor apart from the upstanding, hardworking poor. Discussions of social welfare pitting the deserving versus the undeserving poor gave the clearest expressions of these categories, with the so-called "sturdy beggar"—who was fit but refused to work—providing a useful caricature.[23] Yet as we will see throughout the eighteenth century, despite the constant presence of claims linking contagion to disorder or vice, threats about the pathogenic qualities of the plebeian body consistently crept beyond subgroups like criminals or vagrants to voice sweeping statements about the poor generally. Notwithstanding his claim about taverns, Harvey identified poor bodies as sources of plague elsewhere in ways that had implications far beyond alehouses. For example, he listed a series of "nasty trades" alongside the marshes, dung heaps, and other worrying sources of pestilential filth. As working Londoners and frequently the employers of other men, "Tallow Chandlers, Butchers, Poulterers, Fishmongers and Dyers" probably would have considered themselves a cut above the drunken vagrants and beggars often targeted in plague orders. But as far as Harvey was concerned their filthy environments rendered their bodies just as corrupt and dangerous.[24]

Moreover, Harvey highlighted class in his book's title and structure, offering separate discussions of his "curative medicines both for rich and poor." At first glance, his title seems to promise a range of differently priced medicines suitable for all pocketbooks. And indeed, it does. However, a closer reading shows that Harvey's medical distinctions stem from a deeper sense that classed physiologies differed. Compare his medicines for each.

> *Distinction XIV, Preservatives for the Rich*
> . . . The ingredients being prescribed in their substance do not suddenly exhale or depose their virtues, but maintain the bloud in a gentle fermentation for a whole day and night, actuate the spirits, absorbe the intestinal superfluities, reclude oppilations, mundifie the bloud, oppugn putrefaction, gently expel and work out all contagious Seminaries through the pores, and all this without inflaming the body, which makes it sutable to all temperaments.

> *Distinction XV, Preservatives for the Poor*
> Cacochymies or fowl bodies of the Vulgar, contracted through course and dreggish feeding do require strong Purges, or rather vomits once or twice repeated, among which for its cheapness and excellency in evacuating, deoppilating, and expelling all malignity, we prefer this following . . .[25]

Of course, the cheap availability of the common ingredients like juniper berries, rue, and myrrh that followed the second quotation tells part of the story. However, much more telling is how these bodies needed different treatments. The term *gentle* recurs in Harvey's discussion of medicine for the rich, which mildly cleansed delicate elite bodies. Vulgar bodies, on the other hand, needed much stronger medicine, because—and this is the crucial point—they were "fowl." The term *Cacochyme* stemmed from the Greek words for "bad" and "juices" and referred to the physiological state of possessing corrupt fluids.[26] Plebeian putridity thus remained the key issue.

That Harvey's was a common view is demonstrated by his contemporary Thomas Cock, whose plague treatise *Advice for the Poor* also emphasized powerful cleansing, inside and out, for infected commoners. Cock advised that immediately upon suspecting infection, an impoverished Londoner should begin vomiting, and within fifteen minutes take a sudorific to promote sweating. Poor patients should then repeatedly wash themselves and rinse their mouths with vinegar, then be blistered and cupped to draw out putrid matter even further. Cock's advice amounts to an immediate and full body purge based implicitly on the notion that a pauper's body was full of rotten matter that must be powerfully cleansed. Returning to Harvey, it is also important that when he identified diet as the root of paupers' putridity, he again implicated the poor quite generally—orderly and disorderly poor alike. He would do so again when he warned of spaces that polite Londoners should avoid. As in the cases of Brasbridge's and Bradwell's treatises, one wonders how respectable readers could have thought of anyone but their poorer neighbors when they read: "Avoid passing close, dirty, stinking, and infected places, as Alleys, dark Lanes, Church-yards, Chandlers shops, common Alehouses, Shambles, Poultries, or any places where old houshold-stuff is kept, as musty beddings and hangings, for it is experienced, nothing breeds or retains Pestilent Atoms more than woollen, and feathers." Finally, Harvey confirmed the danger of plebeian bodies' power to generate plague from lesser diseases. Explaining why readers should avoid crowds, he identified the power of human breath to intensify malignity. "Nothing subministrates apter matter to be converted into pestilent Seminaries than peoples steams and breaths, especially of nasty folks, as beggers, and others: whence those houses happen to be soonest infected, that are crouded with multiplicity of lodgers and nasty families."[27] While Bradwell and Hodges suggested dangerous matter was converted into plague *within* a poor body, here Harvey suggested that a pauper merely needed to breathe on it to ignite a pestilential conflagration. Thus, while Harvey clearly had an axe to grind about the disorderly poor in alehouses, his other claims spoke much more broadly, breaking society into two simple groups: "rich" and "poor." Here is Corfield's "rich/poor dualism."

Wear confirms that medical writers typically presented the poor "as an undifferentiated whole." Rather than fine-grained status distinctions, most seventeenth-century plague treatises employed just "two clear categories: the well-to-do people of repute and the disreputable poor." Wear further shows that such thinking colored the thought of other seventeenth-century theorists, including Thomas Lodge, who based his *A Treatise of the Plague* on a sixteenth-century French treatise. Lodge clearly linked plague to poverty, exclaiming, "Where the infestion most rageth there povertie raigneth among the Commons." One of his more telling suggestions was a policy governing travel to be enforced according to status. Lodge instructed the lord mayor and sheriffs not to "suffer[] any of those to enter their Citty that come from such places as are suspected, except they be men of note, of whose prudence and securitie they may be assured. For it is not always a consequent, that all the inhabitants of a Citty are always infected, especially when they are men of respect, who have the meanes, and observe the methode to preserve them-selves . . . but for such as are vagabonds, masterlesse men, and of servile and base condition, for such I say, they ought not to be admitted."[28]

The authorities listened. Although the policing of beggars during epidemics is well known, it is useful to revisit such orders, even if just for a moment, to read them in light of medical theory. Consider, for example, the 1630 orders issued by London's lord mayor. The sheer proximity of rules about vagabonds and those about filth expresses dynamically the underlying medical assumption that paupers' bodies were, like dunghills, sources of dangerous physical corruption.

> First, that all the severall Inhabitants within this City and Liberties thereof, doe from hence forth daily cause their houses to be kept sweet, the streets and lanes before their doores to bee paved, and cleansed of all manner of soile, dung, and noisome things whatso-ever, and the channels thereof to be kept cleane, and washt, by water to be poured down, or let running into the same.
>
> That no Vagrants or Beggars doe presume to come, or presse together in Multitudes to any Buriall, or Lectures, or other publike meetings, whereby to seeke or gaine reliefe as hath beene lately vsed, but that they and every of them vpon every Buriall, doe repaire to such places to receiue the Almes, Charity or Reliefe, as they shall have notice given them by the Officers of the Parish, wherein they doe reside.
>
> That no idle Vagaband, and vagrant Persons doe presume to come, wander or remaine in and about this Citie and Liberties thereof, either to begge reliefe or otherwise. And if any of them shall

be found, or taken to offend therein, Then they and every of them to be apprehended by the Constables and Warders within this Citie, and being punished, to be passed away according to the Lawes and statutes of this Realme, in that case made and provided for.[29]

Ridding the city of beggars' foul blood went hand in hand with removing other rotten substances.

This is not to suggest that the doctors led the way. As Carmichael notes of contagion theory, physicians like Fracastoro trailed behind social policy, offering theoretical justification for practices like quarantine a century after the fact.[30] Still, even if English doctors were merely sanctioning practices that were already moving ahead, by medicalizing the assumptions implicit in plague orders they created a powerful complex, one that took on a life of its own over the next two centuries. However, the inscription of the classed body proceeded even deeper.

Depauperated Blood

We saw that Nathaniel Hodges's *Loimologia* (1671) expressed clear warnings about the plebeian body. However, Hodges published an earlier treatise during the epidemic that invites exploration of a different way that discussions of plague and fever inscribed class on the body. His *Vindiciae Medicinae & Medicorum* (1665) advocated the practice of bloodletting for diseases in which "the blood is depauperated." From the Latin *depauperata, depauperated* was a rarely used term meaning to be impoverished. Hodges thus recommended letting "impoverished" blood. Before 1665, *depauperated* appears to have been used in English almost exclusively in an economic sense. For example, though it is hardly exhaustive, *Early English Books Online* yields just a handful of sixteenth- or early-seventeenth-century vernacular texts using the term or its derivatives, all of which convey literal economic impoverishment. The definitions in Thomas Elyot's 1538 dictionary and Thomas Blount's of 1661 are almost identical, demonstrating that on the eve of the great epidemic its medical definition had still not come into regular English usage: Elyot: "Depaupero, rare, to impoverysshe, or make poore." Blount: "Depauperate (depaupero) to impoverish, to make or become poor."[31] That Blount's dictionary promised to explain the terms of "divinity, law, physick . . . and other arts and sciences" suggests that the term's medical use was rare before the 1660s. That was about to change.

The first English language texts to use *depauperate* in a medical sense appeared during the 1665/6 epidemic. Hodges's treatise responded to a series of critiques of Galenic medicine by members of the Society of Chemical Physicians, especially George Thomson's 1665 *Galeno-pale; or, A chymical trial of the Galenists*, which criticized phlebotomy for plague.[32] Thomson warned that by traditional Galenic treatments like bloodletting "the Malignity [is] detained, the Blood made restagnant, the Vital Spirits depauperated, losing their activity and force, becoming torpid and careless to preserve themselves, and the Morbifick matter more tenacious." In his response, Hodges did not question that blood or spirits could be "depauperated," merely that such patients benefited from bleeding. Determined to have the last word, Thomson countered with his own plague treatise, the 1666 *Loimotomia*, which again described the bodies of plague patients as "depauperated."[33] Three treatises published during the epidemic described the blood of plague or fever patients as impoverished. What did it mean?

A fourth text sheds light on how this economic term was applied to the blood during the great epidemic. Though it does not concern plague directly, John Smith's 1666 treatise on the diseases of old age picked up this new rhetoric that the epidemic seems to have spawned. Smith describes sanguification, the process by which the heart turned the chyle into nutritious blood, blood that was then depleted when it transferred its nutrients to the body. Smith uses economic terms throughout his explanation of the process, employing five different synonyms for poverty to characterize blood bereft of nutrients. He calls such blood poor, low, mean, impoverished, and depauperated. He calls fully nourished blood rich. These phrases all appear in the same paragraph:

> . . . imparting its power and life to the parts that are nourished by it, it becomes weak and much *depauperated*. . . . Such a vast difference there is between the bloud in the Arteries newly brisked in the fountain, and that in the Veins *lowered* and *impoverished* with its journey. . . . He . . . shall call the *rich* bloud going out in the Arteries, Aerial, Jovial, Spiritual; and the *mean* and *poor* bloud returning home in the Veins, Earthly, Saturnal, Gross.

Later in his text, Smith described the elderly body in terms that similarly fused the economic to the pathological. In old age the body becomes predisposed to disease because the blood and humours "become low and much depauperated, they are diminished, and far less in quantity than they were before."[34]

Can it be that in the midst of the last great epidemic, when voices from all corners warned about the pathological bodies of the poor—emphasizing the quality of their blood—medical writers appropriated the language of poverty to describe the physiological qualities that infected bodies took on? It certainly seems the case, and if so, it accords with developments charted by Jonathan Gil Harris, whose *Sick Economies* explores the pervasive intercourse between seventeenth-century rhetorics of mercantilism and medicine. For example, Harris shows that the term *hepatitis* carried connotations of financial depletion that mirror medical claims about "depauperated" blood.[35]

Although Hodges, Thomson, and Smith offer the first English language uses of "depauperated blood," they were slightly anticipated in Latin. Credit for the application of this economic term to medicine seems owing to physician Thomas Willis, who referenced "sanguis depauperatus" repeatedly in his 1659 treatise on fermentation. It is noteworthy for our discussion that this influential book, which launched Willis's career, contained his related text *De Febribus* (On fevers), which contains many of the key references.[36] It is also worth noting that class pervaded other elements of Willis's medical thought, a point illustrated by Robert Martensen's demonstration that Willis used dissections of differently classed bodies for different anatomical purposes.[37] Throughout Willis's descriptions of fermentation—whether of alcohol, the gestation of seeds in plants, or the generation of putrid diseases—he repeatedly employed (simplistic) metaphors of class, contrasting the binaries of rich and poor, which he correlated to attending binaries of strength/weakness or activity/idleness. Noble or rich blood (or wine) was strong and active; depauperated or impoverished blood (or wine) was weak, idle, or inactive. Consider how plants made seeds. "Nature . . . selects from the whole substance of the Plant the more *noble and highly active Particles;* and these being gathered together with a little Earth and Water, she forms in the Seed, as it were the Quintessences of every Plant; in the mean time, the Trunk, Leaves, Stalks, and the other Members of the Plant, being almost quite deprived of the active Principles, are much *depauperated, and are of less Efficacy and Virtue.*" By associating what was impoverished with what was idle, weak, or lacking in virtue, Willis appropriated not just a word for poverty but a whole set of ideas about it—vagrants were said to share the very same qualities—reconfiguring them and inscribing them on bodies both natural and human. He applied the same principles to blood. For example, he here compares diseased blood to oil that cannot sustain a flame. Infected blood becomes "so *depauperated*, that it will not suffice for sustenance to the vital fire: just as it may be perceived in a Lamp, if the Oyl being continually consumed, in its place be put Water, the Liquor is rendered *poor*, and diluted, that it is not able any longer, to cherish at all the flame of the Wick." He connected this medicalized language of poverty to fever and plague with express links to predisposition theory, which we have seen already heavily implicated class. For example, he warned that "by more depauperating the Blood," one acquired a "Feaverish disposition" rendering one more prone to epidemic fevers. Moreover, putrid fever "rarely begins without a . . . previous disposition," and raises an intense heat that "consumes" the blood's vital spirits and sulfur, leaving "the remaining Liquor of the Blood . . . lifeless and poor."[38]

For Willis, this was the essence of plague/fever's effect on the blood. Putrefaction and predisposition remained as important as ever. But the putrefaction caused by these diseases was now thought to raise an intense heat that consumed the blood's sulfur and spirits, leaving it impoverished. The depletion of sulfur was key to Willis's ideas on numerous topics, a point that indicates the influence of iatrochemistry, a body of seventeenth-century medical thought emphasizing the role of chemical substances over humoural balance, which had grown out of the earlier thought of Paracelsus and van Helmont. It became influential in England during the seventeenth century, inspiring upstart "chemical physicians" like Thomson, with whom Galenists like Hodges locked horns. Willis became one of the foremost iatrochemical physicians in England, who, as a member of the College of Physicians, helped make Helmontian principles more mainstream.[39] Emphasis on the role of sulfur in keeping the blood strong in the face of plague probably relates in some way to the common practice of using sulfur and similar substances like gunpowder to ward off plague in the air. Willis liked the example of wine to explain chemical processes, and his advice to vintners on how to replenish depauperated wines showcases the belief that sulfur was a key element of life, an idea again expressed through economic language contrasting rich and poor, activity and idleness, life and death. Willis characterized depauperated wines—those that were "depressed" or "destitute" of sulfur—as "stale and deadish." However, if vintners would add some "*rich tarter*," such wine would be "inspired with Spirit and Sulphur . . . and recover new strength and vigor." Willis perpetuated these links when applying the terminology of depauperated blood in many later texts, including his plague treatise. For example, he sided with the chemists against bleeding plague patients. Phlebotomy should be avoided "because the Spirits being depauperated, are less able to subdue or repel" the plague's "Poisonous Atoms." However, when it came to the larger causes of depauperated blood—and thereby of predisposition to plague—Willis broke little new ground and merely listed the usual culprits, citing alcohol, "a sedentary and idle Life, a Body full of gross Humors, and stuffed with vicious Juices."[40]

For Willis and a generation of physicians inspired by his work, bodies with depauperated blood were dangerously disposed to plague and fevers because they lacked the strength of "rich" or "noble" blood to repel invading disease agents. Willis's descriptions of impoverished blood actually functioned in two mutually reinforcing ways. On the one hand, his accounts of how plague and fever killed used economic metaphors of status to show that the putrefaction of pestilential diseases rendered the blood like that of a pauper. Sapped of its noble components, it took on the qualities of a pauper: it became weak and idle, lazy and inactive, it lacked "virtue." On the other hand, Willis harnessed this economic rhetoric of status to predisposition theory to explain why some were prone to infection. Before plague ever struck, a pauper's blood was believed to have undergone a chemical transformation that rendered it like his class: impoverished, and thus prone to disease. Plague depauperated the blood, and so did poverty. Plague and poverty thus enacted the very same chemical processes. The environments, diets, or lifestyles that "impoverished" the blood made it weak, idle, and stagnant, sapping it of the strength needed to fend off plague. It was so weak that Willis repeatedly described impoverished blood in terms of death; just as depauperated wine was "stale and deadish," plague- or fever-infected blood was "lifeless and poor." Willis would have undoubtedly read William Harvey, who went so far as to say that blood depleted of spirits was as good as dead. (Incidentally, Harvey probably inspired Willis to compare blood to wine.) Wrote Harvey: "In their different ways blood and spirit . . . mean one and the same thing. For, as wine with all its bouquet gone is no longer wine but a flat vinegary fluid, so also is blood without spirit no longer blood but the equivocal gore. As a stone hand or a hand that is dead is no longer a hand, so blood without the spirit of life is no longer blood, but is to be regarded as spoiled immediately it has been deprived of spirit."[41]

Willis's schema thus presented impoverished blood as having progressed toward death. Depauperated blood was closer to death than rich blood. As we have seen, death was itself frequently understood as a process of putrefaction, one that started in life and proceeded after death, with corpses simply continuing the rot that killed them in the first place. It was thus not a coincidence that one of the first vernacular texts to use Willis's language of depauperation was Smith's text on old age, for elderly bodies were similarly situated in an advanced position on a continuum toward death. It is indeed difficult to discern the qualitative difference between Smith's description of elderly blood with that of plague victims. "I cannot exclude hence from that change that befalleth the bloud and natural humours of the body in the time of age: For they become low and much depauperated."[42] Depauperated blood coursed through the veins of the aged, the impoverished, and the plague-ridden, all of whom were understood by way of their proximity to corruption and death.

Depauperated blood entered the mainstream after plague receded. For example, in 1668 George Acton reported experiments involving blood transfusions for fever patients. A fever victim received lamb's blood, believed to invigorate his own by infusing it with vital spirit. In this case, Acton flipped the usual metaphor; instead of using the language of poverty to describe disease, he used the language of wealth to describe a cure: "Surely such an addition of Vital treasure to the depauperated store, must needs enrich it with new strength, quicken all the Vital faculties, and might with very good reason overcome our Patients Fever." Physician Thomas Coxe's treatise of 1669 linked impoverished blood to immorality and infection with further implications for how medical science was moving to essentialize the pathogenic plebeian body. Coxe gave typical if heavily moralized comments about the constitutional effects of intemperance that included lust, idleness, and drinking. However, he warned that these factors could lead to dangerous "depauperated" blood that could became so fixed in the constitution as to become hereditary. Such acts "cannot but leave ill Impressions behind them, to which we may add Hereditary Distempers. For what is more frequent than for weakly diseased Parents to be further tormented by seeing their Children labour under the same Infirmities; which are either rivitted into the Principles of their Constitution, or sucked in with their milk: from which dispositions they are hardly, if ever freed." Predisposition to disease could thus be fixed in the constitution from birth. Children could inherit depauperated blood and be permanently disposed to diseases like plague. Moreover, Coxe emphasized that depauperated constitutions not only caught diseases easily but could intensify them. When he repeatedly warned that they could "exasperate" fevers, he added credence to long-standing warnings about poor bodies churning fevers into plague, suggesting by extension that paupers might possess that dangerous power right from birth.[43] Thus before the 1660s were even out, theories about impoverished blood had significantly amplified the links between poverty and disease that would only grow stronger as the Enlightenment took form.

Putrid Paupers, Menstrual Women, and the History of the Body

Exploring Willis's discussions of other diseases offers a chance not only to see how widely these same ideas—predisposition, putrefaction, depauperated blood, and heredity—recur, but also to begin to reflect on their significance for the larger historiography of the body. Consider plague's not-so-distant relative, scurvy. Both were classified as "putrid diseases," a category that also included pestilential fever, the pox, measles, smallpox, and "the itch." All were said to stem from putrid blood, and all brought nasty skin lesions produced, doctors believed, by the body's attempts to expel such corrupt matter outward. Like plague, scurvy was linked to poverty, filth, and disorder, particularly among sailors, and it was even used as an insult because, as Bernard Capp asserts, it "suggested physical as well as moral uncleanness." It is thus revealing that Willis repeatedly affirmed that scurvy—or more important, a *predisposition* for scurvy—could be passed hereditarily: "Sometimes it is hereditary, and is propagated by traduction from Scorbutick Parents." Willis called this quality a "taint." Infants could inherit a "scorbutick taint" that "for a long time lies hid" but eventually generates disease. He described the permanence of this disposition, which he located squarely in the body's fluids: such taints "becoming indeed permanent arise by reason of the Blood or nervous Juice." As with plague, its predisposition arose from corrupt food, foul air, idleness, or an "evil crasis of the blood, vitiated by former disease." Thus, again, such inner putridity could generate disease all by itself. More important, Willis applied classed language to scorbutic blood, repeatedly calling it "depauperated," "poor and liveless," exclaiming that it "declines from a noble and spirituous, into a poor and thin Juice." Highlighting filth, he called scorbutic blood "poor and feculent."[44]

We finally learn why the idle were believed so prone to putrid diseases. Perspiring was one of many ways to purge foul matter, making sweat an essential form of excrement, a point that explains why physicians often prescribed sudorifics for plebeian plague patients. However, according to Willis, the lazy were predisposed to putrid diseases like scurvy because their "long Idleness" meant that they did not sweat out bodily waste, which then putrefied. The idle didn't work, thus they didn't perspire enough. In his history of social policy Paul Slack notes that idleness became "the Mother of all vice" during this tumultuous period when the English economy transformed and attitudes toward the poor hardened. The logic of that position directly informed so many of the policies that addressed poverty over the next century, most important the workhouse.[45] And here was one of England's most renowned physicians offering a mechanism to medicalize it.

Willis attributed other lowly diseases to faulty perspiration arising from idleness. Of the skin disease known as the itch he said, "Wherefore, not only they that have been long in prison, but also those who being of a sedentary life, are used to nastiness and sluttishness, do live obnoxious to the abovementioned maladies; inasmuch as the cutaneous humour being not at all eventilated, is corrupted by mere standing, after the manner of putrefying water."[46] Although he does not name the poor specifically, they are heavily implied by the references to prison, idleness, and filth. The point was not lost on later commentators, who quoted this very passage and tacked on the subsequent claim to which it pointed: "which is the true Reason, why the Poor are most obnoxious to Disasters of this Kind." Moreover, if Willis did not specify the poor here, he did when discussing other ailments caused by a failure to purge corruption, and those that were also potentially hereditary, for example madness.

> As the foregoing Cause of Madness sticking in the Blood, is often-times innate or original, so sometimes the same is by degrees begotten, either by an evil manner of diet, or by the suppression of usual evacuations, or by reason of a Feavour going before, or for some other causes, and at length being brought to maturity, breaks forth into Madness. It is an usual thing in great want of sustenance, that some poor people, being constrained to feed only on very disagreeing meats, and of ill digestion, become at first sad, with an horrid aspect, louring and dark, and a little after Mad. The

Hamorrhoids, and the after flowings of Women in Child-bed, being restrained in their flux, or some evil and foul running Ulcers being suppressed, dispose some towards this Disease.[47]

Among numerous things that stand out here is the comparison of the pauper's putridity with that of women with obstructed afterbirth. He made the same connection for scurvy, linking it both to low living and "to usual excretions, as the Piles and monthly Courses being suppressed." Such thinking was not novel. Theophilus Garencières's 1665 plague treatise cited both poverty and suppressed menstruation as causes of plague and tellingly advocated a medication to strengthen the "noble" parts of the blood, which both cured plague and promoted menstruation. An anonymous 1652 treatise was written in lockstep, warning that "women which have not their natural course on them are most prone to receive and take the infection," offering a medicine that promoted menstruation as prophylaxis. This thinking almost certainly inspired Bradwell's attribution of heightened predisposition to plague to pregnant women, for their halted menstruation would have caused them to retain the "excrementitious juices" that he anxiously cited. That physicians categorized the putridity of the poor alongside obstructed women speaks volumes, for it allows us to begin to reflect on some of the larger historiographic implications of the classed body.[48]

Historians of the body have argued that Willis's period of the mid- to late seventeenth century lies at the center of modern constructions of the gendered body. While Laqueur and Schiebinger have suggested that the later Enlightenment marked the point when we see a more fixed, essential female body emerge in the biomedical science of anatomy, a range of scholars have pushed the chronology of that development back to the seventeenth century, including Robert Martensen, whose analysis emphasizes Willis's theories to divergent gender constructs. Mary Fissell's *Vernacular Bodies* is also pertinent, making a convincing case that during the seventeenth century women's bodies were cast not just as different from men's but as frightening. The gendered body was increasingly tied to danger, disorder, and disease in the seventeenth century, the period when Fissell says "the womb went bad." Theories on the improper flow of bodily fluids, menstruation primary among them, provided seventeenth-century doctors with key conceptual tools to essentialize and pathologize the female body. My own work on late-seventeenth-century theories about the generation of syphilis supports that picture. Doctors theorized that lascivious women (often but not always identified as prostitutes) manu-factured the disease by having sex with multiple men, thereby taking in het-erogeneous sperm, which putrefied in their filthy, overheated wombs, much like suppressed menstruation. It is not coincidental that the same mechanism of putridity—and specifically Willis's theories about it—was influential here.[49] Indeed, when Willis theorized about suppressed menses or retained afterbirth, he referenced his wider theories of putrefaction, forging direct connections with his doctrine of fevers and explicitly linking the pathogenesis he associated with depauperated blood to that caused by disrupted menstrua-tion. Just as in prostitutes who retained multiple men's semen or lazy paupers who didn't sweat, obstructed menses, Willis argued, putrefied, and an "enven-omed taint is impressed on the Mass of Blood which . . . produces grievous, and almost malignant Distempers." We should remember that "malignant" fever was one of several names for pestilential fever; the adjective's presence here is no accident. Neither is Willis's description of putrefying afterbirth as a "cadaverous substance," a claim that again linked putridity with death. When different sections of Willis's work are read together, we see that the improp-erly menstruating woman and the inadequately perspiring pauper (and in the work of other doctors the lascivious prostitute) had the same chemical proc-esses occurring within them.[50] Thus doctors at the same moment deployed the mechanism of putridity to forge morally charged constructions of both the gendered body and the classed body.

Historical work on the body has, for the period under question, undoubtedly focused to a much greater degree on gender than on other cate-gories, with race more recently receiving attention.[51] I wish to argue now that medical theories on the plebeian body are no less important to that historio-graphic project. Willis's seamless drift from the putrid plebeian body to the putrid female body should signal that class not only deserves a body-centered history of its own, but that it interacted dynamically with other identity cate-gories that were just then emerging as scientific facts. The work of Gail Kern Paster, in particular, offers extensive analysis of physicians' thinking on women's blood with tantalizing insights for how gendered and classed studies of the body might intersect. She shows, for example, that one of humoural-ism's key distinctions was that women's blood was more inclined to corrup-tion than men's. A tendency toward corruption—with a direct bearing on disposition to disease—thus simultaneously characterized medical thinking about women and paupers. Moreover, the language of class crept into gendered formulations of blood, though in ways that have until now been largely overlooked. It is likely only after considering the cultural import of "depauperated blood" that one can appreciate the subtle importance of early modern claims that men's blood was "richer" than women's. Moreover, Paster's analysis of literary texts occasionally shows that gender and class informed each other, as in cases where plebeian characters were feminized. She is undoubtedly correct that "meanings attached to blood . . . could not be isolated from the inevitably hierarchical structures of social difference."[52]

Just as Enlightenment anatomists would graft gendered and racialized qualities such as nurturing or intelligence upon skeletons, and as physicians would inscribe female irrationality and delicacy on the nerves,[53] I contend that seventeenth-century pathologists inscribed class—understood simplistically according to contemporary rich/poor dualism—onto the body, primarily on the blood. By emphasizing the moral failures of the poor—idleness especially, but also through discussions of hygiene, diet, and environment—Stuart-era physicians did not merely issue warnings to avoid or police the potentially infectious poor. At a deeper level they crafted a coherent set of principles that accorded with widely held medical opinion and that made a strong case for the biology of class. I must note, with apologies, that coming chapters will largely have to explore class independent of other identity markers like gender. Specifically female forms of fever like puerperal (childbed) fever, or treatises on sexual diseases like the pox, which we know continued to emphasize putridity and advance powerful moralizing agendas, may afford future scholars opportunities to probe medical connections between gender and class in the Enlightenment.[54] However, while my task at hand prevents me from pursuing a fuller intersectional study within the body of this book, I will return to the issue in the Conclusion, where I sketch how my findings for class might be integrated dynamically with a category like race.

It is also beyond the scope of the current book to advance confident claims about the timing of developments or their underlying causes. The chronological coincidence of Fissell's picture of the gendered body's turn toward the pathological and my own of a similar turn for the classed body may suggest that the processes were linked. However, we also must read theories about plague and the poor in light of the hardening of attitudes toward poverty that historians have suggested for the period. Population boom in the sixteenth century, economic depression in the seventeenth century, and rapidly advancing urbanization fueled harsher attitudes toward the poor, especially in cities, and there is every reason to presume that these forces powerfully influenced how doctors discussed paupers. Scholars have also made a case for the Reformation, transforming the structures of poor relief and changing ideas about work, poverty, and charity.[55] However, when it comes to medical constructions of poverty, one must also consider plague as itself a catalyst for change.

Plague forced doctors to think and write about the poor more than ever before. As the body count mounted in poor parishes, an obvious question presented itself, and physicians scrambled for answers. Nor were their theories about plebeian bodies hidden away in obscure academic debates; they were voiced in discussions of the most pressing medical problem of the day. From their available intellectual tools, whether those of Galen, Fracastoro, or emerging chemical theories, English physicians reconfigured the plebeian body, making its predisposition to putrefaction its most essential feature. Despite numerous developments in medical theory, no discernable debate raged on the putridity of the poor or their responsibility for epidemics. Core issues like putrefaction and predisposition were mainstays of contagionist and miasmatic thinkers, as well as traditional Galenists and upstart chemists, all of whom advanced a surprisingly coherent set of ideas about the plebeian body, a vision that coming chapters will show continued virtually unchanged despite major scientific development during the next century and a half.

Moralizing claims colored these theories, but I have been at pains—quite by design—to resist emphasizing the policing elements of these discourses. It is vital to stress that the implications of the pathogenic plebeian body reached well beyond specific criminalized groups. Explicit claims and implied assumptions suggested that putridity was an essential quality of plebeian bodies generally. The subtle impact of ideas like predisposition or "taints" lurking in the blood meant that plebeian putridity was merely a *tendency*. It represented a characteristic of bodies that existed independently of epidemics. It was, after all, *pre*-disposition. Moreover, it need not be patently obvious; it lurked in the blood even if no one could see it. Seemingly healthy commoners were thus implicated. Merely living in a small house or crowded neighborhood, being assumed unable to afford quality food or a rich wardrobe, or having been born to parents who could have passed on the remnants of disease—any of these factors implied the possibility, nay probability, of harboring putrid blood. And by that logic, the entire underclass was implicated, a point supported by the lazy manner in which doctors discussed classed bodies in plague texts, using the simple binary of "rich" and "poor" rather than more finely grained distinctions.

That point established, it is clear that concerns about disorder influenced these ideas. The fusion of the physical and the moral in plague discourses dates back centuries and marks a persistent theme in plague studies. It is especially clear in spiritual constructions of plague in which divine wrath dominated explanatory schemata. Spiritual concerns never disappeared from plague treatises, but as the early Enlightenment began to take form, medicalized claims about disorder assumed a greater policing potential as spiritual discourses started their slow fade. Regardless, when physicians discussed the poor, they constructed what I have elsewhere termed a moral biology, the sense that moral action transformed physiology in lasting ways with particular importance for disease risk.[56] Claims about hygiene were never disinvested with moral import; nor were assertions about the sexuality, alcohol consumption, or other forms of intemperance of the urban poor. However, the clearest expression of the moral biology of poverty may have come in assertions about idleness. Seventeenth-century physicians developed a science of idleness, medicalizing the cardinal sin of the late-Stuart poor. Not only did they seize upon a process—faulty perspiration—by which they could imagine idle bodies growing putrid, they compared them to another long-pathologized caricature, the inadequately menstrual woman. Physicians thereby enhanced the credibility of theories about the plebeian body by harnessing them to a much older but culturally powerful complex of ideas. But doctors like Willis did even more. By embedding the language of status in the new science's jargon about disease and blood, they deepened the corporeal inscription of class considerably. Here the impact of the emerging science of chemistry may be important. What doctors like Willis or Thomson said about the plebeian body was not new; how they said it may have been groundbreaking. Depauperated blood had particular qualities: most notably, it was idle. When physicians described "noble" or "rich" blood as active, strong, and full of "vital spirits" and compared it with "impoverished" blood that was inactive, weak, and stagnant, they presented idleness as a feature so essential to plebeian bodies as to characterize their very fluids. So weak and inactive was depauperated blood that doctors repeatedly employed the language of death. Impoverished blood was "lifeless."

It mattered little whether a physician stressed one predisposing factor over another, whether diet, hygiene, or environment. Physicians usually invoked several in concert. By the end of the 1660s physicians had a new term. In some ways it expressed an idea that was already decades old: the poor were predisposed to plague. But it conveyed that idea in a novel and compelling way. Chemically speaking, the poor's blood was like plague-infested blood, even when plague was absent. London paupers walked around daily with a mild form of the same corruption that typified an epidemic. Hodges spoke volumes when he said that paupers' corrupt blood presented "so great a Similitude to the pestilential poison."[57] The difference between poor blood and plague-infested blood was a matter of degree, not kind. And indeed, as Bradwell and others showed, plebeian blood could become plague-infested blood all by itself. Its natural corruption needed merely to intensify. While Hodges was a traditionalist who still spoke in terms of humours, chemists like Willis galvanized the idea by creating an altogether new way of speaking about blood.

There was thus an essential difference that set off the bodies of the poor in a dangerous way, which by the time of the great epidemic found expression in increasingly trendy terminology.[58] Moreover, the application of this term to the poor as a whole, and certainly the speculation that a putrid constitution could be fixed hereditarily, meant that even respectable workers who shunned intemperance could harbor depauperated blood. Two related fears—that the horrors of plague would return, and that the bodies of the poor represented the most likely source of that crisis—carried these ideas into the eighteenth century, as we will now see.

2. Reframing Plague after 1666

Despite reports of its demise, plague was alive and well in eighteenth-century Britain. One of the less-celebrated features of Paul Slack's seminal book is that it offers one of the few studies of plague in England to continue past 1666. However, the title of his relevant chapter, "The End of Plague, 1665–1722," signals that while Slack extended the analysis beyond its usual endpoint, he only postponed plague's inevitable death, moving the goalposts so that the anxiety during the Marseilles epidemic of the 1720s now marked plague's narrative conclusion.[1] Chronologically, this chapter emulates that one, with the variation that I hope not to close plague's story but rather to keep it open. For considerable evidence will demonstrate that plague remained a major concern throughout the eighteenth century. And when early Enlightenment Britons commented on plague, they relied heavily on the ideas we just encountered.

Plague in the Press

Newspapers provide a useful glance at just how frequently plague presented itself in mainstream English culture long after the calamity of 1666. A survey of London newspapers for the latter 1690s reveals a society still on edge about plague, even though it was three decades removed from its horrors firsthand. Britons kept a close eye on plague, monitoring its movements all over the world. In their reportage we can detect if not anxiety, at least palpable caution.

The 1690s do not stand out in the history of plague. Indeed, they were chosen at random for this exercise. However, they do offer a useful period to survey. Roughly three decades after the great London outbreak and three decades before the Marseilles scare, the latter 1690s fall roughly midway between these two larger touchstone events and thus offer a convenient moment to take stock. On the surface, at least within England, it seems as if little regarding plague occurred during the decade. Nevertheless, London readers encountered the disease as a regular feature of their news in the years 1695–1700. Plague would be remembered in works of history, of course, with major epidemics cited among important national events.[2] But as the eighteenth century dawned, plague was hardly a thing of the past. It remained very much a current event.

The most common reports about plague concerned foreign epidemics, newsworthy for their threat both to merchants' lives and businesses and to domestic safety should a ship carry the disease into port. Consider how widely the journalistic eye scanned for such epidemics. Readers were kept apprised of plague in Poland in 1696 and Romania in 1697 and 1698, and of outbreaks as far afield as Colombia and Mexico in 1697, 1700, and 1701. However, epidemics in three locales commanded the lion's share of attention. One was Turkey, where in April 1696 the *Post Man* reported, "Plague sweeps away many thousands there every Day." Plague continued to strike the Turks that summer, and then a series of reports detailed high mortality through late 1697. The safety of Christians in Constantinople was of particular concern. They fled the city in December, by which time it reportedly lost six hundred people daily and the disease had spread throughout the Ottoman Empire. "The Consternation is very great here," wrote a correspondent in February 1698, though one imagines the claim would have also applied to the story's readers, who soon learned that the epidemic had spread even farther. By January 1700, reports of a ship transporting plague to Venice must have been frightening, especially when read alongside reports that it was ravaging islands in the Aegean and was rumored to be in Croatia. Reports on plague in northern Africa parallel these. Articles on the disease in Cairo, Alexandria, Algiers, and the Barbary appeared in 1696 and then again from 1698 to 1700. Mortality rates were frightening: seventy-eight thousand were reported lost in Alexandria and Cairo in July 1696, while two hundred to four hundred people were said to die daily in Algiers by July 1698.[3]

Reports of plague closer to home must have been even more disturbing. Judging by the papers, Londoners monitored an epidemic in northern France closely during the autumn of 1699. Reports demonstrate that some of the ideas about plague that had emerged by 1666 continued to be influential three decades later. For example, the first news that something was amiss was the following late-September report in the *Post Man:* "Some advices say that the Gates of Mezieres, Rocroy, and Charleville are shut up, because of the contagious Distemper that rages therein, and as the Spotted Fever sweeps away a world of people at Amiens, and several other places, they are afraid with much reason of the Plague." (Spotted or "petechial" fever was another common name for pestilential fever.) Thus still current was the fear that a form of fever could intensify into plague. If plague did not yet rage in Amiens, spotted fever deaths signaled that it soon might. There soon followed a more detailed report with a telling correction that further highlights the continued relationship between plague and its usual forerunner, pestilential fever: "The Governor of Namur having received repeated advices, that a violent spotted Fever, or rather the Plague, rages at Charleville, Philippeville, Mezieres, and other Frontiers of France." When Charleville's governors replied, they again underscored the fuzzy relation between plague and fever. The city's physicians denied the presence of plague; "They own however that they have had some Fevers."[4]

Journalists kept readers abreast of the French epidemic for weeks. The outbreak was chiefly attributed to "the Famine the poor People have laboured under in that part of France, for ill food cannot but occasion distempers, and a long experience has convinced the world, that as War begets Poverty and Famine, so Famine produces Plague." Newspapers thus continued to present plague as a fever that started in impoverished bodies and intensified until it broke forth more viciously. If medical theories on poverty and pathogenesis were previously confined to learned treatises, by the 1690s they were mainstream assumptions circulating in the popular press. In these and other ways—including numerous reports of servants infecting their employers and the steady appearance of advertisements for plague medicines[5]—plague continued to occupy the minds of Englishmen as the eighteenth century dawned, and it did so in ways that underscored the idea that socially inferior bodies were potentially dangerous.

Marseilles, 1720–1722: Open Disputes and Silent Agreements

Although reportage on plague was common throughout the late seventeenth and early eighteenth centuries, anxieties spiked in certain periods, none more than when plague struck Marseilles in 1720. As Slack and others have shown, the fear of importing the epidemic spurred the government to quick action, and it passed the Quarantine Act in the winter of 1720–1721. The legislation was controversial for its implications on trade and liberty. The quarantining of ships would remain in place, but public controversy and political pressure led to the gutting of some of the act's domestic policing powers in 1722. Scholars such as Arnold Zuckerman have explored the debates between contagionists, who felt sure that controlling the movement of people and goods was vital to public health, and a small but vocal group of anticontagionists, who countered that such actions were moot because the disease was climatic in nature, spread by miasmatic air, against which the shutting up of houses was pointless.[6] There is no doubt that the Marseilles panic brought debates between contagion and miasma theories into stark relief. However, other debates have received less attention, for example, whether plague could be generated in England at all. While such positions had significant ramifications for policy directives, when it came to depictions of the poor, commentators staking out different positions typically advanced strikingly similar pictures.

Medical and lay commentators relied on two connections made by seventeenth-century doctors: plague's link to pestilential fever and its fundamental connection to poverty. A report in *Applebee's Journal* illustrates both. The reporter explained two claims then circulating about the source of the French epidemic: that infected cotton bales had carried plague from the Levant, or, alternatively, "that it was occasion'd principally by the dearness of Provisions, and the Bad Diet, which the poorer sort of People have been oblig'd to live upon, and that at first this made them sickly; that it began with a new kind of Fever, but that it encreased with the Cause, and at length became Contagious." Such reiteration of seventeenth-century ideas—that plague morphed out of a lesser fever within lower-class bodies—probably owes much to the fact that the Marseilles panic encouraged new editions of seventeenth-century plague treatises. Looking for strategies to protect themselves, Britons in 1720–1721 eagerly consumed old books. For example, a new edition of Hodges's *Loimologia* was advertised just two months into the epidemic. It identified plague as a "pestilential fever," as did the 1721 edition of Willis's *A Preservative from the Infection of the Plague*.[7]

Newly written works propagated the same links. As its title suggests, Richard Blackmore's *Discourse upon the Plague, with a preparatory account of Malignant Fevers* (1721) treated plague and malignant fevers interchangeably. Likewise, the author of *The Great Bill of Mortality: or, the late dreadful plague at Marseilles* (1721) called plague "a continual malignant burning Fever," while the author of a 1721 treatise calling himself only "Phil-anthropos M.D." claimed that his new book "gives an Account of the Nature and Effects of the Plague, Pestilence, Malignant, Contagious, Putrid, and Pestilential Fevers; shewing the Affinity that each have with one another; proving, That they only differ in Degree of Malignity and Contagion."[8] Sydenham's ideas were alive and well in the early 1720s. However, an important authority raised questions.

Richard Mead was the preeminent British physician of his day. Not only did the government turn to him to help craft its quarantine policies, but his *Short Discourse on Pestilential Contagion* went through eight editions between just 1720 and 1722.[9] Although his book strongly connected plague to poverty, one of Mead's theories had the potential to undermine efforts to blame the English poor for epidemics. Mead presented plague as a unique disease in ways that appear to challenge its basis in lesser fevers. In the event, however, Mead ended up largely confirming precisely the point he sought to refute.

Mead believed that plague could not be bred in Britain. "*Plagues* seem to be of the Growth of the *Eastern* and *Southern* Parts of the World, and to be transmitted from them into colder Climates by the Way of *Commerce*. Nor do I think, that in this *Island* particularly there is any one Instance of a *Pestilential* Disease among us of great Consequence; which we did not receive from other *infected* Places." Mead advanced this claim throughout his original treatise, citing histories of imported epidemics and detailing quarantine procedures for ships traveling from exotic locales. He repeatedly identified Africa and Turkey as the most common sources of epidemics, calling the latter "almost a perpetual Seminary of the Plague." His clearest refutation of Sydenham's theory came in his revised eighth edition, in which he condemned as "erroneous" the notion that "plague differs from a common fever" only in "its greater violence." He emphasized specific symptoms—the skin eruptions and buboes associated with plague—as clear marks proving that plague was distinct: "This in particular shews us the difference between the true plague and those fevers of extraordinary malignity, which are the usual forerunners of it."[10]

Mead's claim rested mainly, though as we will see, not exclusively, on climate. Like the human body, the air was said to have a "constitution" and thus possessed its own "predisposition" for disease. According to Mead, excessive heat in Asia and Africa rendered the air putrid, allowing diseases there to rise to much greater heights of destructive power. The cooler English climate could sustain an imported plague, but only until its temperate weather gradually weakened it. England was simply not hot enough to breed plague. Mead considered it "a satisfaction to know, that the Plague is not a Native to our Country," though this was probably cold comfort considering Britain's heavy exposure to the disease via trade. Mead's theory placed him among a growing chorus of voices that used climatic theories to argue that many diseases had exotic origins in the so-called Torrid Zone, where excessive heat and moisture bred danger. His comments are important for our purposes because they stood at odds with long-standing warnings that locally grown fevers could intensify into full-blown plague. Potentially, Mead might exonerate the English urban poor from responsibility for plague. However, the matter was not so simple.[11]

For starters, plague's uniqueness was less clear in Mead's work than some of his seemingly categorical claims suggest. In his unrevised first seven editions, he repeatedly compared plague to pestilential and malignant fever and included plague in discussions of "pestilential fevers." Mead was entirely in line with earlier theorists like Willis when he emphasized putridity and the corruption of the blood as causes of plague, as here, when presenting plague as a kind of malignant fever that intensified out of control.

> The Blood in all *Malignant Fevers*, especially *Pestilential* ones, at the latter End of the Disease, does like Fermenting Liquors throw off a great Quantity of active Particles upon the several Glands of the Body. . . . These, in *Pestilential* Cases, although the Air be in the right state, will generally infect those, who are very near to the sick Person; otherwise are soon dispersed and lost: But when in an evil Disposition of *This* [the air] they meet with the subtle Parts; its Corruption has generated, by uniting with them they become much more active and powerful, and likewise more durable and lasting, so as to form an *Infectious Matter* capable of conveying the Mischief to a great Distance from the diseased Body, out of which it is produced.

Indeed, readers of Mead's 1720 treatise were encouraged to continue seeing plague and pestilential fever as related diseases occupying different points along a continuum. His interpretation of the sweating sickness of the sixteenth century is revealing in this regard. He considered it an example of plague in decline, calling it "a *Plague* abated in its Violence" and "a *Plague* with less-ened Force," claims that barely differed from Sydenham's assertion that pesti-lential fever was "a species of plague but a degree below it." In 1720 Mead had made these claims to support that plague was only ever bred abroad. He recast his claims about the sweating sickness, however, in his eighth edition two years later. Mead now backtracked and allowed that the English sweat might provide an exception to the rule. "Whoever examines the histories of plagues in all times . . . will find very few that do not agree in these essential marks, whereby the plague may be distinguished from other fevers. I confess an instance or two may be found to the contrary: perhaps the history of our own country furnishes the most remarkable of any," that example specified in a footnote: "The Sweating Sickness." Try as he might, Mead could not sever the ties between plague and fever. Moreover, corruption remained essential; plague was "generated chiefly from the Corruption of a Humane Body."[12] Thus by keeping alive the links between fever and plague, and by emphasizing the role of bodily corruption in pathogenesis, Mead sustained lines of thought that were indispensable to the pathogenic plebeian body.

He did so in other important ways, particularly by emphasizing poverty. Climate was merely one factor in his explanations of plague generation in foreign lands. By 1722 Mead had become convinced that Africa was the seat of plague worldwide, repeatedly pointing to Egypt and especially Cairo. Although he wrote at length about North Africa's hot climate and such sources of putridity as animal carcasses rotting on the African plains, Mead advanced a picture of urban poverty quite like those drawn by English writers on plague throughout the previous century. Explaining why Egypt was the "great seminary of plague," he began: "Grand Cairo is crouded with vast numbers of inhabitants, who for the most part live very poorly and nastily; the streets are very narrow and close." For Mead, environmental factors played a greater role than did diet, which we saw was one of the most common mechanisms by which doctors attributed plague to the poor. But this matters little, for the message was clear. Poor urban dwellers, again depicted as overcrowded and filthy, provided the bodies that generated plague. Mead largely transferred to Egyptians many of the seventeenth century's ideas about the plebeian body, including that its fluids were akin to plague-infested fluids and that it shared an affinity with corpses. "It is very plain, that animal bodies are capable of being altered into a matter fit to breed this disease: because this is the case of everyone who is sick of it, the humours in him being corrupted into a substance which will infect others. And it is not improbable, that the volatile parts with which animals abound, may in some ill states of air in sultry heats of Africa be *converted by putrefaction into a substance of the same kind:* since, in these colder regions, we sometimes find them to contract a greater degree of acrimony than most other substances will do by putrefying . . . as in those pernicious and even poisonous juices, which are sometimes generated in corrupted carcasses." Mead supported this point with the example of similar pathogenesis in domestic sites of crowds and filth, notably in the lowly bodies of prisoners and soldiers. "Nay more, we find animal putrefaction sometimes to produce in these northern climates very fatal distempers, though they do not arise to the malignity of true plague: for such fevers are often bred, where a large number of people are closely confined together, as in gaols, sieges and camps." (His ability to move so easily between African bodies and poor English ones showcases an intriguing tendency to compare the two, a phenomenon that we will explore further in the Conclusion.)[13]

But it was in his suggestions for public health strategies that Mead advanced his most direct claims about plebeian bodies. Plague policies, he wrote, should focus their attention on poor neighborhoods. For example, when authorities fear an epidemic, they should immediately send physicians to inspect houses "especially of the *Poorer* sort, among whom this Evil generally begins." Later, addressing the need to remove causes that "breed and promote Contagion," he similarly instructed officials to inspect "the Dwellings of all the meaner sort of the Inhabitants," and to evacuate and cleanse those they found "stifled up too close and nasty." Although he held to his line that true plague was exotic, Mead followed this last point with a claim that again emphasized the nearness of fevers born in domestic slums to plague itself, and which stressed the role that corrupt bodies played in generating disease: "For nothing approaches so near to the first Original of Contagion, as Air pent up loaded with Damps, and corrupted with the filthiness, that proceeds from Animal Bodies." It is furthermore revealing of how he considered such bodies to be forms of hazardous filth that he included the arresting of "Beggars and Idle Persons" within his advice to keep the streets "clean from Filth, Carrion and all Manner of Nuisances."[14] On this score we know he was hardly breaking new ground.

The class implications of Mead's claims should have been clear enough. He identified the poor as targets of policing and specified the benefits of such policies for elite Londoners, noting that they should become standing rules not only during epidemics, but "at all times." One would have thought that the well-heeled would have been satisfied to read Mead's lament that laid bare the role of class in his scheme: "I am sorry to take Notice, that in these [cities] of London and Westminster there is no good police established in these respects; for want of which the Citizens and gentry are every Day annoyed in more ways than one." Yet in his revised edition two years later Mead felt the need to clarify even further that his policing strategies were only ever meant to apply the poor. Mead had critiqued the shutting up of whole families together, and instead advocated speedily removing the sick from their homes to isolated pesthouses. However, the power to remove citizens from their homes was precisely the sort of policy that worried Whiggish critics. Mead's 1722 clarification makes clear how firmly he ascribed to the medical belief that the poor represented a uniquely contagious threat, and also that their liberty was more expendable than that of the more affluent readers of his learned treatise. The Preface to his revised edition addressed the issue directly.

> It has hardly ever been known, when the disease did not first begin among the poor. Such therefore only will be the subject to this regulation, whose habitations by the closeness of them are in all respects very incommodious for diseased persons. So that my advice chiefly amounts to the giving of relief to the poor, who shall first be infected, by removing them to more convenient lodgings. . . . This observation, that the plague usually begins among the poor, was the reason why I did not make any difference in my directions for removing the sick, in regard to their different fortunes, when I first gave my thoughts upon this subject: which, however, to prevent cavils, I have at present done; and have shewn what method ought to be taken, if, by some unusual chance, the plague should at the beginning enter a wealthy family.[15]

In other words, when Mead first wrote in 1720, he considered the fact that plague began among the poor to be so well known that he felt no need to specify that policing should be applied according to status. He trusted that readers would naturally understand that his strategies were meant exclusively for the poor. It is difficult to assess which provides more powerful evidence of the doctrinal belief in the epidemic danger of the plebeian body, Mead's explicit clarification of 1722, or his silent assumptions of 1720.

Mead was the most authoritative physician of his day. Yet his was but one voice. A host of lesser known commentators writing during the epidemic—from a range of different perspectives—advanced similar ideas about the poor, even when they disputed other issues. The stakes were high in 1720–1722. Doctors and politicians debated many things; whether the poor bred disease was not one of them.

For example, writers disputed the origin of the Marseilles outbreak. The translation of Pichatty de Croissainte's account, published in London while the crisis was still raging in 1721, attributed the plague to the arrival of the merchant ship the *Grand-Saint-Antoine*. At first only a few people connected with the ship sickened. Two weeks of quiet followed, and locals began to rest easy that the trouble had passed. But then, English readers learned, the true crisis ignited, predictably, in the slums, "in the Street of *Lescalle,* a Part of the old Town inhabited only by poor People." Local physicians initially denied that it was plague, though they tellingly dismissed it as "a contagious pestilential Fever, occasioned by bad Food, which Want had long forced those poor Creatures to live upon." Croissainte detailed the spread of the epidemic through the Lescalle slum, emphasizing the two to three thousand beggars in the city and the deepening crisis of poverty and famine as the epidemic worsened.[16]

But not everyone agreed that the disease came by ship. Physician Richard Blackmore thought that account a myth and argued, *pace* Mead, that it was locally born. He had it on good authority that plague had circulated in Marseilles—"under the name of a Malignant Infectious Fever"—for at least two months before the *Grand-Saint-Antoine* sailed into port. Either way, the infection undoubtedly intensified in the bodies of the poor: "The Force of the Contagion was wonderfully improv'd and augmented, by its reception into a Place where the Inhabitants by a Malignant Distemper were so much prepared and dispos'd to entertain and spread it, which might not have been able to have made such Impression and produce such Mischief, had not the Bodies of the Poor ill nourished People been so much dispos'd to receive the Infection."[17] Blackmore here encapsulates the central ideas that had long made the plebeian body so frightening, its predisposition to pestilential diseases and its ability to transform bad diseases into worse ones. Thus although Blackmore and Croissainte differed starkly in their opinions on the origin of the outbreak, their texts advanced the same vision of plebeian physiology.

Blackmore also challenged Mead's position that northern countries always imported plague. Epidemics in inland European communities must prove, he argued, that outbreaks could initiate in "one person, who first bred that poison in his own bowels." Under what circumstances? The requisite "Viscious Humours" were generated in the bodies of those suffering "Famine . . . Dearth and Scarcity of Provisions." Blackmore found support in the pseudonymously penned *Distinct Notions of the Plague* (1722), in which "The Explainer" agreed with Croissainte that Marseilles's plague started in the slums of Lescalle street, but that finally "the Sheriffs could not confine it to that Quarter, nor any longer to that Rank of people; for it now began to rage, and to attack all, without Distinction." A similar treatise emphasized Marseilles's natural advantages, including airy country surrounding it and plentiful clean water. Its population, however, was another matter. "As for the Inhabitants they are for the most part, Poor and uncleanly . . . nor do they take any Pains to clean their Streets. . . . Necessary Houses, they are utter Strangers to, but the Terras of their Houses are made the Repositories of all their Ordour, where it lies for some time, before it is carried away, being no otherways remov'd, but by the Force of the Rains which washes them down into the Streets."[18] Mead's influence notwithstanding, the danger of domestically generated plague remained a frightening possibility not so easily blamed on Africa.

Assumptions about poor bodies also spanned the well-studied debates between those who viewed plague as contagious and those who stressed miasma. It is important to note, as DeLacy has advised, how difficult it often is to categorize eighteenth-century doctors according to a neat contagionist/anticontagionist divide. Nevertheless, the Marseilles crisis brought out stark positions. And though the anticontagionists were a small minority, some made their voices heard.[19] On the central concern of this book, the role of the poor in epidemics, it has to be said that the contagionists tended to advance clearer statements linking plebeian bodies and disease. Critics of contagion like George Pye or John Pringle often emphasized nonhuman, usually environmental, factors, and so implicated the poor less directly. Nevertheless, even their treatises advanced some of the most important tenets underlying the association between plague and poverty. Anticontagionism worked to undermine policies like quarantine, but it did little to undermine ideas about plebeian physiology.

Although Pye never uses the term *miasma*, his vision bears the inheritance of that theory. Pye set himself at odds with Mead right in his title and argued that emissions from the sick were not toxic and that unwholesome air caused plague. This did not restrain him, however, from repeatedly supporting key pillars of the pathogenic plebeian body. For example, he underscored plague's foundation in putridity, noting that poorly drained land "becomes rotten and putrid," sending forth "noxious Effluvia." Moreover, Pye argued that plague could be generated by "unwholesome diet," and he repeatedly pointed to the "manner of living" as a prime cause, opening the door for class to play a role in his scheme. He advanced standard claims about predisposition and variances in human constitutions to argue that bodies were not uniform. When he then proceeded to discuss what might produce "extraordinary Aptness and Disposition" to plague, he highlighted poverty, via diet: "A great Want or Scarcity of good and wholesome Provisions is oftentimes wont to precede a Pestilence, and may in some measure contribute to the producing it." Moreover, he inscribed class on the fluids, as when excessive drinking "impoverishes the Blood" and invites disease. Most pointedly, however, he deployed discourses of cleanliness and urban geography to highlight the danger posed by paupers. The suburbs— where the poorest Londoners lived—demanded attention, especially their sewage: "I would recommend it to the Persons, whose proper Business it is to take care that the Streets, *especially in the out-Parts of the Town*, be kept more clean than heretofore." At this point Pye says something that coming chapters will show was prophetic, moving seamlessly from a discussion of slums to another context in which lowly bodies congregated, prisons: "The Goals [*sic*] and Prisons too should be better and more frequently cleansed, so as to be freed and preserved from all noisome Smells and Stenches." And though he opposed the shutting up of the infected, he admitted, "It may be proper to provide some Places for the Reception of the Poor."[20] A similar pattern emerges from physician John Pringle, who also opposed contagionism vehemently (and who should not be confused with the physician of the same name discussed in Chapter 4). Yet he similarly argued that in epidemics "the poor Suffer'd most," that foul bodies "encrease the malignity" of plague, that susceptibility hinged on one's "manner of living," that authorities should target such sites of poverty such as "Hospitals, Gaols, publick Slaughter-Houses, and Streets," and that confinement should be avoided as a social policy—except for the poor for whom institutions should be built.[21] The contagion-miasma debate did little to undermine assumptions about poor bodies.

One other theoretical stance warrants mention. Insights from micros-copy produced animalculism, the theory that diseases were caused by invis-ibly small insects. Popular in the late seventeenth and early eighteenth century, animalculism provided an alternative explanation for a range of diseases, notably two ailments that were categorized alongside plague as putrid diseases, namely the pox and the itch. The latter of these was often probably scabies, and the discovery of the scabies mite by Italian micros-copist Giovanni Cosimo Bonomo gave animalculism considerable credibility as an explanatory model. Indeed, it was Mead who was responsible for publishing Bonomo's account in 1702. Although animalculism accounted for disease in a new way, in practice it had close associations to contagionism because discussions often highlighted the migration of insects from body to body as a means for the sick to infect the healthy.[22] Whatever the case, animal-culist accounts of plague in the 1720s only lent further support to medical constructions of class.

The anonymously written *A New Discovery of the Nature of the Plague* suggested that plague was a minuscule insect. It advanced a number of intriguing arguments, including that the plague spread too rapidly for it to be anything but a living being. Conceiving of the disease as a microorganism is a noteworthy idea, one noted by scholars exploring the genesis of modern understandings of disease,[23] not least because of what we now know about the role played by fleas spreading plague. But as novel as this paradigm seems, it quickly reverted to long-accepted principles, including the centrality of putridity to epidemics and of poverty to putridity. For example, when the *New Discovery* posited that plague's insects subsisted on "virulent Matter" in the body, it perpetuated mainstream thought on predisposition: bodies with greater levels of putridity were predisposed because they provided more food for the insects. The plague insect "succeeds according to the Virulency of the Humours in the body to support it."[24]

Predictably, poverty led to such corruption. History had shown, said the author, that episodes of extreme poverty prompted epidemics. Describing the 1688 siege of Derry, he stressed, "It was common with the poorer sort of People all over that Kingdom, in those Black Times, to have the Flesh of Horses and rotten Cows, and Sheep, for their daily food." And the same factor now prepared the ground—or, to avoid speaking metaphorically, the bodies—in Marseilles. "In the late War, that Kingdom was reduced to the lowest Streights of Poverty," forcing commoners to survive on "worse Nourishment . . . [which] brought on them all Kinds of Sickness and Distress; Often very Malignant Fevers," and eventually plague itself. And though rotten food was the primary cause of paupers' putridity, the *New Discovery*'s repeated claims about vice demonstrate that moral constructions of the poor continued to frame medical theory. The cadence of such claims set the tone for discussions throughout the treatise. "Intemperance and Debauchery . . . open[ed] the Slucies of all manner of Vices," rendering bodies prone to plague. Elsewhere: "Plague makes prey of those, who have been most intemperate, and irregular in their Oeconomy." Like many before him, this doctor stressed idleness. Rates of sickness in Italy, France, and Spain were high because those nations were "inhabited by careless, nasty idlers, who live always on the Fruits of Laziness, [and] the most loathsome Food." Closer to home plague ravaged "indulgent, indolent Livers, slothful and easy, [and] exercised in licentious Pleasures." It is important that here was also leveled a critique of licentious elites who ruined their natural physiological advantages through luxury. To make the case, the author employed the comparatively rare rhetorical strategy of comparing scandalous elites to the diligent workers who are uncommonly presented here as healthier. However, in practice this merely again underscored the danger of impoverished bodies, as once again scarcity and diet drove the poor toward inevitable pestilential ends. "The part of Mankind inur'd to Labour, whose Necessities make indifferent Food habitual to them find it [plague] much less severe, except it be in a very Extraordinary Case, as when circumstances bring them to live on worse Food than they were used to; then, indeed, a Languishing follows in proportion and leaves them remediless." Moreover, vice wrote itself on the blood permanently. The *New Discovery* repeatedly advanced the possibility that predisposition to plague was hereditary, offering one more way that understandings of moral biology were gaining a harder, more fixed essence in the early eighteenth century. Although people usually acquired diseases though their own ill behavior, blameless were those who "have a *Distemper* descended with his Inheritance" from immoral parents.[25]

When its author came to his clearest statement on the ultimate and most important source of plague, he was unequivocal. "But when all this is done . . . [we reach] the true Cause of the Plague's raging in Cities, which is the great Number of poor People pent up together." The author's animalculist stance demanded the presence of what he elsewhere called the "prolifick reptile," but paupers' living conditions were nonetheless vital; he punctuates the claim thus: "So bad are their Circumstances, that were the *Plague* deriv'd from Putrefaction [alone]"—which, we must remember, the vast majority of physicians believed was the case—"it could never fail of being among them and consequently with us."[26] This final line is revealing, for it signals, on the one hand, the possibility that the conditions of the urban poor could render them *perpetual* sources of epidemic danger—a stance that later chapters will show became increasingly common—and on the other, that physicians like this one frequently assumed a class affinity with their audience. Despite earlier proclaiming a desire to educate "all ranks," this statement makes clear that this doctor and his assumed readership understood themselves to occupy a different zone from that of the dangerous slum dwellers, here described in stark terms of alterity: literally as "us" and "them." Thus despite a range of policy stances and theoretical frameworks, seventeenth-century ideas about class and disease were alive and well in the 1720s.

Defoe's Master Plan

One final text from the Marseilles crisis deserves attention both for what it says and for who said it. Daniel Defoe's *Journal of the Plague Year* is the best known of all the plague tracts produced during the Marseilles crisis. It has received extensive analysis for its novelistic form, which straddles the line between historical fiction and journalism.[27] Yet on the questions pertinent to the current study a more revealing text is his lesser known *Due Preparations for the Plague* (1722), published several months before the *Journal*. Unlike the latter book's narrative form following a London saddler through the turmoil of 1665–1666, the *Due Preparations* assumes the shape of a medical treatise. It is directly didactic, laying out a strategy for medical police in London. We know that Defoe researched seventeenth-century sources to write his *Journal*, but the *Due Preparations*' discussion of pathology may make that point even clearer. Defoe's commentary is often contrasted with Mead's because the two differed on the all-important issue of quarantine, which Defoe opposed but Mead recommended. Appealing to Whig sensibilities, Defoe raised the specter of absolutism in Mead's plan to enforce quarantine with troops, criticizing it as a "French model."[28] However, an investigation of the *Due Preparations* shows once again that ideological opponents were usually in lockstep when it came to plebeian physiology.

Defoe was not a physician, but he had clearly done his homework. The centrality of putridity, the role of filth in generating plague, the ability of bodies to intensify diseases, the importance of predisposition, and vice's role in paving the way for infection all find repeated expression in the *Due Preparations*. A few examples must suffice. Reflecting on the 1665/6 epidemic, Defoe explained that plague raged more forcefully after it gathered strength in impoverished bodies; inhabitants of crowded suburbs "being Poor and wanting Conveniencies . . . died in heaps and stengthen'd the Contagion." Discussing why poor suburbs had suffered the worst in 1665/6, Defoe invoked physicians' theories on how bodies imbibed their filthy environments, citing "the Opinions of the Physicians concerning Nastiness and Nauceious Smells, that they are Injurious and Dangerous, that they propagate Infection, and are a means to encrease the Plague." Predictably, he advocated cleaning slums, the "abominable sink[s] of publick Nastiness." He then asked rhetorically: "But what a Sink and Receptacle of Filth is the Body of Man?," arguing that cleaning the body's fluids—a process he called "cleansing the jakes"—was one of the most vital of his "due preparations." (The term *jakes* referred in the period both to latrines and to human excrement itself.) "People ought to turn their Thoughts to cleansing a worse Jakes than that of the Tide-Ditches in *Southwark* or *Fleet-Ditch,* &c. and that is, that the People, especially such as are to stay here at all Adventures, should Universally cleanse themselves, cleanse their Bodies of all Scorbutick Distempers, ill Habits, and especially Digestures, gross Distempers, and the like." A sense of moral biology recurs in the text as Defoe augments his discussions of filth and poverty with warnings about vice. Like Willis before him, he presented infection as a battle occurring within the blood, cautioning that "Intemperance in Drinking . . . is a most dreadful Induction to the Plague; when the Spirits are attack'd by the Venom of the Infection, they being already Exhausted, are in no Condition to Defend the Body." Echoing generations of physicians, Defoe called vice "a dreadful kind of Fuel for a Contagion [that] miserably prepare[s] us for a Plague upon our Bodies."[29] And although he made time to condemn luxury and the high diet of the rich, the *Due Preparations* presented the bodies of the urban poor as unquestionably the most dangerous source of contagion. Notwithstanding the place of the *Journal of the Plague Year* in the history of English literature, Defoe's advice for what to do about those bodies represented one of his most creative contributions.

Where Mead recommended quarantining the sick, Defoe advocated emptying London of its poor. It stood to reason. If plague preyed upon poor bodies, and if poor bodies strengthened the disease, then an absence of such bodies should stop the disease in its tracks. Pauper removal thus represented the central strategy of the *Due Preparations. A Journal of the Plague Year* depicted London as it had been, the *Due Preparations* as how it might be. One reported the past; the other looked to a future. The *Due Preparations* presented a stunning vision, a poverty-free London. Anyone who could suspend the obvious questions about the plan's practicality must have been struck by its utopian nature: London, free of paupers. It must have appealed to polite readers who daily made their way through ever more crowded streets. The plan is so ambitious in scope, so unthinkable in terms of logistics, that it seems worthy of comparison with the satirical visions of Swift or Mandeville. Yet Defoe was absolutely serious.

In many ways his plan represented a logical extension of some of the oldest plague policies on record. As Pullan, Carmichael, Slack, and others have shown, banishing beggars was one of the most common policies in times of plague. But why stop there? Surely, medical theories made it plain that it was not merely the *homeless* poor who generated, intensified, and spread plague. The settled and working poor also posed a risk. Defoe suggested that virtually all of them must go. The author of the animalculist *New Discovery* had depicted paupers' blood as food for the disease. Defoe offered only a slightly different metaphor: "These Evacuations of People, would greatly lessen the Numbers of the Poor in London, and consequently take away the Fuel which the Fire of the Pestilence generally Feeds upon."[30] Plebeian bodies were plague's fuel. Ergo, clearing away that fuel would protect the city. Defoe's plan comprised thirteen proposals, eight of which— numbers two, three, four, seven, eight, nine, eleven, and twelve—identified specific segments of the poor to be removed. By his estimate the measures below would alleviate London of two-thirds of its population:

> *First,* That upon the Approach of the Infection, Proclamation should be made, that all People that intend to remove themselves and Families, should do it within a certain time.
>
> *Secondly,* All reasonable Encouragement should be given to the poorer sort of People, who had any Friends or Relations to receive them, to remove with their Families, even to the giving them reasonable Allowances for their Travelling that as many poor Families as

possible may quit the City and separate, which would be their safety, and Contribute much to the Safety of the whole City also.

Thirdly, That all such Persons as have no legal Settlement in the Parishes within the City and Liberties, &c. should be forthwith pass'd away by Authority, and sent home to the Parishes and Counties from whence they came; no Beggars, Vagabonds, or loose People to be suffer'd in the Streets.

Fourthly, All the Parish Pensioners Alms poor, and Poor chargeable upon the Parish, as also all the Hospital poor, should be immediately remov'd at the Expence of the Parishes respectively, to such Places as each Parish cou'd procure for them, at least 20 Miles from *London,* and to be maintained there at the Charge of the Publick Parishes to which they belong.

Fifthly, All Occasion of bringing people to *London* by the necessity of Business should be as much as possible prevented; to which purpose the Terms must be Adjourn'd, the Inns of Court shut up; no Man should be arrested for Debt, so as to be put in Prison above a certain Time; but that if he cou'd not give Bail or some Pledge for his Appearance, such Debtors should be remov'd to such publick Places as the Officers of the City should be oblig'd to prepare, at the Distance of 15 miles at least.

Sixthly, That all the Prisoners for Debt should be immediately removed to the same Places as above.

Seventhly, That all Criminals, Felons and Murtherers, should be forthwith Tried, and such as are not Sentenc'd to Die, should be immediately Transported or let out, on Condition of going 40 Miles from the City, not to return on pain of Death.

Eighthly, That all the Children of *Christ-Hospital,* call'd the *Blew Coat-Boys* and *Girls,* be immediately removed by the Governours of the said Hospital to *Hertford* and *Ware,* where they have Houses for their Reception.

Ninthly, That all *Work-house* Children, Charity Children, and all the Children of the Poor, as are not in Condition to maintain them, should be remov'd into the Country, at least 30 Miles from the City, and be maintained there by the Publick.

Tenthly, That all Masters of Families, who purpose to abide the Extremity, be Exhorted to send all their Children that are under Fourteen Years of Age into the Country; and if any of them are

destitute of Places and Friends to send them to, on paying a reasonable Sum to the Common Treasure of the City, care should be taken
to provide Accomodations for them in the Country at the publick
Expence, where they should be well provided for, for a Year.

Eleventhly, That the Governours of the *Blew Coat Hospital*
should undertake on the Payment to them of a reasonable Sum of
Money by the City, to provide Maintenance for all such Children as
the City should recommend to them; and to be kept in the terms of
the Hospital; that is to say, as they now keep other Children, not
exceeding the number of twenty Thousand.

Twelfthly, That the Governours of the *Work-Houses,* do the like
in Proportion, so that in short, all the Children in the City and
Suburbs should be sent away. These Evacuations of People, would
greatly lessen the Numbers of the Poor in *London,* and consequently
take away the Fuel which the Fire of the Pestilence generally Feeds
upon.

Thirteenthly, That after the Time limited for all People, that please
to remove, if any Person after that should desire to remove, He
should not be hinder'd otherwise, than on the Conditions following:

I. On bringing good Testimony of his Body being Sound and not
Infected: This Testimony to be given by some able Physician or
Surgeon, or other Person, after their having search'd the Person
three Days successively.

II. On the Persons performing a Vinctine [quarantine], that is to
say, a Restraint of 20 Days, in such Barracks or Houses as shall be
appointed by the Magistrates of the City, at some Place Five Miles at
least from the Suburbs; after which, and no Sickness appearing upon
him, he shall have Testimonials of Health, and may go whether he
pleases.

All of these Measures being taken at the Beginning of the Infection, or at the first Approaches of it, we might reasonably hope,
Gods infinite Mercy concurring, that the City would be in a Posture
to bear the Visitation, much better than ever it was before; for tho'
there would still be many Thousands of Inhabitants left, yet they
would live at large, be unincumber'd with Poor, and with Children,
and with all the Stench and Filth that attend those who want Conveniencies, and who would in such a Calamity only serve to Infect one
another, and strengthen the Contagion in general.[31]

According to point 2, the poor should be "encouraged" to leave. However, it is immediately clear that most removals would be compulsory: the unsettled and beggars (3), parish pensioners, recipients of poor relief, and all inhabitants of hospitals and almshouses (4), prisoners (7), children in charity schools, workhouses, and other institutions, and the children of people too poor to maintain them (8, 9, 11, and 12). Defoe's concern with saving children is palpable and perhaps laudable. And Defoe is hardly the worst bigot when it comes to class. His touching portrayals of the bravery and compassion of the poor in *A Journal of the Plague Year* offer one of its most notable features. Moreover, Andrew Wear gives a sympathetic reading of Defoe's plan. He suggests that the above strategies promised to save the rich and poor alike, and that when Defoe discussed the origin of plague he did not go as far as some who suggested that poor bodies could generate plague *de novo*.[32] Perhaps. However, Defoe went nearly as far, as we have seen, arguing that the poor's putrid constitutions predisposed them and allowed their bodies to intensify the disease—a point that Defoe used expressly to punctuate his proposals. One need not dispute the honesty of Defoe's sympathy for the sufferings of the poor to point out the influences of medical theory on his thinking or the powerful support his plan lent to the now well-established belief that, in terms of biology, poor bodies were dangerous.

Further details of Defoe's plan demonstrate the extent to which such medical theories framed his vision. Overlooked to this point have been the distances that Defoe suggested removing differently classed bodies. Not everyone had to travel equally far. Indeed, the distances of Defoe's removals allow for a kind of calculus of risk, expressed geographically. Beggars and the unsettled poor were to be removed to their parishes of settlement. This made sense because it would allow authorities to use legal mechanisms of the poor law to remove such people and pay transportation costs. Simple enough. However, the settled poor were a different matter. The outdoor poor, such as pensioners, or residents in almshouses and hospitals had to go twenty miles. However, the indoor poor—those in workhouses—as well as the children of the extremely poor ("those not in a condition to maintain them"), had to travel farther, thirty miles, roughly the distance to Hertford and Ware, where Christ Hospital's orphans would be placed. Felons in prison had to go even farther: across the ocean if possible, forty miles if not. Debtors, however, were a different matter. These polite offenders had to travel only fifteen miles. This applied equally to imprisoned debtors, even though many would have inhabited some of the same prisons as the felons. In other words, a debtor in Newgate who had been exposed to the same filth, effluvia, and contagion as Defoe's most dangerous bodies (felons) still posed less risk than an old-age pensioner, who would be expelled five miles farther from the city, or a child from a workhouse, who had to go twice as far. It is further curious that respectable citizens who chose to leave after the epidemic had begun (13) had to travel a mere five miles. Remember that Defoe's pauper removals were to occur *before* an epidemic hit. These were due *preparations* for plague. By Defoe's logic, then, the poor in his many categories posed a greater risk *before an epidemic hit* than a respectable citizen exiting a city in which the plague raged. A temporal reading augments the geographic one, for while these latter polite bodies did have to undergo a process of isolation and inspection, it was not a full *quarant*-ine, which, as its name implies, was forty days, but a period merely half as long. Defoe's concern for the safety of children might make one think that these differing distances reflected his urge to protect these various groups, sending some to zones farther removed from the dangers of the epidemic, suggesting a plan inspired by protection *of* these groups, rather than the dangers *from* them. However, that reading does not bear scrutiny, for it poorly explains why felons would be sent the farthest.

ᗞᙓᑕ

Defoe's plan was never implemented. How could it have been? However, notwithstanding his sympathy for the poor who had suffered in past epidemics or his desire to prevent replication of that suffering, his *Due Preparations* offered one of the clearest iterations of the pathogenic plebeian body in the early eighteenth century. When panicked Englishmen learned of developments in Marseilles, they scrambled to inform themselves, returning again and again to the literature from London's last epidemic. Defoe is only the best known of many writers who researched seventeenth-century plague in the early 1720s and carried early modern insights into the next century.

By the second decade of the eighteenth century the danger of plebeian bodies was a matter of medical fact, one that was beyond debate. The unanimity on this position is noteworthy because medical men were divided on so many issues, whether concerning theory, policy, or treatment. But doctors' various positions in these debates mattered little when it came to their stances on the poor. Whether they thought that plague was exotic or local, spread by contagion, miasma, or tiny insects, whether they supported or opposed the practice of quarantine, doctors with vastly different agendas agreed that plebeian constitutions were uniquely dangerous.

This chapter can conclude with a question that may have struck readers a moment ago. Why did Defoe recommend banishing prisoners farthest? We saw that Mead, Pye, and Pringle had also each singled out prisons for special comment. As the ensuing chapters will show, medical worries about the plebeian body would soon shift to focus on jails as the most worrying site of pathogenesis.

3. Prisons, Debtors, and Disease in the Early Eighteenth Century

Defoe's plan suggested that prisons posed a special risk. The idea was neither new nor incidental. Despite the continued presence of plague in the early eighteenth century, both as a material threat and as a monster of the imagination, worries about the pathological dangers of the poor increasingly came to focus on diseases born in prisons. Britain's carceral institutions would eventually become primary targets of public health strategies, strategies that are usually explored under the heading of prison reform.[1] In various ways these developments will be the focus of the next four chapters.

It will not be news to historians of crime or prisons that the squalid conditions in eighteenth-century jails figured prominently in debates on how to reform them. So-called jail fever (later typhus) has received regular attention from scholars studying prisons since at least the time of the Webbs, with depictions of overcrowding, filth, and mortality rates providing seemingly requisite elements of any discussion of English jails in the age before the penitentiary.[2] In the coming chapters I seek not to put jail fever on the historiographic map but rather to begin tracing in new detail its implications for eighteenth-century culture by exploring how discussions of prisons helped craft and perpetuate important claims about plebeian bodies well beyond the narrow realm of medical science. I hope to move beyond humanitarian narratives that so often use snapshots of the filthy, diseased prison as starting points in teleologies that celebrate late-century reformers like John Howard. Indeed, the reforms associated with Howard so dominate the historiography of prisons that a goal of the next several chapters is to explore discussions of bodies and disease in earlier penal discourses so that the developments of the 1770s and 1780s can be more richly contextualized.

Of course, other than humanitarian narratives characterize the historiography on prisons, as the seminal work of Foucault makes clear. Yet even critical studies of the penitentiary have yet to reveal what debates about disease might teach us. Michael Ignatieff, in *A Just Measure of Pain*, makes one of the fullest attempts to integrate contemporary medical theories with prison-reform discourses. However, like many penal historians, Ignatieff concerns himself more with order than with health. Like Foucault he was primarily concerned with exploring the penitentiary as a technology for producing orderly men. Ignatieff's insights about medicine orient toward illuminating Enlightenment theories on the mind-body connection and how reformers sought to address prisoner's souls through technologies aimed at their bodies. Medicine thus remains a handmaiden to order, with disease playing its traditional role as a component of the "before" picture set against the "after" snapshot of the orderly (and therefore healthier) Pentonville. The point here will not be to challenge that the penitentiary was a technology of modernity. Rather, by setting the story of penal reform in the longer history of ideas about epidemics that this book charts, I wish to make the case that public safety—by which I mean the safety of propertied Englishmen, not the safety of prisoners—was a more essential component of penal debates than is often allowed.[3]

In doing so, this analysis builds on the insights of several historians in particular. Margaret DeLacy's study of prison reform in Lancashire made a number of valuable contributions, especially concerning regional variation and local processes. One of her more important arguments, that prison reform was motivated by fear of fever epidemics, has been less heralded. Throughout her chapter explaining the driving forces behind reform, she is unequivocal: "It was the growing fear of typhus that was the decisive factor in determining the timing of new prison construction." As DeLacy lays bare, by the 1780s personal safety, rather than humanitarian or sentimental affect, drove propertied citizens to commit to gaol reform. She found support in the work of Roy Porter, who concurred in his study of Howard that "typhus proved the best prison reformer." Moreover, architectural historian Robin Evans's *The Fabrication of Virtue* devotes a chapter to establishing that fever epidemics not only provided a major impetus to reform jails but informed the physical forms that new penitentiaries eventually assumed.[4]

In the coming chapters I hope to augment these works by expanding the chronological framework considerably and by orienting the material toward different questions. On the one hand, I intend to use debates about prisons for reasons other than to explain what eventually happened to English jails, which has been more than capably achieved by the works cited above. Rather, I mean to read debates about prisons as a gauge of how widely felt and communicated were anxieties about the plebeian body. It is a central contention of this book that class-driven contagion anxieties constituted a deeper element of eighteenth-century culture than is usually acknowledged, and prison reform, which at points became a movement of national concern, can demonstrate this point powerfully. Moreover, I intend to explore these debates for what they said about bodies. Evans and the many historians who have joined him to chart the well-known story that modern prisons became cleaner and better ventilated have tended to focus their attention on the quality of air and the structures of buildings. Both elements were vital. However, a focus on air, walls, and windows can easily obscure how claims about prisons forever advanced claims about bodies. The close integration between physicians and prison reformers that Ignatieff, Evans, Porter, and DeLacy have all stressed suggests that debates about prison reform offer fruitful possibilities for exploring how ideas about the plebeian body made themselves felt far beyond the realm of medical literature. Finally, and in keeping with the thrust of this book concerning long continuities, I wish to make the case that there is much to gain from setting eighteenth-century developments within the much longer history of ideas about epidemics. Even those historians, like DeLacy, who have stressed health concerns as a catalyst of reform tend to focus on the last third of the century. In a like manner, histories of prison medical services similarly take 1770 as a rough starting point. Penal reform undoubtedly accelerated in the late eighteenth century, but it would be a mistake to suggest that debates about prison conditions began then. Far from it. And early debates, as we are about to see, were frequently structured by class.[5]

Debtors and Their Bodies

"This City seems to encourage nothing, that may lay it open to the Rage of the Plague, but Prisons." So wrote the author of *A New Discovery of the Nature of the Plague* at the height of the Marseilles epidemic. London was doomed, the anonymous doctor warned, because every quarter of the city had a prison, and prevailing air currents promised to sweep their deadly fumes from jail to jail, intensifying the poisonous vapors along the way and leaving no one safe. His pestilential tour of city jails is worth quoting at length. Even neighborhoods with clean air "are certain of being depriv'd of it,"

> by the Prisons of Ludgate, and the Fleet; Newgate continues the bad Air along the Hill to Smithfield: Wood-street and the Poultry Compters bring their Smells to the Places of greatest Concourse, in the Heart of the City; the Goals of Clerkenwell, and Whitechapel are to the chief Gates a Nuisance; the King's bench Prison, and that Den of miserable, starv'd helpless Creatures, the Marshalsea infects the Borough, with London-Bridge. That other Kennel of bad Air, Custom's Darling . . . the Mint, prevents the Good the Fields joining might bring the City, by its Nastiness hastening the Death of several. Nor does Westminster with its Gatehouse, down in a Marsh, avail of acting its Part; the soggy Mists, and Goal Steams, but ill accommodate the Court end of Town. Thus we see Prisons are so plac'd, that let the Wind set in what Point it will, it can never allow Good to the People; and if there be no Wind stirring, that Force by which the bad Air is expell'd, is sufficient to disperse it all abroad.[6]

Prisons were the perfect breeding grounds for epidemic disease, combining all of the requisite ingredients—plebeian bodies, filth, and material want—pent up in close confines. And London had them everywhere.

When he lumped together so many different institutions, this doctor inadvertently conveyed something quite important for our study. Many different types of carceral institutions could be found in a place like eighteenth-century London. The author indicted eleven jails, but could have easily doubled that number, for just three years later Defoe listed twenty-two. That London needed so many jails may surprise us, since imprisonment was not a primary punishment for serious crime throughout much of the eighteenth century. Jails generally held offenders only until their trials, where they tended to receive punishments like transportation, banishment, forms of corporal punishment, or hanging. John Beattie has shown that it was only after the 1770s that imprisonment itself began to be used more commonly as a punishment for serious crimes. For example, in only five years between 1690 and 1775 did incarceration account for more than 5 percent of punishments handed down at London's Old Bailey courthouse. That said, Beattie also demonstrated that from the first decade of the century incarceration at hard labor became an increasingly common punishment for petty offenders, and Shoemaker has noted that the ability of local justices to commit such lesser offenders to jail without a jury trial helped expand the prison population in this period. Periodic crises of overcrowding can be detected from the 1690s, especially when levels of prosecution spiked or transportation was interrupted.[7]

Thus London had jails of many shapes and sizes. Newgate, its most notorious prison, was the primary jail for serious offenders, often holding upward of three hundred prisoners at a time. Petty offenders and vagrants were locked in bridewells, or houses of correction, such as Westminster's Tothill Fields, or London's bridewell, which dated from medieval times. Although bridewells employed work as a reforming corrective and were sometimes thought of as workhouses, they should not be confused with the parish workhouses that started cropping up all over London beginning in the 1720s. These latter institutions were primarily for poor relief, with paupers usually applying to get into them rather than being committed there against their will. The Savoy Prison held army deserters and other military offenders, while small lockups like the Wood Street and Poultry Compters jailed prisoners committed by the lord mayor, which in practice often meant debtors. This last class of prisoners had several institutions devoted to them, such as the Marshalsea, Fleet, and King's Bench prisons. However, debtors also ended up in numerous other jails (including Newgate, as we will see), especially in smaller communities that could not run multiple jails for different categories of prisoners. While terms in jail tended to be short—just a few months to a year for vagrants or petty offenders, and merely until their trials for accused felons—debtors could find themselves locked up for lengthy stays, typically incarcerated until their creditors were paid. But although contemporaries would have understood important distinctions between compters, houses of correction, debtors' prisons, and Newgate, the author of *A New Discovery* notably conflates them. There is no distinction between the "Goal Steams" emanating from these very different jails. Just as doctors tended to speak vaguely about the undifferentiated "poor," they similarly painted with broad brushstrokes when discussing prisons. One thing all jails had in common was that they housed lots of poor people. And this, stressed the *New Discovery* author, was key to their contagion. Speaking at once about all of the above jails, he claimed, "Throngs of poor People press'd into them, send forth Smells very prejudicial." Authorities as important as Mead concurred. Addressing the dangers of the "corrupted . . . Filthiness" that he associated with the poor, Mead generalized thus: "Our common *Prisons* afford us an Instance of this, in which very few escape, what they call the *Goal Fever,* which is always attended with a Degree of Malignity in proportion to the *Closeness* and *Stench* of the Place."[8]

Proximity to jails thus spelled danger. However, propertied Englishmen did not merely fear that disease would seep out of prisons to strike them in their homes. Too often they found themselves or their companions locked up as debtors, prisoners whom we might anachronistically consider the white-collar criminals of the early modern age. English law allowed creditors considerable power over those who owed them money. People alleged to owe forty shillings or more could be imprisoned until trial if they could not make bail; if they lost in court, they could be held indefinitely until the debt was paid. Creditors had significant discretion and often used the threat of imprisonment as a key collection tool in an age when credit transactions were ubiquitous. Many criticized the practices by which Englishmen could be deprived of their liberty merely on someone's word and by way of scant processes that Joanna Innes has described as "a system of legalized bullying." However, the perception that creditors needed some kind of leverage, along with the eighteenth-century drive to use the force of law to protect property, ensured that the debt laws stayed on the books. As a result, a huge number of Georgian Britons were touched by them throughout their adult lives. Living in a web of debits and credits, they knew all too well that the specter of prison—a threat that we will see was powerfully framed by contagion—haunted so many of their transactions. And not a few of them were actually locked up. One scholar estimates that between one in thirty and one in twelve eighteenth-century Englishmen would have spent some portion of their adult lives incarcerated for debt, and that this figure would have been much higher for London, where "virtually every adult male member of the lower middle class would have been vulnerable to arrest at some point in his life, and as many as one or two in four actually jailed." Even late in the century, when imprisonment had become more common for serious offenses, John Howard noted that debtors still represented fully half of the entire English and Welsh prison populations.[9]

Although creditors held the whip hand, we know that some debtors used the debt laws creatively, for example, choosing to enter prison rather than liquidating assets to pay their debts. Thus while some debtors entered prison because they were without resources, many hailed from the propertied classes, continuing to negotiate with their creditors and participate in some economic activity. Craig Muldrew concluded of England's incarcerated debtor population that "most of these poor prisoners had, in fact, once been wealthy tradesmen who had become insolvent." That said, many working people also found themselves locked up for debt. The mixed nature of their population thus contributed to the confusion surrounding debtors as category. By 1786 Josiah Dornford tried to clarify the picture by sketching a literal class structure: "Debtors may be considered of three classes. The first under the description of Merchants and capital Traders. The second Tradesmen, Mechanics and Artificers, in the middle walk of life. The third, of the lower orders of Journeymen, of Labourers and Domestics." But as Ian Duffy has shown, such a neat classification belied reality. As a result of their clientele, debtors' prisons had to provide accommodations worthy of respectable men, with spacious furnished apartments on the "Master's side" of jails, and even such amenities as racket courts and wine clubs. Such frills did not come cheaply. Keepers charged considerable, many said extortionate, fees for privileged room and board. However, once a debtor's resources were exhausted, he was cast to the sparser, crowded, and usually grim "Common side" of the prison. In some places better-off debtors also had their pick of so-called "spunging houses"— Defoe claimed there were more than one hundred in the neighborhoods surrounding London's prisons—where they could serve their sentences within private homes. But as their name implies, their fees were steep.[10]

    Debtors present a fascinating example of liminality for class that would reward more attention. Were they rich or were they poor? Like cross dressers or mixed-race people, debtors traversed a culturally constructed boundary and offered a puzzling hybrid for the eighteenth-century public. The schizophrenic response to their plight is highly suggestive of the confusion they engendered. Incarcerated and imperiled, but literate and organized, debtors frequently made the loudest and most effectual calls for the reform of England's jails. Innes has explored the political organization of eighteenth-century debtors, a group on whose behalf there was far more agitation than for any other class of criminal throughout the period under study. It is clear that the questions raised by their incarceration reverberated loudly. Seventeenth- and early-eighteenth-century discussions of prison conditions overwhelmingly addressed those faced by debtors. According to Sean McConville, "Such nationally ordered ameliorations of prison conditions as there were in the first part of the [eighteenth] century affected only debtors."[11] Debtors had much to complain about; one of their most pressing concerns was their forced proximity to the potentially infectious bodies of commoners. Within prisons, polite bodies and rotten bodies were forced to cohabit; this was a problem.

A fascinating text that showcases vividly the contagion anxieties associated with such class-mixing is Moses Pitt's *Cry of the Oppressed* (1691). Pitt was a publisher whose overambitious project for an atlas left him in debt and eventually confined in Fleet Prison in 1689. Appalled at the conditions, he corresponded with debtors incarcerated elsewhere, collecting their complaints and publishing a compendium of prison oppression, complete with illustrations. Debtors protested numerous practices, and although DeLacy and Wayne Sheehan have issued important reminders that corruption did not uniformly characterize early prisons, *The Cry of the Oppressed* includes such common complaints as physical abuse, the lack or poor quality of food and bedding, and extortion. Such criticisms provide common components in histories of prereformed English jails, but less attention has come to fall on the profound claims made by Pitt's correspondents about bodies—theirs and those of others—throughout the book. And while Pitt's agenda—to press for parliamentary action to redress these grievances—demands that we keep in mind the possibility of exaggeration, *The Cry* remains a fascinating collection of texts contributed by debtors themselves. Whether they accurately reflect late-seventeenth-century prison life is somewhat beside the point. What matters is that Pitt and his colleagues addressed issues that they felt were vital and which (and this is the important point) they believed would inspire members of the respectable reading public to lobby for them. In this regard, the repeated claims that these recently propertied men were locked in dangerously close proximity to the infectious bodies of lowly prisoners offered some of the most common, graphic, and frightening claims of the book.[12]

Pitt opened with an epistle to Parliament: "In this small Book we here present to your View our Wounds and our Distempers, our Boils and our Carbuncles, the Briberies and Perjuries, the Oppressions and Extortions, we Groan under. You are not only our *Princes*, but our *Physicians*, unto whom should we Complain and Cry (next to *God* and their *Majesties*,) but to *You* for Healing?" He was speaking metaphorically, of course. But in the plague sore—the carbuncle—Pitt chose a telling metaphor. A page later he made clear that the choice was no accident. Putting metaphor aside, he highlighted

the tragedy that debtors should "lie Starving, Rotting with Soars and Carbuncles, Devour'd with Vermin, Poisoned with Nasty Stinks, Knock'd on the
Head, and that for no Crimes, but for their Misfortunes, Miscarriages, and
Losses, by Trade and Merchandizing." The last line makes clear—not that
seventeenth-century readers needed help understanding the point—that the
victims for whom Pitt spoke were polite men of the mercantile class. He did
not advocate on behalf of the common felons or vagrants who shared so many
of the institutions discussed in his text. Rather, the tragedy lay in these victims
of circumstance whom the harsh market had ruined, and who now lay "rotting"
(note the term) with carbuncles that were not metaphors. Pitt thus opened his
book by stressing the physical corruption of debtors' previously healthy bodies
that resulted from being pent up with paupers. Indeed, Pitt highlighted his own
proximity to such a rotten body by noting that the bed adjoining his held "a
Burst Man, of a Corrupt Body, and Full of Vermin," who soon died.[13]

Pitt did not spare details. He was at pains to emphasize his banishment
from the "Gentlemen's Side" of the prison. Like so many debtors, Pitt was
initially housed separately from vagrants and felons until the keeper extorted
his funds through excessive and possibly illegal fees, then summarily cast
him from his private room into "The Wards." Describing it as "miserable"
and a "dungeon," Pitt found himself sharing a room with twenty-seven poor
men. It was here he was forced to sleep next to the abovementioned mendi-
cant with the "corrupt body," a phrase he used twice. The keeper's greatest
crime may have been his repeated efforts to prevent Pitt from availing
himself of the amenities of the gentlemen's side after his banishment.
Consider Pitt's description of his efforts to delouse himself. (He speaks in
the third person.)

> He was not able to keep himself clean from Vermin, being forc'd to
> Louse himself most commonly Twice a Day, wither in the open
> Yard, or in the House of Office; for at any time if the said *Pitt* had
> the use of any of the Gentleman's Chambers for his Devotions,
> Study or Lowsing himself, if the said *Warden* came to hear of it,
> both he and his Wife should be very Angry with the said Gentlemen,
> and would hunt him thence as a Partridg upon the Mountains. And
> that the reader may be satisfied, that it was impossible for the said
> *Pitt* to keep himself clean from vermin, whilst he continued in the
> said *Wards* of the *Fleet* Prison, he doth Assure his Reader, that many
> of his Chamber-Fellows were so Lowsie, that as they either walk'd,

or sat down, you might have pick'd Lice off from their outward garments; but enough of this lest my Reader Scrubs and Scratches at the Reading of it.

Pitt's apology at the close hints strongly at the assumed class of his readership. However, as an apology it was entirely disingenuous, for Pitt surely included gruesome details precisely to invoke a passionate if unpleasant response in readers he hoped to jolt into action. Moreover, he made sure to emphasize that his plight represented a matter not just of discomfort but of life and death for propertied Englishmen like himself, warning that a debtor cannot occupy such jails "without danger of his Life."[14] It is here worth noting that despite copious details about lice, filth, corruption, and death, Pitt never advocated cleaning the prison. The villainy here is not that common prisoners were subject to such conditions but that *gentlemen* could be thrust into them through a keeper's extortion.

Pitt's compatriots from jails across the country echoed his story, presenting the need to separate debtors from felons and vagrants as self-evident and the failure to do so as egregious. The debtors in Salop can speak for those incarcerated in Leicester, Exeter, Derby, and Halifax who all stressed the same point: "Prisoners of all sorts, as Murderers, Felons and Cutpurses, have not only been daily kept, but also continually Lodged, among Debtors, without redress." They wore their social status as a badge of honor, one that cold-hearted wardens stripped from them. For example, these same Salop debtors complained of a lack of servants, bemoaning that they had to clean their cells with "their own pains and labours," while their brethren in Devonshire's Stock Gaol objected that their laundresses were prevented from entering the jail to serve them. The debtors in Lincoln may have expressed this sense of wounded class privilege most clearly when they described being thrust "into a stinking Cave; not fitting for Persons whose Extraction is Laudable, and Education is Ingenious." It is telling that the threat of disease was almost never absent from claims that class boundaries had been breached. Debtors in Derby protested that the keeper lodged with them prisoners who "ought not to come amongst the Debtors," a practice "very prejudicial to the poor Debtors, in respect of their Health, and hereby also they are in great danger of Diseases to breed among them by the Noisome smell that is occasioned by the croud." They held plebeian prisoners in such low esteem that they even compared them to swine, literally. When the warden allowed his pigs to lodge in their quarters, they complained of the hogs and felons in the same breath: "the Swine ran in upon us; in like manner, he hath Abused us, by putting Felons amongst us."[15]

Others also protested the presence of animals and their excrement, but when the Derby debtors complained about their lavatory facilities, they expressed one of the most commonly voiced (and for our purposes most telling) criticisms. Human waste appears in *The Cry* repeatedly, and as no laughing matter. Debtors presented their close proximity to ordure as one of the most dangerous features of prison life. Debtors in Lincoln bemoaned that they were not granted "liberty to ease nature, whereby the Prisoners do oftentimes become Offensive to each other." Those in Appleby, Rothwell, and Halifax concurred. However, it was the felons' waste, rather than their own, that most frightened the debtors. If putrid corruption lay at the heart of medical thinking about classed bodies, and if bodies purified themselves by excreting corrupt matter, then it stood to reason that the excrement of felons and vagrants was toxic stuff. As evidence that medical thought on this matter pervaded the lay public, consider the complaints of the debtors in Exeter's Southgate Prison. They, too, were forced to live among common prisoners. And although they retired to separate rooms at night, their bedchambers communicated dangerously with the felons' privy: "Also here is a house of Office in it, which Ten or twelve Men do Ease themselves in, so we that are close Confin'd do suck the ill Air that doth proceed from their Excrements, and the Nastiness of the House of Office, so that we are suffocated with ill Air, which makes us very Sick, and are broken out with *Boils, Carbunckles,* and *Botches*."[16] These men thus made direct reference to plague sores that stemmed, they believed, from exposure to felons' waste. It is further telling that this episode is one of a handful that Pitt chose to illustrate. The engravings in *The Cry of the Oppressed* showcased numerous travails that debtors suffered, such as being forced to catch rodents for their sustenance or suffering physical abuse. The plates conveniently include page numbers to identify which stories they illustrated. The plate titled "Debtors brook out with Boyles Carbuncles and Botches" (Figure 1) referenced the account above.

Here the debtors' skin did all the talking. Their sores revealed their inner corruption, corruption that had made its way out of felons' bodies (as waste) and into their own by way of fumes that seeped through the windows displayed prominently on the back wall. The man at the desk is still healthy, for he is not yet marked. However, he holds his head in his hands in a posture that typically conveyed melancholy, for he knows that all who breathe this

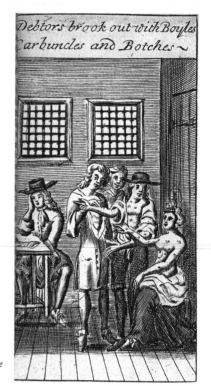

Figure 1. "Debtors brook out with Boyles
Carbuncles and Botches," Moses Pitt, *The Cry of the
Oppressed* (London, 1691), Granger.

fetid air face a similar fate. The presence of the infected woman also raises
important questions. She was probably included to represent the danger of
prison-born infections to the families of debtors, who we know entered
prisons to visit relatives and sometimes even lodged therein. Indeed, the
debtors in Southgate prison warned that such visitors faced grave dangers and
often neglected to visit them for that reason, a point confirmed by Sheehan.[17]
Again stressing their proximity to common criminals' excreta, they observed
that their room "looks out into the common Goal where Criminals are kept
. . . which with the Air that doth proceed from their Room and House of
Office, and our House of Office, doth quite take away our Breath. Our Friends
. . . often refrain to come to us by reason of the ill scents, for fear of Infection." The same problem was voiced by debtors in another Devonshire jail,
the Stock Gaol, where only one privy served seventy prisoners, rendering the
jail "noisome" and the target of strong complaints by visitors. Petitions from
Bury St. Edmonds, including one by a medical man, surgeon John Suckerman,

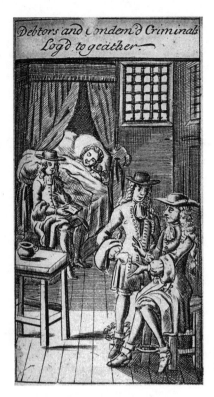

Debtors and Condem'd Criminals Log'd togeather.

Figure 2. "Debtors and Condem'd Criminals Log'd togeather," Moses Pitt, *The Cry of the Oppressed* (London, 1691), Granger.

echoed these complaints. Warded with commoners and forced to stay "next door to the House of Office," Suckerman charged that the gaoler "well near Poisoned me with Noisome Scents, that I had broke out with Boils, and Lameness." His fellow prisoners shocked readers with even more gruesome details, again stressing as the salient crime that they were forced to share space with more lowly inmates. "This is not enough but some of those that Lodg in the Houses, or Fore-Chambers, as they call them, are set into this our Ward-Yard, in the Night Season, when we are Barred up in our Room, and there some of them do Spew and Shit to Ease themselves; and some of us the aforementioned Prisoners, the next Day are Locked up in the said Yard, and are denied to come to the Pump for Water . . . such is their cruelty, that it may and will breed all manner of Diseases, if it cost not some of us our Lives."[18] These men also had their plight sketched in an illustration, although thankfully one not as grimly detailed as it might have been. The image was captioned: "Debtors and Condem'd Criminals Log'd togeather" (Figure 2). Though the bodies here appear healthy, the chamber pot on the table would have ensured that viewers kept the vile details of the accompanying petition well in mind.

Because *The Cry* was a published text, it is open to the criticism that perhaps Pitt wrote it himself and that its form as a collection of unique petitions is a ruse. However, a series of surviving manuscript petitions by contemporary debtors locked in a variety of London jails suggests *The Cry* is representative.[19] Pitt petitioned Parliament, but these London debtors addressed their concerns to the lord mayor and the Court of Aldermen. While Innes and Margot Finn have emphasized the political agency of eighteenth-century debtors to secure decent conditions, recent analyses of early- to mid-eighteenth-century petitions point to quite poor conditions for imprisoned debtors.[20] London petitions certainly support that view. Again, the threat of infection loomed large.

The lack of clean water, for example, marked a consistent problem. No fewer than seven petitions, two each from prisoners in Newgate, Ludgate, and the Poultry Compter and one from those in the Wood Street Compter, begged authorities to address their water needs and warned of potential epidemics, repeatedly linking plumbing crises to contagion. Ludgate petitioners warned that they were "utterly Choackt up & Poysonned" and "must be incurably lost through contagious Distempers," while Newgate debtors predicted "ye Want of Water may Cause a Contagion." Moreover, whether because they believed it to be true or were simply playing a strong card, petitioners structured their claims to highlight that it was not just their own lives at stake but those of London citizens more broadly. Debtors in the Poultry Compter invoked full-blown plague: "Such is the Contagious Noisomness of the Place in generall that when a Warmer Season Approaches we have great reason to dread a pestilence." Ludgate petitioners confirmed Pitt's claims that polite friends and families feared visiting them. Discussing contagion, they lamented "the violent Scents of the Prison does annoy. Deter, & keep back their friends from coming to see them." The hint that such visitors might carry disease out with them was not subtle. If they veiled the threat of a citywide epidemic, Newgate debtors were explicit: "Yo[u]r Petition[er]s most humbly prayeth thy Hon:ble Court to give ord:s to bee done As well to prevent Infection amongst them a[n]d the adjacent Inhabitants who are very Sensible of the noisome Smells sent from the said Goale and if an Infection should once Seize the Neighbourhood God knows what part of this hon[oura]ble Citty itt might terminate." Moreover, such warnings again made explicit links to bodies and their waste. Ludgate petitioners warned that damaged lavatories exposed them to filth and threatened "infection and mortality . . . if not timely prevented." Their counterparts in the Poultry Compter complained of the toilet facilities there, warning that "Nautious Stench of the Vaults wch Wantt empting . . . when the Weather grows Warmer is very likely to Breed a Contagion."[21] Manuscript petitions thus offer strong evidence against dismissing *The Cry of the Oppressed* as merely the product of Moses Pitt's imagination.

Such sources also make it hard to agree with penal historians who have asserted that before the late eighteenth century "the problems of gaol fever did not cause concern." Indeed, even by its publication in 1691 the concerns voiced in *The Cry of the Oppressed* were not novel. In fact, the Insolvency Acts, for which Pitt and his colleagues lobbied—which created avenues for some debtors to leave jail before their debts were fully paid—had their roots in contagion fears. If Pitt and other petitioners were strategic in emphasizing biohazard, it may have been because they were familiar with England's first Insolvency Act, passed in 1670, the preamble of which highlighted the threat of prison-born epidemics as a primary motive for freeing jailed debtors: "Forasmuch as very many persons now detained in prison, are miserably impoverished, either by reason of the late unhappy time, the sad and dreadful fire, their own misfortunes, or otherwise, so as they are totally disabled to give any satisfaction to their creditors, and so become, without advantage to any, a charge and burden to the kingdom, and by noisomness (*inseparably incident to extreme poverty*) may be come the occasion of pestilence and contagious diseases, to the great prejudice of the kingdom." Coming on the heels of 1665/6 the warning embedded in this legislation was dire. Indeed, it was this very act that established as law the need to separate debtors from felons, though if *The Cry* is to be believed, it was often flouted. Such actions suggest on the one hand that health concerns loomed large in discussions of prisons a century before John Howard, and on the other hand that the act of moving genteel prisoners away from potentially contagious plebeian ones constituted an important component of prison reform in the age before the large-scale restructuring of England's jails. Indeed, legal historian Paul Hess Haagen suggests a link between the first Insolvency Act and a specific epidemic at the Poultry Compter that killed a third of that jail's debtors in just seven weeks. He writes: "Strong was the association between disease and prison, and particularly the common side of debtors' prisons, that virtually every effort to reduce the size of the imprisoned population was justified on the ground that it was in the interests of public health."[22]

The Oglethorpe Committees

This line of argument is supported by the fact that it was nothing other than the infection and death of a debtor that inspired England's most important prison reformer before Howard, James Oglethorpe. In 1728 Robert Castell, a personal friend of the member of Parliament Oglethorpe, found himself incarcerated for debt in the Fleet. An architect, Castell spiraled into a debt of more than £900 to multiple creditors. Oglethorpe is believed to have assisted him to the tune of £125, funds that may have helped Castell initially stay in the privileged confines of a sponging house external to the prison run by a Mr. Underwood. But Underwood expertly relieved Castell of his remaining funds, and this, along with the rumor that Castell might flee the country, drove authorities to transfer him to a more secure residence, a lowlier sponging house called Corbett's. The problem was that a prisoner there named James White had just died of smallpox. Castell reportedly begged not to go there, stressing that his body was poorly prepared for the environment, never having had the disease, but to no avail. Transferred on November 14 and given the same bedding as White, he contracted the disease by about December 1 and died December 12. Outraged at the treatment of his friend, and probably acting in concert with Castell's widow, who pressed for murder charges, Oglethorpe persuaded Parliament to form a committee to inquire into the state of prisons. That committee delivered three reports in 1729–1730, one each on the Fleet, Marshalsea, and King's Bench debtors prisons.[23]

Oglethorpe's investigations mark one of the most important moments in early English prison reform. The committee's reports were published, led to two high-profile trials, and inspired newspaper articles, pamphlets, and even some laudatory poetry. Sheehan credits them with instigating a pivotal moment in London prison reform, because the City of London was spurred to action if only to keep Parliament from fiddling in its administrative domain. Oglethorpe, of course, is better known as the founder of the American colony of Georgia. However, these episodes were related, for the movement to establish a colony for released debtors was a natural outgrowth of his prison efforts.[24]

What is useful for our purposes is to see how Oglethorpe's reports and the writings they inspired amplified discussions of the concerns about debtors raised by Pitt and others and drew on medical theories about class and the human constitution. At first blush it is easy to miss this point, because so much of Oglethorpe's reports focused on forms of financial extortion. However, a close reading demonstrates what was at stake when keepers extorted debtors. As both Castell's and Pitt's cases showed, extortion led directly to polite men being banished from zones of security into biohazardous zones characterized by proximity to lowly bodies and their filth. According to testimony, Castell (whom Oglethorpe described as a "Gentleman" and "a Man born to a compe-tent Estate," lest MPs miss the point about his class) expressed his fear of relo-cation in terms of constitutional vulnerability: "The said Bambridge [the keeper] ordered him to be recommitted to *Corbett's,* where the Small-Pox then raged, though Castell acquainted him with his not having had that Distemper, and that he dreaded it so much, That putting him into a House where it was would occasion his Death." Here notions of predisposition matter, because Castell framed his protestations around his body's lack of suitable prepared-ness for this harsh new environment. If Oglethorpe is to be believed, wardens like Bambridge used the threat of contagious disease as a strategy to frighten debtors into paying up specifically to avoid the dangers of the dreaded common side. He related the tale of a formerly wealthy merchant named John Holder who similarly had feared that his respectable lifestyle rendered his constitution unfit to live among paupers, a fear the warden manipulated. "He feared Bambridge's cruel treatment of him would be the Cause of his Death: the Miseries of the Common Side, which he dreaded, had such an Effect upon him (being a Man of an advanced Age, and accustomed to live in Ease and Plenty)." Notions of class and predisposition shine through here, and an inev-itability is implied as this delicate body almost immediately sickened once banished to the live among the poor. Oglethorpe sketched the decline of such polite bodies further. "When the miserable Wretch hath worn out the Charity of his Friends, and consumed the Money which he hath raised upon his Cloaths and Bedding, and hath eat his last Allowance of Provisions, he usually in a few Days grows weak for want of Food, with the Symptoms of a *Hectick Fever;* and when he is no longer able to stand, if he can raise 3*d.* to pay the Fee of the common Nurse of the Prison, he obtains the Liberty of being carried into the Sick Ward, and lingers on for about a Month or two, by the assistance of the abovementioned Prison Portion of Provision, and then dies."[25] Debtors had little hope under these conditions, as biological forces took over and, to borrow from modern gender commentators, biology became destiny.

Oglethorpe prefaced that passage by noting that "the Goal Distemper" pervaded in the Marshalsea because of inadequate toilet facilities, high-lighting the hazardous nature of plebeian excreta along lines we have seen.

The stench was "noisome beyond Expression, and it seems surprising that it hath not caused a Contagion." Common prisoners' waste was dangerous, but it was the failure to quarantine polite debtors from that danger that was most concerning: "Generally a very desperate and abandoned Sort of people, are suffered to mix with all the unhappy Debtors of the Common Side . . . [where] a Day seldom passed without a Death." Some rooms were so foul that Oglethorpe confessed that he and his fellow inspectors feared entering them. The stench in one "was so intolerable, that Your Committee could not continue in the Room six Minutes." The situation was no better at the Fleet, where debtors cast from the master's side were put in dungeons "adjoining to the Sink and Dunghill where all the Nastiness of the Prison is Cast."[26]

If that were not bad enough, this was also where the prison stored dead bodies. Proximity to rotting corpses presented serious danger. Marshalsea keeper William Acton, who found himself on trial as a result of the investigations, was accused of using corpses in his reign of terror. One debtor was confined for six days with two corpses that were already four days dead. Imagine the impact on MPs and polite readers when Oglethorpe described the scene: "Yet was He kept there with them Six Days longer, in which time the Vermin devoured the Flesh from the Faces, eat the Eyes out of the Heads of the carcasses, which were bloated, putrifyed, and turned green." Of course, such language of putrefaction would have rung bells for anyone familiar with plague discourses, which, given the Marseilles epidemic just a few years earlier, would have been most people. Other debtors were forced to lodge with the sick, which was almost as bad. Several at the Marshalsea pleaded to remove a sick woman named Mary Trapps, to no avail: "At last she smelt so strong that the Turnkey himself could not bear to come into the Room . . . and they were forced to lie with her, or on the Boards, till she died." When the committee inspected this prison, it found other debtors confined with a sick man despite having paid rent of two shillings and sixpence each per week, "submit[ing] to such Rent and Usage rather than be turned down to the Common Side." This last claim is intriguing for two reasons. First, it implies the horror of the common side for these propertied prisoners, who would rather lodge with a sick polite body than be cast among the crowds of paupers. Second, Oglethorpe's emphasis on their rent highlights how he, members of Parliament, and his polite readership interpreted the keeper's malevolence. These debtors' rent should have procured the safety that members of their class expected. It should have purchased safe quarantine from a menacing biohazard. An even worse complaint was leveled against Bambridge at the Fleet, who cast debtors to the common side "tho they have paid the Master's Side Fees."[27] The indignation that comes through in so many passages in the Oglethorpe reports is not for the conditions of commoners, who by all accounts lived in filthy and hazardous environs. Rather, the repeated criticism is that polite bodies had not been properly protected. In the above instances, the clearest marker of class—money— does not procure protection. This, to Oglethorpe, was the height of treachery. Corrupt wardens literally stole debtors' class from them. They extorted whatever money these polite men had and thrust them into poverty, expressed by starvation, filth, and crowding, all of which brought the biologically inevitable results of disease and death. However, these last examples are potentially even more vicious, since these men were not yet out of cash. They held a few shillings and could thereby still lay claim to some measure of privileged safety, procured through the payment of rent. Bambridge took their money yet still thrust them into dangerous proximity to foul bodies. If Oglethorpe seems particularly outraged, it is at least in part because what has been threatened here is not just the health of these particular men but something much more vital, the foundation on which much eighteenth-century bourgeois identity rested and the mechanism by which it was attained: the contract.

Oglethorpe's efforts have been simultaneously hailed as the most important prison-reform activity of the age and declared a failure. On the one hand, he succeeded in casting a spotlight on London's prisons. His reports stirred up considerable concern, and in ways that foreshadowed how Howard would be received, he was cast as a hero. Poems like *The Prisons Open'd* by Samuel Wesley employed the imagery of plague and rot ("Piecemeal alive they rot, long doom'd to bear / The pestilential foul imprison'd Air"), while simultaneously lauding Oglethorpe's courage for entering such hazardous spaces, ("Despising no Man's Danger but his Own"). James Thomson similarly applauded the committee's courage and humanity for braving "the horrors of the gloomy jail . . . Where misery moans; Where Sickness pines."

Hogarth captured the spirit of the moment in his painting *The Gaols Committee of the House of Commons* (1729), which portrayed Oglethorpe's committee interrogating a shifty-looking keeper while a prisoner in rags pleads on bended knee. Like so many of his paintings it would be reproduced

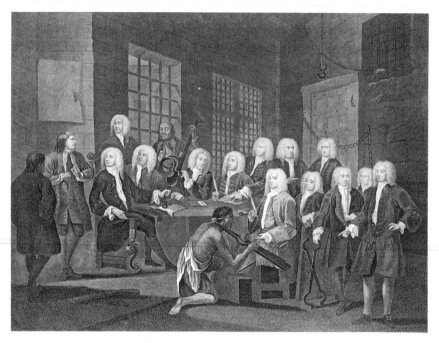

Figure 3. "Bambridge on Trial for Murder by a Committee of the House of Commons" (1803), based on William Hogarth, *The Gaols Committee of the House of Commons* (1729). Engraved by Thomas Cook. Photo: Tate London, 2017.

as engravings throughout the century (Figure 3). The ragged dress, supplicating position, near nudity, and dark skin of the prisoner even seem to mirror eighteenth-century portrayals of New World indigenes and even later abolitionist depictions of African slaves. The wide cultural response to Oglethorpe's work has led such scholars as John Bender to proclaim 1729 "a signal date" in the history of prison reform.[28]

Yet little reform followed. Bambridge and Acton were charged with felonies and their trials were actively followed by the press. Testimony makes clear that the concerns about bodies raised in Oglethorpe's reports resonated. For example, the court inquired about minute details like the precise proximity of the deceased's room to the sewer. Both keepers were acquitted, however. Scholars like Alex Pitofsky argue that the City of London, the body that ran the institutions in question and for which Oglethorpe's reports presented high-profile criticism, had little stomach for reform. Moreover, Oglethorpe aimed his critique too narrowly upon individual corruption rather than wider structural problems. Nefarious keepers, rather than the debt laws or the prisons themselves, took the blame. Moreover, Pitofsky suggests that the same culture that supported the Bloody Code stood by the idea that prison should be unpleasant in order to deter crime. McConville concurs, citing anxieties about perceived spikes in street crime leading to tough attitudes and undercutting support for prison reform. Quoting Howard biographer William Guy, Pitofsky notes that "between 1729 and 1773 prison reform 'seems to have fallen asleep' " and asserts that "virtually nothing changed as a consequence of Oglethorpe's investigations."[29]

Such claims overstate the case. There was a quite telling parliamentary response: Insolvency Acts. Parliament created the conditions that allowed for the release of lots of debtors from lots of prisons. Under these acts any debtor jailed for more than six months could petition for release. He had to present a copy of his estate to the Quarter Sessions, swear to its veracity, and publish notice of the proceedings in the newspapers. If a debtor's claims were accepted, his property would be divided among his creditors, and he would remain liable for outstanding amounts. But he would be released from jail and could not again be imprisoned for the same debts. Having passed two Insolvency Acts in 1728, Parliament quickly passed another in 1729. By the time of Oglethorpe's report on the Fleet in 1730, he was able to boast that nearly six thousand debtors had been recently released from prison. Even this relief, it seems, was not enough, for the following year Parliament passed another act. Four Insolvency Acts had been passed during the first twenty-seven years of the century, but the decade beginning the year of Castell's death (1728) brought the passage of six more. If this seems unimpressive, consider that by 1735 Parliament made previous Insolvency Acts into standing orders. The *Act to explain and Amend . . . An Act for the Relief of Debtors with respect to the Imprisonment of their Persons* (1735) extended the provisions of the 1728 and 1729 acts to 1740, at which time Parliament passed another statute extending these provisions for another seven years. The ad hoc and occasional nature of Insolvency Acts had been replaced by ongoing, standing laws that provided debtors with perpetual channels out of jail. Even during these extensions Parliament passed further Insolvency Acts in 1736, 1737, and 1742, then two more in 1747. Moreover, in 1738 a law was passed to enforce an Elizabethan statute enabling debtors to collect monies from the poor rates, which would have helped sustain them in jail. In all Parliament passed no fewer than thirty-seven Insolvency Acts between 1670 and 1800. Duffy has argued that concerns about conditions in jail had a direct bearing on this legislation, and that acts often emerged during periods of overcrowding.[30]

There was thus considerable legislative activity following Oglethorpe's actions. It would seem a semantic quibble to debate whether this legislation counts as "reform." If for reform one seeks rebuilt prisons, the seventeenth and early eighteenth centuries will disappoint. However, the removal of select bodies from prisons may represent not a lack of reform but simply a different approach to it. This legislation offers evidence of high levels of concern for the bodily safety of debtors. Time and again, petitioning debtors employed the language of poverty, corruption, and disease bequeathed by plague. They feared for their lives when forced to live like paupers, or worse, among them. Oglethorpe became a loudspeaker broadcasting that language to a national audience. And MPs listened, up to a point.

They did not react as later prison reformers and historians may have thought they should, namely calling for the root-and-branch restructuring of jails. MPs still showed little concern about the conditions facing felons and vagrants. They did, however, realize that men like themselves could easily see their fortunes take an unexpected turn. The threat of debtors' prison was all too real. Wealth might be fleeting, and fortunes could turn on a dime in this emerging market economy. Had not the South Sea Bubble—so firmly fixed in propertied men's minds during the 1720s—taught this very lesson? MPs stood by debt laws, of course. Creditors were hardly to be left in the lurch. But the public health menace presented by jails worked to soften the hard line on debt. So MPs moved not to let debtors off the hook but to help establish greater separation between them and more lowly criminals. They ensured that debtors received levels of support in jail that could help prevent them from slipping classes, to remain fed rather than starving, clothed rather than naked, and safely housed away from rotten bodies. More important, creating channels for debtors to get out of jail while still owning up to their responsibilities allowed thousands of once-respectable men to escape the biohazardous zones of filth described in such vivid detail by Pitt and Oglethorpe. It was not merely that debtors might die, but as petitioners always stressed, visitation practices meant that respectable family members and friends could become frightening vectors unwittingly spreading contagion beyond prison walls. Charting the coincidence of prison epidemics and the timing of so many Insolvency Acts is beyond the scope of this chapter, though it is tempting to suggest it as a future research topic, given that an even earlier attempt to address the problem of insolvent debtors tellingly followed an outbreak of fever in the Upper Bench prison.[31]

Moreover, there was some actual prison building. For example, in 1736 Parliament authorized officials in Kent to build a new jail. The act's preamble makes clear that two concerns drove the legislation: the threat of epidemic to the wider community and the desire to protect debtors.

> Whereas the common Gaol for securing the Prisoners of the Crown at *Maidstone*, in the Western Division of the County of *Kent*, is in great Decay, too strait for the safe keeping of the Prisoners, and standing in the middle of the said Town, is often, from Distempers of the Prisoners, both offensive and dangerous to the Inhabitants of the said Town, and to such as resort thither; and there being no Prison for confining of Debtors, great Charge, Expence, and Hazard are thereby occasioned to the Sheriff of the said County . . . And whereas there is no Scite of Ground to enlarge the said Gaol, or to erect a Prison and other Conveniences for the safe keeping of Debtors . . .[32]

The extensive concern about debtors' bodily safety offers a glimpse at how plague doctors' warnings about poverty had nourished the growth of wider fears, ones that expressed themselves through claims about class and the body and found expression far beyond medical genres. The plight of the debtor struck at the heart of tangible bourgeois anxiety in the early eighteenth century. All too often the propertied would have heard stories about incarcerated friends, relatives, and neighbors and must have imagined themselves in similar straits. Finn has shown how commonly narratives of debt and imprisonment appeared in both fictional and autobiographical texts of the period, while Muldrew has noted how fears of debt and prison literally haunted propertied men's nightmares.[33] Among their greatest fears, it seems, was that they would never survive the ordeal. Plunged into an environment of poverty and filth, a debtor stood to catch infection from an inmate or descend into poverty until his own body took on the qualities of malnourishment and corruption that led to deadly disease. After all, is this not what generations of doctors had said about the biological effects of poverty? Class was not an unbridgeable divide, as nineteenth-century formulations of categories like gender or race later became. The propertied knew that their bodies could degenerate into the rotten bodies of the very poor. Debtors thus present fascinating liminal figures. Thinking of them in this way can help us make sense of the schizophrenic response to their plight. It is worth bearing in mind that the Insolvency Acts were passed by the same legislative body that enacted so many laws to protect property with the death penalty, laws that have spurred the accusation of a class conspiracy by some criminal historians.[34] If the Bloody Code protected property, Insolvency Acts protected the propertied. Parliamentary activity demonstrates the strong affinity that propertied citizens had for debtors. They saw themselves in them. And yet in his *Due Preparations for the Plague* Defoe warned that public safety required that debtors be cast out from the city with the rest of the paupers—although strangely, and tellingly, they did not have to go quite as far. Debtors were thus like hermaphrodites for class, neither fully polite nor fully plebeian. Indeed, debtors' petitions and Oglethorpe's reports presented two very different presentations of them, often simultaneously. Oglethorpe invited polite readers and MPs to identify with victimized debtors whose cases he highlighted, humanizing his reports by providing their names and personal details. Yet he presented debtors on the common side as a frightening anonymous mass lurking with disease and danger. Of course, that amorphous crowd would have included men who just weeks or months earlier had been quite like the propertied protagonists of his stories. Oglethorpe's reports thus convey this hermaphroditical quality: the debtor as polite, the debtor as pauper. Hence we see not a clear stand on the issue of incarceration for debt in the early eighteenth century, but rather a perplexed, conflicted response whereby MPs worked to soften the enforcement of laws that they themselves had passed. The political class stood by the laws that cast debtors into jail, while simultaneously passing other laws to help them get out.[35] The confusion of that response has its basis in the confounding, liminal figure that the debtor presented to early-eighteenth-century culture. Simultaneously poor and respectable, debtors received a mixture of scorn and sympathy that demonstrates that no one was sure quite what to do with them. Though they are rarely considered in this light, Insolvency Acts thus represent public health strategies, ones that aimed to protect patrician bodies from plebeian bodies by creating distance between them.

જ⁊૯

Throughout the first third of the eighteenth century, then, there was considerable dialogue about the epidemic dangers of prisons. Whether in plague treatises, debtor's petitions, parliamentary reports, or the popular press, there was a strong sense that jails represented a pressing health concern. These debates helped spread key ideas about the plebeian body, voicing them beyond medical treatises and generating ever more anxiety among respectable Britons. At times, commentators even referenced a new disease. The typographically challenged Mead called it the Goal Fever, while in the trial of William Acton it was known as Gaol Distemper. Prisons had a disease all their own, a disease related to plague, but one that would soon step from the shadows and assume the reins as the primary driver of anxiety about the plebeian body.

4. Jail Fever Comes of Age

On April 25, 1750, London's Old Bailey courtroom was more than usually crowded. Twenty-three men stood trial for an assortment of typical eighteenth-century crimes: highway robbery, coining, and various forms of theft. Among the defendants was a naval man, Captain Edward Clark, accused of killing fellow officer Captain Thomas Innes during a duel. Their dispute had grown out of words spoken at another tribunal, a series of courts martial in December 1749 related to behavior during a naval battle near Cuba. Clark shot Innes in March, and by the time he stood at the bar in late April the case was a cause célèbre. The space allotted in the *Old Bailey Proceedings* was apparently not sufficient to meet the demand for details, so a pamphlet on the case quickly emerged, and newspapers kept the public informed about efforts to obtain the pardon that allowed Clark to evade the death penalty he received.[1] Clark was saved. The same cannot be said for many of the well-heeled Londoners who craned their necks from the gallery during the five-hour trial.

It was two weeks before people realized that something was wrong. London newspapers typically reported the deaths and serious illnesses of well-known citizens, so it was not out of the ordinary when the *London Evening Post* reported that alderman Sir Daniel Lambert had succumbed to a "violent fever" on Sunday, May 6. However, a string of notable deaths quickly commanded attention. During the week that started May 12, readers of various papers learned of the deaths from "violent" or "malignant" fever of Baron of the Court of the Exchequer Charles Clarke, Judge of the Court of Common Pleas Sir Thomas Apney, attorney and Clerk of the Papers John Sharpless, and

Common Councilman William Hunt, as well as a Mr. Beardsmore, who was deputy marshall to the lord chief justice of the Kings Bench, an "eminent Barrister" named William Baird, a councilor named Otway, and the attorney and under sheriff Robert Cox, Esq. The connections of these men to the Old Bailey raised suspicions of an epidemic that can be detected by about May 20. The bad news kept coming, manifested by the deaths of several jurors in the Clark trial and then the fever, sickness, and death of Samuel Pennant, the lord mayor of London. Early reports that "we do not hear that the supposed Infection communicates itself" were probably unconvincing, for the same paper reported that the mayor's doctor "continues dangerously ill," surely suggesting that the disease was contagious. The 25 percent spike in fever deaths reported by May 29 must have amplified fears.[2]

The first paper to forge a link between these deaths and the Old Bailey may have been the *Whitehall Evening Post*. Its issue for May 17–19 reported that officials had ordered the courtroom to be rendered "more airy"—"it being conceived, that the Stench of the Prisoners, and the Court being generally much crouded, may endanger the Health of the Judges, &c." The subsequent issue then followed Mayor Pennant's obituary by proclaiming an epidemic and centering it squarely on the courtroom. Chief Justice William Lee, whose deputy marshall was one of the first casualties, soon sent an envoy to the Court of Aldermen demanding reforms of Newgate prison (the jail adjacent to the court, from which the defendants had been transferred), exclaiming that it was "dangerous for Persons to attend the Business of the Sessions." Lee underlined the epidemic's cause, listing twenty men killed by "the noisome Stench of the Prisoners." At least three papers printed the same report verbatim on May 26, ensuring that within a month of the trial and just a few weeks of the first casualties citizens across London were reading that the epidemic fit a very old pattern, whereby elite bodies were infected by lowly ones. Orders for cleaning Newgate and washing prisoners before they entered the court quickly followed.[3]

Notwithstanding the health hazards long associated with jails, it would be this epidemic that galvanized fears surrounding an emerging disease that would be called jail fever. In this chapter I seek to chart the history of this disease and demonstrate how it drew upon the medical traditions that we have explored. We shall leave to the next chapter the task of exploring Londoners' reaction to the epidemic itself.

The words and actions of late May suggest that Londoners made up their minds quite quickly about what the disease was and where it came from:

a malignant fever emanating from the bodies of prisoners. The possibilities they rejected are worth considering. For example, they did not attribute the disease to climate, despite mention of the coming summer season and the importance of medical environmentalism in the eighteenth century.[4] Nor did sheriffs limit the number of spectators in the court, even though the crowded nature of the courtroom was noted repeatedly. Polite bodies seem not to have been seriously considered, if considered at all, as possible sources of this disease. The washing of *prisoners'* bodies and the spaces that those bodies inhabited point clearly to the presumed source of the "noisome stench" believed to kill so many civic leaders. It is also telling that no report implicated the gentleman defendant Clark as a source of the disease. Rather, unnamed accused felons bore the accusation. In their early days epidemics often breed shock and confusion. In this one, however, opinion coalesced remarkably quickly. It did so because of history.

The Black Assizes: Oxford, 1577

One explanation for the long continuities in ideas about epidemics that this book charts is the ongoing practice of researching old epidemics to make sense of new ones. This happened with stunning efficiency in 1750. Between May 24 and 26 three newspapers ran the following story, which included a passage from Mead.

> As the Deaths of several Persons who were at the last Sessions at the Old Baily, have been attributed to the noisome Stench of the prisoners, we have, in Confirmation of the said Opinion, quoted the following from one of Dr. Mead's Books.
>
> "In our common Prisons many have what they call the *Gaol Fever*, which is always attended with a Degree of Malignity . . ."
>
> The *Black Assize* at Oxford, held in the Castle there, in the Year 1577, will never be forgot; in which the Judges, Gentry, and almost all that were present, to the number of 300, were kill'd by a poisonous Steam, thought by some to have broken forth from the Earth; but by a noble and great Philosopher, Lord Bacon, more justly supposed to have been brought by the Prisoners out of the Gaol into Court.

There then followed a passage from Richard Baker's *Chronicles of the Kings of England* (1643) detailing this 1577 epidemic using uncannily similar language to news accounts from earlier that week. It blamed the Oxford disease on the "Pestilent Savour" and "noisome Smell" of prisoners and similarly listed its high-profile victims. "There died Robert Bell, Lord Chief Baron; Robert D'oyle, Sir William Babington D'oyle, Sheriff of Oxfordshire, Harcourt, Weymen and Fettiplace, the most of them Men in this Tract, Barham the famous Lawyer, almost all the Jurors, and three hundred others, more or less."[5] Londoners trying to make sense of the sudden death of judges and lawyers in 1750 thus had keen instincts for precisely where to look for relevant knowledge. By turning to writers like Mead and Baker they at once connected their crisis with the plague scare of the 1720s, with older plague epidemics (given the historical thrust of Mead's book), and with this specific episode of 1577. The 1750 Old Bailey epidemic was thus framed in real time in a profoundly historical way, a practice that would help update and reinforce ideas about the pathogenic plebeian body nearly a century after 1666.

The so-called Oxford Black Assize of 1577 was itself a touchstone event that would be recast in medical and historical works throughout the two centuries that followed it. It claimed at most just a few hundred lives, which—relative to England's more vicious plague epidemics—may hardly seem worthy of such commemoration. Yet it was clearly a story worth telling and remembering. To this day employees at the County Hall in Oxford eat in a cafeteria beneath a plaque commemorating it, one notably hung in the late nineteenth century (Figure 4). Literary scholars like Priscilla Wald have called attention to the structures, themes, and formats of so-called "outbreak narratives," in which stories of epidemics demonstrate revealing patterns.[6] Such an approach is useful for thinking through some of the elements that became fixtures in how the stories of 1577 and, later, 1750 would be told and retold over a long time.

In 1577, as in 1750, it was not the sheer number of victims but the quality of those victims that mattered most. Modern epidemiologists gauge epidemics' ferocity numerically; the worst kill the most. However, in the tale-telling that characterizes how epidemics are culturally framed, unique circumstances or patterns of transmission can have particular narrative force to shape how a disease-event is registered and remembered. Often, an issue that matters more than the cold body count is the question of who constituted the source and who the victims. The figure of Typhoid Mary, the poor immigrant cook who unwittingly spread disease to her wealthy employers, or of Gaétan Dugas, the handsome Canadian flight attendant framed as

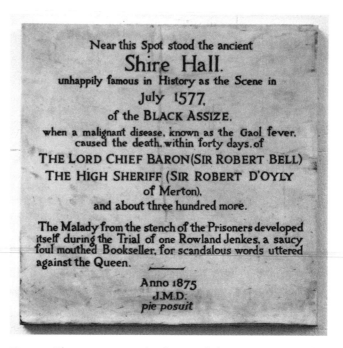

Near this Spot stood the ancient
Shire Hall.
unhappily famous in History as the Scene in
July 1577,
of the BLACK ASSIZE.
when a malignant disease, known as the Gaol fever,
caused the death, within forty days, of
THE LORD CHIEF BARON(SIR ROBERT BELL)
THE HIGH SHERIFF (SIR ROBERT D'OYLY
of Merton),
and about three hundred more.

The Malady from the stench of the Prisoners developed
itself during the Trial of one Rowland Jenkes, a saucy
foul mouthed Bookseller, for scandalous words uttered
against the Queen.

Anno 1875
J.M.D.
pie posuit

Figure 4. Plaque commemorating the 1577 Black Assizes, County Hall, Oxford. WikiCommons, photo: Motacilla, 2015.

Patient Zero in the AIDS epidemic, offer two of the more notorious examples of how outbreak narratives can hinge on particular story elements that fascinate or terrify. Laura McGough has similarly explored how early modern Italians framed the Renaissance syphilis epidemic around rich tales of dangerously beautiful prostitutes.[7] In similar fashion, the 1577 Oxford epidemic captured the imagination not because of how many people died, but because of who died and how they got sick. And in the panicked weeks of May 1750 its story reached through time and imparted vital lessons to Enlightenment Londoners.

The central figure in 1577 was a prisoner named Rowland Jenks, a Catholic bookbinder on trial for something he had said. Later texts called him foulmouthed and seditious, suggesting that he had insulted the queen. Early sources reveal a profound Reformation context that would fade over time. It is not known what Jenks said, but early accounts craft him as a Catholic martyr even though he did not quite die for the cause. (Instead, he had his ears nailed to the pillory and was made to cut himself free.) Robert Parsons' 1582 *An Epistle of the Persecution of Catholickes in Englande* called the infection of judges and jurors "a wonder full Iudgement of God" for such brutal treatment of his coreligionist. Predictably, Protestant writers took a different view. According to Oxford historian Anthony Wood, rumors swirled that the disease was the result of Catholic "Art Magick." As late as 1741 Jeremiah Whitaker Newman could quote a story portraying Jenks in the frame of an early modern plague spreader, purposely fomenting the disease by igniting a poisonous candle in the courtroom.[8] These were minority opinions. In the versions that would dominate memories of the Black Assizes, Jenks's punishment was warranted and the disease just a tragic coincidence, stemming not from Jenks but from the other filthy prisoners who stood trial that day.

It was not physicians but chroniclers like Baker and Wood who offered the more commonly cited depictions of the epidemic. In his *Chronicles* Baker dropped the religious nature of the case. Written in 1643, versions of these words followed Mead's in London newspapers in May 1750:

> About this time, when the Judges sate at the Assizes in Oxford, and one Rowland Jenkes a Book-seller was questioned for speaking approbrious words against the Queen, suddenly they were surprised with a pestilent savour; whether rising from the noysome smell of the prisoners, or from the dampe of the ground, is uncertaine, but all that were there present, almost every one, within forty hours died, except Women and children; and the Contagion went no further. There died Robert Bell Lord chief Baron, Robert D'Oylie; Sir William Babington: D'Olye Sheriffe of Oxford-shire, Harcourt, Weynman, Phetiplace, the most noted men in this Tract; Barham the famous Lawyer; almost all the Jurours, and three hundred other, more or lesse.[9]

The immunity of women and children would be occasionally mentioned as part of the epidemic's lore, but it had little influence on later formulations of jail fever. Indeed, eighteenth-century experts on a specifically female form of fever—puerperal or childbed fever—argued that poor women were highly susceptible to the disease for the same reasons that paupers were prone to other putrid fevers (even comparing puerperal fever to jail fever and mentioning the black assizes).[10] It is in Baker that we find reference to the "noysome smell" of prisoners, the precise phrase repeated in 1750. His use of the term *pestilent* suggested links with plague.

On this last point Baker was following Francis Bacon, the greatest scientific authority to address the disease and one whom we saw Mead quote directly. That Bacon would become the leading authority on the 1577 Black Assizes is odd because he didn't actually mention Oxford. Rather in his *Sylva Sylvarum: or A Natural History in Ten Centuries* (1627) he included a general discussion of diseases spreading from prisoners to judges within his larger discussion of the transmission and properties of immaterial forces. The most frequently cited early modern passage on the disease that became jail fever exclaimed: "The most pernicious infection next to the plague is the smell of the gaol, where prisoners have been long and close and nastily kept; whereof we have had in our time experience twice or thrice, when both the judges that sat on the gaol, and numbers of those that attended the business, or were present sickened upon it and died." Like Sydenham, who would call pestilential fever a slightly weaker species of plague, Bacon situated jail fever adjacent to plague as the second-deadliest disease. This connection becomes even clearer when we consider that the above passage immediately followed three paragraphs on plague and was directly followed by discussion of putrefaction and the danger of human odors: "such Foule Smels . . . consist chiefly of Mans Flesh, or Sweat, Putrified." Bacon's doctrine of sympathy also resembled Nathaniel Hodges's theory that plague's poison possessed a great "similitude" to putrid predisposed blood. Although he spoke of immaterial airs and spirits (rather than blood and poisons), Bacon's claim is nearly identical: "For they are not those Stinckes, which the Nosthrils streight abhorre, and expell, that are most Pernicious; But such Aires, as *have some Similitude with Mans Body;* And so insinuate themselves, and betray the Spirits." His comments on predisposition's role in contagion demonstrate even further how firmly Bacon's ideas about the disease that became jail fever drew on plague discourses that we encountered in Chapter 1. Furthermore, Bacon signaled that the Oxford outbreak was not a singular event. Wood, who quoted Bacon directly, pondered which outbreaks he had meant. The Cambridge Assizes of 1521–1522, after which judges and other "gentlemen" in the courtroom sickened and died, was one possibility. However, Bacon probably had in mind the 1586 Exeter Assizes, described in Raphael Holinshed's *Chronicles,* perhaps the first text to register a name for the disease "commonlie called the Gaole Sicknesse."[11]

Holinshed addressed another key feature found in the outbreak narratives about both 1577 and 1750. In version after version prisoners whose status rendered them unworthy of note were imagined to infect men whose status demanded that their deaths be publicized, the nation's loss itemized, by listing their names and titles. Although Holinshed acknowledged that most deaths in the Exeter epidemic were of "plebeian and common people," he named the many judges, knights, and justices of the peace who died and asserted that their elevated statuses literally made their lives more valuable and their deaths more costly. His words suggest a kind of sliding scale of national loss: the higher the class, the greater the loss. "The losse of everie of them was verie great to the commonwealth of that province and countrie. ... The more worthie were these personages, the greater losse was their deaths to the whole common wealth of that countrie." It was thus the tragedy that great men could be killed by lowly ones that invested the story of 1577 with imaginative force, rendering it a cautionary tale that would be told again and again. Mead was not hyperbolic when he wrote 143 years after the fact that "the *Black Assizes* at Oxford . . . will never be forgot."[12] This was so because the story was not relegated to the pages of physicians' treatises but was registered by historians and chroniclers as a touchstone event in the national memory.

Gaol Fever Takes Form, 1720–1750

It was during the Marseilles plague scare that we begin to see the "Gaol Distemper" or "Gaol Fever" increasingly discussed by name. Before then such terms were fairly rare. Although Holinshed used such a term in 1586, none of the accounts of the Oxford Assizes followed suit. Nor, it is useful to note, did any of the sixteenth- or seventeenth-century books currently available for full-text searching in *Early English Books Online*.[13] By 1700 we find an account of last words uttered by condemned criminals, claiming that a John Cooper was "seiz'd with the Jayl-Distemper, which is a violent Feaver."[14] It is potentially notable that it was identified as a violent fever, one of the terms used to characterize the epidemic in 1750. Nevertheless, terms like *jail fever* remained rare before the 1720s, at which point physicians, rather than historians, stepped forward to frame the disease.

Here again Mead emerges as a key figure. He solidified the jail sickness as a form of fever, repeatedly calling it "Goal Fever" both in the passage explored earlier and again in his revised eighth edition (1722) during a description of one of Sydenham's plague medicines that he considered useful "in Illnesses of the same kind with the *Goal Fever,* which approaches the nearest to the *Pestilence.*" Thus Mead identified jail fever as Sydenham's pestilential fever, the disease most closely related to plague. He also framed it so as to highlight class. It is important that his account of the Oxford Assizes that would be so widely quoted in 1750 was sandwiched between statements about poverty, firmly situating "Goal Fever" within his larger claims about plebeian bodies that we explored in Chapter 2. For example, we will remember that he urged authorities to inspect houses of the poor because "nothing approaches so near to the first Original of *Contagion,* as Air pent up, loaded with Damps, and corrupted with the Filthiness, that Proceeds from *Animal Bodies.*" It was precisely here that Mead places his claim about jail fever. Because the wording differs slightly from that in newspaper accounts thirty years later, here it is once more: "Our common *Prisons* afford us an instance of this. In which very few escape, what they call the *Goal Fever,* which is always attended with a Degree of *Malignity* in Proportion to the *Closeness* and *Stench* of the Place: And it would certainly very well become the Wisdom of the Government, as well with regard to the Health of the *Town,* as in Compassion to the *Prisoners,* to take care, that all *Houses of Confinement* should be kept Airy and Clean as is consistent with the Use to which they are design'd. The *Black Assize* at *Oxford,* held in the Castle there, in the Year 1577, will never be forgot." Set in the context of the claims that surround this passage, Mead's use of the definite pronoun *this* in the first sentence is important. Jail fever affords us an example of *"this"*—that is, the danger of pent-up plebeian filth, of the poisons that impoverished bodies emit and the toxicity of such poisons when accumulated. Moreover, Mead then followed his paragraph about 1577 with further claims about class, shifting immediately back to the issue of urban medical police. His transition reminded readers of three important points: first, that jail fever was not unique to jails but simply one example of the danger that attended *any* congregation of poor bodies; second, that such bodies were inherently rotten; and third, that cross-class infection from "beggars" to "citizens and gentry" was an explicit threat. "The proper Officers," he wrote, "should be strictly charged to see that the *Streets* be washed and kept clean from *Filth, Carrion,* and all Manner of *Nusances.* . . . *Beggars* and *Idle Persons* should be taken up, and such miserable Objects, as are neither fit for the common *Hospitals,* nor *Work-houses,* should be provided for in an *Hospital of Incurables.* . . . I am sorry to take Notice, that in *these* [cities] of *London* and *Westminster* there is no good *Police* established in these Respects; for want of which the Citizens and Gentry are every Day annoyed more ways than one."[15] In Mead, then, we have one of the earliest, most influential, and most authoritative framings of this new disease, jail fever, a disease that was linked to both plague and poverty from the very start.

Mead wasn't alone. Surgeon Peter Kennedy, who published two treatises during the Marseilles crisis, also identified "Goal Distemper" as a common fever that descended into a malignancy. He bound his discussion of prisons to poverty, underscored by a classic formulation of pauper predisposition. "Contagious maladies most commonly . . . rage amongst a crouded and penn'd up Herd of Creatures, who by Poverty do wallow in their Dirt and Nastiness. . . . Such poor miserable People will be much more liable, and their Bodies more dispos'd to receive, harbour and nourish the malign Atoms of a contagious Malady, than any else."[16] Thus during the Marseilles scare doctors slipped quickly into and out of discussions of jails in the midst of making larger claims about the dangers of filth and poverty. Jail fever was clearly identified by physicians in the early 1720s, but the discussion was fitful and brief.

Textually speaking, jail fever then remained fairly dormant between the Marseilles epidemic and the 1750 Old Bailey outbreak. References pop up only here and there. A 1724 newspaper reported a death in the Marshalsea prison, noting, "Twenty die Weekly of the Goal Distemper (which is the *Spotted Fever*)." We saw that the 1729 trial of William Acton referenced the disease by name, as did the following year's roguish account of the criminal and amorous adventures of John Evert. A 1736 Dublin paper reported that a petty con man contracted "goal distemper," while the *Englishman's Journal* two years later reported the sad tale of a woman who caught the disease in bridewell and conveyed it to her family. A condemned felon died of "the Jail-Distemper" in 1743 before he could reach the scaffold.[17]

The paucity of references to jail fever in the period 1722–1750 is somewhat surprising, given that there was a notable outbreak in 1730. The events closely parallel those in 1577 and 1750. Sir Thomas Pengelly, lord chief baron of the Exchequer, fell ill while on the Western Circuit. Starting April 7, newspapers described his illness as a fever, noting that physicians had "little or no Hopes for his Life." By April 16 Pengelly's clerk and groom were both reported dead, as was Sir James Sheppard, sergeant at law and member of Parliament for Hointon. Sheppard died in Exeter, where an "Epidemical

Fever" was said to rage in the town. The *Monthly Chronicle* soon reported the deaths of other court officers. Notably, these reports set the epidemic in its historical context: "On this melancholy Occasion, it may not be improper to insert the following Paragraph out of *Baker's* Chronicles," followed by the same account of the 1577 Oxford Assizes that 1750 papers would reprint again and again.[18] Thus the epidemic that would come to be associated with Taunton (the town where Pengelly was said to be infected) was framed as an episode of jail fever—though without using that precise phrase—deploying many of the same historical resources that Londoners would deploy twenty years later.

Nevertheless, the 1730 Taunton epidemic did not register nearly the same cultural impact as would the 1750 Old Bailey incident, and a few probable reasons suggest themselves. First, the 1730 epidemic did not directly threaten London. It had the potential to do so, but voices quickly worked to play down the danger. The "epidemical fever" proclaimed in Exeter was swiftly denounced, presumably by Exeter authorities worried about the impact of such rumors. Whereas the Old Bailey was centered in the heart of London and potentially threatened a repeat of 1665/6, the Taunton epidemic affected smaller communities and posed a lesser danger. Although later accounts would claim that hundreds died in Taunton, Creighton could find no support for the claim.[19] The 1730 Taunton episode had many of the same features as the 1750 Old Bailey epidemic: elite men were infected by the noisome effluvia of common prisoners. However, whether we consider it in terms of sheer body count or, more important for this study, psychic terror, its epidemic was more limited.

Jail Fever in 1750: John Pringle
Frames an Eighteenth-Century Terror

The Old Bailey outbreak presented a monster of a different scope. If jail fever was not born in 1750, it certainly came of age then, for the second half of the century looks altogether different to scholars analyzing the disease. Consider that not a single book was devoted to the topic prior to 1750. Before then, one must scour works of history for the occasional paragraph, often finding the same few passages reiterated again and again. By contrast, entire treatises on the disease appeared in the second half of the century, written by such medical men as John Pringle, James Lind, James Carmichael Smyth,

John Heysham, Robert Robertson, Daniel Peter Layard, and John Mason Good. Digitized texts reveal patterns that are so clear as to assuage the healthy methodological concerns about the imperfections of current search engines. Consider that of the 185 eighteenth-century newspaper items that the *Burney Newspaper Collection* identifies containing variant spellings of "Jail/Gaol/Goal Fever" or "Jail/Gaol/Goal Distemper," only 5 (2.7 percent) appeared before 1750. The same searches of the more than 100,000 books in the *Eighteenth Century Collections Online* produces the same picture. Of the 452 books in which any of the above terms appear, just nineteen (4.2 percent) predate 1750.[20] But even that figure is bloated, for nearly half were editions of Mead. Jail fever became a different cultural force after 1750.

What is remarkable is how quickly after the Old Bailey incident this shift happened. On May 29, just twelve days after the first reports of the epidemic, newspapers advertised that physician John Pringle had published the first (and, we will see, perhaps the most important) treatise on jail fever. The lord mayor was dead barely a week before printers in the Strand had *Observations on the Nature and Cure of Hospital and Jayl-Fevers* on their shelves. It is fitting that it was written by a disciple of Mead, to whom the book was addressed. Such a quick response signals both the level of concern in London and the remarkable agility of the eighteenth-century market, something demonstrated equally well by advertisements for patent medicines. Within days of Pringle's advertising his new book, the *Whitehall Evening Post* included lengthy testimonials trumpeting the efficacy of "Dr. James's Fever Powders" for the epidemic. With a separate ad for the medicine elsewhere on the page, the newspaper ran what looks at first glance like a news story. "At this Juncture, when every body is alarmed at the frequent Deaths of Numbers of People who attended at the late Sessions at the Old Bailey, and when most people seem alarmed lest the Contagion should spread still farther, it may be some Satisfaction to the Publick to be informed that no one, who contracted a Fever in Consequence of that Attendance, and took Dr. James's Fever Powders, has died." Then followed accounts of an insurance clerk and a bookseller who allegedly attended Clark's trial. In narratives that will appear typical to those familiar with the promotional materials of eighteenth-century empirics, both men were given over as lost by eminent physicians before this patent medicine saved their lives. London's medical marketplace has been well studied, so the appearance of a nostrum seller tailoring his pitch to current events should not surprise us.[21] But an eminent physician producing a learned treatise within two weeks of the outbreak—a treatise that would stand as the authoritative account of the disease for decades and that cannot be dismissed as a flimsy quack pamphlet—this is a more remarkable turn of events, one that surely signals that the Old Bailey incident had indeed set London and the medical world on its ear.

Sometimes people are just in the right place at the right time. Pringle, a highly regarded Scottish physician who studied under Boerhaave and became a disciple of Mead, had extensive military experience treating soldiers during the Jacobite rebellion.[22] Physician-in-ordinary to the duke of Cumberland by 1750, he was already at work on a major study of the diseases of soldiers when the Old Bailey epidemic broke. Witnessing the spread of fever in military hospitals, he came to believe that such fevers represented the same condition as those prevailing in jails, ships, and similar contexts. The revelation that hospital, jail, and ship fevers might all be the same disease occurred to him during a 1746 epidemic involving jailed prisoners of war. Observing that their disease mimicked fevers in hospitals, he concluded that "these prisoners . . . brought with them the jayl-distemper," and that he therefore "consider[ed] the two diseases as one." Pringle was thus already engaged in a research project on jail fever at the time of the Clark trial. Whether it was opportunism or public spirit that drove him to publish his findings sooner than he intended—his *Observations on the Diseases of the Army* would not be completed for another two years—matters little. His preface captures vividly the pressing sense of fear and confusion, as well as the profound demand for medical advice in May 1750. Framing his book as a letter to Mead, he wrote,

> Whilst I was revising the notes I had made on the diseases most incident to an army, the jayl distemper having broke out in such a manner as to alarm the town, I thought I could not comply more seasonably with your [Mead's] desire of having them published, than by communicating at present, that part of my observations which relate to this disease. . . . Yet as people may justly be under some apprehensions as long as this distemper lasts, though I thought it my duty, to offer these few sheets to the publick; that whatever be the consequence, I might not hereafter have reason to upbraid myself with having suppressed any useful discovery my experience may have furnished in these matters, from the consideration that they were to go abroad, in a loose and unfinished manner. And I the more willingly embrace this occasion of writing, that at this time

every body is inclined to listen to the subject, those whose special business it is to take care of jayls and other publick places, which neglected, produce malignant and contagious distempers.[23]

Over the course of fifty-two pages Pringle then framed jail fever in its most extensive form to date, offering a theory of the disease deeply indebted to long-held medical ideas that would provide the foundation for all subsequent eighteenth-century discussions of the disease. What did he say?

Much will be familiar to anyone who has looked at the broader history of fevers, penitentiary reform, or Enlightenment-era public health, each of which has incorporated the eighteenth-century fascination with so-called "crowd diseases." Jail, ship, hospital, and camp fevers now all referred to the same disease—pestilential or malignant fever—a disease that will later be called typhus, and which eighteenth-century doctors believed was generated by a basic set of conditions: too many bodies confined in too little space. Without a source of fresh air, the atmosphere in crowded spaces became poisonous. This was jail fever. The need to keep such spaces clean, to manage the relationship between the number of bodies and the amount of space, and above all to ventilate: these kernels of advice flowed from the pens of doctors and reformers throughout the second half of the century, as medical and penal historians have shown and as coming chapters will explore.[24] What matters for our purposes is not to reiterate that reformers championed clean and airy institutions but rather to chart the implications of those discussions for the history of the plebeian body. After all, only jails with bodies in them generated disease. Empty jails posed no threat. I thus contend that claims that initially appear to address the structure of buildings often advanced deeper claims about the structure of bodies.

For starters, Pringle emphasized putridity. In spite of continuing theoretical development within medicine, the role of putrefaction in theories of epidemic fevers remained as strong as ever. The language of corruption, rot, and putridity everywhere adorns his text. "The hospitals of an army, when crowded with sick, or when the distempers are of a putrid kind; or at any time when the air is confined, especially in hot weather produce a fever of malignant nature, always accounted fatal." Pringle here points to the quality of the air. However, as in the case of plague, something had to corrupt the air. Again and again Pringle identified the emissions from putrid bodies as the most dangerous source of corruption. Explaining the passage above, he noted that institutional air became poisonous when it was "particularly vitiated with perspirable matter. Which, as it is the most volatile part of the humours, is also the most putrescent." Thus it was not the *building* that corrupted the air but the effluvia, in this case the sweat, from the bodies within it. Consider further: "This fever is proper to every place that is the receptacle of crowded men, ill aired or kept dirty; or *what is the same,* wherever there is a collection of putrid animal steams, from dead or even diseased bodies. . . . And upon this account, jayls and military hospitals, are most obnoxious to this kind of pestilential infection; as the first are kept in a constant state of filth and impurity; and the last are so much filled with the poisonous effluvia of sores, mortifications, dysenteric and other putrid excrements." Pringle here moves back and forth between bodies that were officially diseased (those in hospitals) and those that were essentially similar—"what is the same"—the impure bodies of prisoners. Here is another notable echo of Nathaniel Hodges's claim about the "similitude" between plebeian blood and plague-infected blood. Prisoners' impurity parallels that of the diseased and (as we also saw in the seventeenth century) even the dead. The breath, sweat, and bodily waste of either the officially sick or the simply putrid were again presented as fundamentally similar. Pringle stressed this point. The intensity of a fever's malignity depended on one of two things: 1) "the long continuance of putrefaction in the same place" or 2) "the degree and quantity of it." The first factor typified jails where "the putrid ferment is exalted" (intensified) by "the long succession of animal filth." Hospitals exemplified the second case, "which tho' of no long standing, yet by the great quantity of putrid exhalation, will produce *the same effect.*" The putrid emissions of a diseased body in a hospital might be stronger and thus capable of sooner reaching the infectious tipping point than those of a nondiseased (yet putrid) prisoner, sailor, or soldier. Nevertheless, the nature of their emissions differed only in "degree"—Pringle's exact word—not in kind: they produced the same disease. Moreover, the blood, not the nerves or fibers, remained the foundation for understanding putrid diseases. The worst fevers were those in which the blood reached "the highest state of putrefaction."[25]

Pringle's discussions of symptoms and treatments further highlighted putridity. In the same manner as his forebears had searched for signs of plague, Pringle instructed physicians to use their eyes and especially their noses to detect putridity. Sweat, for example, was important. "The sweats are always fetid; and at all times of fever, the patient, if delicate, complains of an ill taste of his mouth, and an offensive smell." Feces told the same tale. "If there are ichorous, cadaverous, and involuntary stools, it is a sign of certain death." The adjective *cadaverous*, which we saw Willis employ a century earlier, is telling. Long used to describe the stench of plague-infected bodies, it would become an increasingly common way of describing bodily emissions in putrid fevers, one that strengthened the conceptual links between putrid plebeian bodies and corpses. Pringle warned doctors not to allow fever patients to remain constipated "lest an accumulation of *faeces* in this putrid disease prove a new *fomes* of corruption." Moreover, he told physicians to sniff urine and stool, warning that feces "of a cadaverous smell . . . [is] the sign of approaching death." The *petechiae*—the spots on the skin that prompted yet two more names for the disease, "spotted fever" or "petechial fever"—represented another sign of inner putridity, following on a long tradition of reading skin lesions in this manner. Pringle's approach to treatment highlighted putrescence further: "We shall still be more convinced of its putrid nature, since all the remedies prove to be of the anti-septic kind." He also held putridity's theoretical partner, predisposition, as doctrine, emphasizing that certain bodies were "much more susceptible" and that contagion "depend[s] on the constitution of the person." Finally, he reaffirmed jail fever's links to plague, emphasizing "the similarity between this fever and a true pestilence."[26]

Thus, throughout the first treatise devoted to jail fever, Pringle voiced virtually all of the claims that doctors had advanced about poor bodies and epidemics for a century: jail fever was a form of pestilential fever, intimately related to plague, generated by putrid blood, the possession of which increased one's level of predisposition. In terms of their constitutions, corrupt bodies continued to exist on a spectrum, fundamentally similar and differing only in degree: from the putridly predisposed, to the putrescent sick, to the rotting corpse. However, Pringle never actually named the poor. Class is heavily implied, of course. The cohorts he describes—soldiers, prisoners, and hospital inmates—were all understood to hail from the lower orders, and he twice warns of slums.[27] Moreover, anyone reading his treatise with a knowledge of plague discourses, or whom Pringle had inspired to read Mead's book (which had recently come out in a new edition), would have easily connected the dots and concluded that jail fever was a classed disease.

Nevertheless, if Pringle's stance on class had to be inferred in 1750, it was crystal clear by 1752, when he finished his larger project on military medicine. *Observations on the Diseases of the Army* laid out in much greater detail the basic formulation that he had rushed to sketch two years earlier. If Pringle overlooked mentioning the poor by name when writing for a deadline in 1750, his magnum opus afforded him plenty of space. What would stand as the leading authority's foundational text on jail fever explained the point. His clearest claim came in a chapter on dysentery, which he presented as one of the many forms that putrid disease could take among soldiers: "This malady is most frequent in hot, close, and moist seasons, when bodies are most subject to putrefaction; and . . . it prevails chiefly among such as are of a scorbutic habit, or the meanest and poorest people, who, from foul air, bad diet and nastiness, are most liable to putrid diseases."[28] Putridity. Predisposition. Poverty. We have seen that these three features characterized plague and fever texts throughout the seventeenth and early eighteenth century. From Bradwell, Harvey, Hodges, and Willis in the seventeenth century to Mead, Defoe, and a host of doctors in the 1720s, we can now add Pringle at midcentury.

Jail Fever: Theory to 1800

Indeed, this line of thinking would be perpetuated throughout the literature of fevers and epidemic disease for the rest of the century. It is worth using this chapter's remaining pages to chart medical ideas on jail fever for the remainder of the century so as to establish them to be taken as read for coming chapters. That strategy is relatively easy because we will see that the ideas were remarkably durable. However, the point is also historiographically pressing, because Hamlin takes a somewhat different view in his recent history of fever. Hamlin does much to acknowledge the central role of putridity in theories of fever, charting the concept back to Galen. However, despite this long pedigree he argues for discontinuity, suggesting that theories of putridity were "rare after 1650," and that we witness a "renewed interest" in them in the mid-eighteenth century. We have seen that this was clearly not the case. His position, which is asserted rather than investigated, may stem from his reading of the Victorian sanitarians, for he hints elsewhere at seeing as novel their links between environmental and internal putridity. Before Pringle, he suggests, "internal, pathological putrefaction had not usually been equated with external putrefaction." This, of course, would have been news to the legions of seventeenth- and early-eighteenth-century doctors who railed about environmental filth and the tendency of the urban poor to internalize it. Although DeLacy addresses slightly different issues, her thesis about medical thought on contagious diseases during the century after 1650 seems apropos: "Claims that this period saw an abrupt break with the past or future are exaggerated or misplaced."[29]

For example, writing a few years after Pringle, physician Dale Ingram asserted that it was "well know[n] that the poor in general are the first to receive the original attacks of any contagious distemper, for a depravity of the blood, coarse diet, uncleanliness, &c. contribute not a little to such diseases." Meanwhile, major authorities like Edinburgh physician John Gregory, best known for his foundational work on medical ethics, promoted such ideas as doctrine to his students at Europe's top medical school. Gregory's *Elements of the Practice of Physic*, published in 1772 and reprinted as late as 1788, stood alongside William Cullen's textbook as an essential teaching text. We saw Gregory's comments at the start of this book: "Predisponent Causes: Whatever increases the putrescency of the system, want of exercise and usual labour, especially in the lower class, who are accustomed to it, and, in consequence of this to perspire copiously; living on putrid animal food; want of fresh vegetables, good bread, sugar, wine and other antisceptics; foul air, in consequence of nastiness, and the want of free ventilation, which is seldom found in the houses of the lower class of people, among whom this disease is most frequent and fatal." It is notable that Gregory kept alive medical assumptions about idleness and perspiration well over a century after Hodges and Willis commented on the issue. Moreover, like Pringle, Gregory did not limit his comments to prisoners but put forth a wider claim about the putrid blood of the poor generally.[30]

The real explosion of medical publishing on jail fever occurred during the 1770s and 1780s, for reasons we will explore in the next chapter. But although one could now choose from numerous treatises on the disease, when it came to theory, these works largely reiterated orthodoxy. In fact, physician Daniel Peter Layard began his *Directions to Prevent the Contagion of the Jail Distemper commonly called the Jail Fever* (1772) by eschewing theory altogether. Why bother repeating what everyone knew, his opening paragraph reasoned: "Sir John Pringle's and Sir Stephen Theodore Janssen's accounts are almost in the hand of every one, whether of the faculty or not." Layard thus took Pringle as read and quickly moved on to practical matters. He split his book into two parts, treating the disease as it related to prisoners and court officers separately because these sections "relate to different persons." When he discussed the former, his debts to Pringle's ideas about putridity and poverty were obvious, for example when he described paupers' pestilential impact on prison air. More influential was Scottish physician James Lind, whose work on the diseases of sailors was foundational to both naval and colonial medicine. His earlier work on scurvy helped establish the putrefactive theory of that disease as the dominant interpretation throughout the century. Like Pringle before him, Lind's work in naval hospitals allowed him to forge links between institutional medicine and military concerns. Indeed, the admission of prisoners and workhouse inmates into the navy meant that the connections between these two fields were never merely theoretical. Lind, who included his "Observations on the Jail Distemper" within his 1774 treatise on naval medicine, addressed the health risks of impressing vagrants and felons into the navy and in so doing demonstrates his faith in the by-now classic picture of the putrid plebeian contagious threat: "That there is a disease of a contagious nature, the produce of filth, rags, poverty, and a polluted air, which subsists always in a greater or less degree in crowded prisons, and in nasty, low, damp, unventilated habitations loaded with putrid animal steams, is now well known, and has been too often fatally experienced, by taking such persons into our ships." Indeed, when discussing the role of putrefaction in Lind's thought, Mark Harrison has noted that he attributed fevers to "a process akin to the decay of corpses." Even animalculist tracts on fever in the period, which appear theoretically distinct in historically important ways, continued to stress putridity and warn of the infectiousness of the "poorer sort."[31]

It is important to emphasize this continued role of putridity, because important developments influenced medical theory during the last third of the century, with significant implications for theories of fever. I mean, of course, the growing emphasis that fever was a disease of the nerves. G. S. Rousseau's work has done much to bring to light the importance of the nervous body in eighteenth-century culture. In Britain, the aforementioned Edinburgh physician William Cullen (1710–1790) was the most prominent of those doctors Hamlin refers to as "nervicentric." Cullen's position as the leading clinical teacher of his day, and his popular nosology that categorized diseases taxonomically for generations of students, ensured the influence of his ideas well into the nineteenth century. Cullen first sketched his nosological categories in his *Synopsis nosologiae methodicae* in 1769, expounding on these ideas in his most famous work, the four-volume *First Lines of the Practice of Physick*. He defined five classes of diseases, with fevers as one of the orders within the class of "Pyrexiae." Such was his emphasis on the nerves that Bynum has suggested that for Cullen "all diseases were neurotic." So-called debility of the nervous power took on increased significance in explanations of many diseases, fever included, and the nerves provided the key mechanism for physicians' contributions to the Enlightenment's great mind-body question via speculation on the physiological pathways connecting the two.[32] However, fever remained complicated, and Cullen was not dogmatic. He continued to believe in multifaceted causation and included room for environmental, constitutional, and behavioral factors as well as the role of specific *contagia*.

While historians have rightly emphasized Cullen's influence driving attention to vital and nervous properties, they have less frequently noted the sustained emphasis on putridity in spite of Cullen's ideas. DeLacy has helpfully pointed out the direct influence of thinkers like Pringle on his thought. Emphasis on nerves had the potential to displace putridity, which we have seen was usually thought to be rooted not in the body's solids (like fibers or nerves) but in its fluids. However, Cullen himself warned of putridity often. Effluvia responsible for fevers had two sources: human bodies or marshes. Both were putrid. "To render our doctrine of fever consistent and complete, it is necessary to add here, that those remote causes of fever, human and marsh effluvia, seem to be of a debilitating or sedative quality. They arise from a putrescent matter. Their production is favoured, and their power increased, by circumstances which favour putrefaction; and they often prove putrefactive ferments with respect to the animal fluids." Much had changed, yet much remained the same. Here Cullen demonstrates his continued support for several key ideas. First, fever-generating effluvia were produced by rotten bodies. Ergo, bodies that shared the qualities of a marsh—putrescence—emitted dangerous toxins. Second, he shows his support for notions of predisposition by claiming that circumstances favoring putrescence favor fever production. Third, he argues that putrid bodies can intensify fevers, a belief that we have dated back to at least Sydenham. And finally, the effects of such effluvia on the system were still seen as putrefactive on the body's *fluids*. This is why doctors like John Alderson, who pinned epidemics on poor neighborhoods in the 1780s, could quote Cullen directly. If anyone needed proof that jail fever was generated in plebeian homes, there was no greater authority. Said Cullen (and quoted Alderson): "The late Observations on the Jail and Hospital Fever, have fully proved the Existence of such a Cause; and it is sufficiently obvious, that the same virulent Matter may be produced in many other Places."[33]

The Moral Biology of Paupers and Prisoners

Thus jail fever, under a plethora of names,[34] was the disease that, more than any other, provided the vehicle to express medical worries about the biohazardous plebeian body in the second half of the eighteenth century. It is worth asking: of all diseases, why this one? Part of the answer lies in the specific epidemics that seemed to point to prisons as dangerous sites of pathogenesis. But the phenomenon may also owe to the unique ability for jail fever to merge moral claims with medical ones, impregnating the disease with wider conceptual power, and inviting medical treatises to weigh in on social issues during a period marked by increasing class tensions.

Of course, discussions stretched beyond prisons, as we have seen and will continue to explore. For example, doctors like Pringle and Lind said much about "Camp" or "Ship" fever. But it was the jail, far more than the army barrack, that loomed as a site of danger. Compare for a moment the threats posed by prisoners and soldiers. England had no standing army. Mobilization of soldiers was thus episodic, whereas prisons presented a perennial threat. Moreover, military men were frequently deployed elsewhere. Epidemics among them could have security implications within the realm of geopolitics, and soldiers could end up in domestic military hospitals. But 365 days a year, prisoners threatened to ignite disease right in the hearts of English cities and towns, diseases that doctors continued to believe could morph into full-blown plague. Indeed, the most pressing predicament associated with soldiers came after wars when they demobilized and transformed back into so many working-class men who streamed into port towns looking for jobs that often weren't there. In other words, society's biggest problems associated with soldiers commenced when they ceased being soldiers. Thanks to John Beattie, we know that spikes in crime following wars were common, a pattern that contemporaries noticed and that helped intensify concerns about the shiftless poor in key periods.[35] During these perceived crime waves some soldiers literally transformed into prisoners, as hard economic circumstances drove survival strategies that landed them in jails.

Indeed, it may matter that jail fever burst on the scene in 1750 precisely during one of these periods, namely during demobilization after the War of the Austrian Succession. Nicholas Rogers has recently presented the period of 1748–1753 as a time of heightened anxiety and social strain. Falling real wages, high unemployment, increased poor relief expenditure, and a spike in crime (or at least in prosecutions) characterized London in these years. A range of topics from crime to gin drinking provided opportunities for respectable Britons to express their intensifying worries about the urban poor. Indeed, one of the most famous depictions of how anxious eighteenth-century patricians imagined the deplorable underclass, Hogarth's famed *Gin Lane*, emerged just nine months after the Old Bailey epidemic, coincident with Henry Fielding's widely read treatise blaming social disorder on moral decay, *Enquiry into the Causes of the Late Increase of Robbers* (1751).[36] The jail fever crisis thus broke out during a period of palpable class tensions, pressures that Tim Hitchcock and Robert Shoemaker have shown intensified as the century progressed. On the one hand, rising numbers of prosecutions—Beattie shows that 1751 showed the highest numbers for a century[37]—meant that more bodies crammed into jails, presenting a material issue that we will see came to a head by the 1770s. But so, too, did they help make institutions like prisons an increased focus of popular attention. Moreover, the actual population within carceral institutions was magnified by the stark increase in the use of workhouses throughout London and beyond. That an *institutional* disease would capture the imagination in the second half of the eighteenth century makes much sense, given that urban Britons saw buildings filled with paupers cropping up all around them. Many of these, especially jails and workhouses, carried a heavy moral taint.

Jail fever may thus have been a potent cultural tool because it invited moral discourses to merge with medical ones. It could do so precisely because the people said to produce the disease were those who, by virtue of being in jail, were unequivocally, nay *officially,* immoral. Prisoners, more than any other fever carrier, thus offered a tantalizing fusion of poverty, filth, and wickedness, a heady brew that cried out for commentary. And so physicians wishing to lend their voices to the growing chorus complaining about the ne'er-do-well poor after 1750 found in jail fever a pregnant opportunity indeed. However, little they said was all that novel, for they typically perpetuated ideas about the moral biology of the poor that had been embedded in plague discourses long ago: transgressive behaviors wrought constitutional damage that enhanced levels of predisposition.

John Huxham provides a good example. Like Pringle, the Plymouth physician published his treatise on fever within weeks of the Old Bailey epidemic, a book that stood as an authoritative text for decades. His bona fides to do so rested on his 1739 Latin treatise on epidemics, and his new *Essay on Fevers* promised discussions of "Putrid, Pestilential, Spotted Fevers," and how such fevers "depend[] on different Constitutions of the Blood." He held to putrefactive theories and repeatedly deployed examples of prisoners to prove points about fever. For example, he asserted that violent fever raged among prisoners not so much because of the air they breathed, but because of the preexisting state of their bodies and lifestyle: "Malignant Fever was chiefly owing to the high scorbutic Habit of Body, Manner of Life, Confinement, &c. to which the above Set of people were subject." Prisoners' confinement clearly mattered, but no more so than the state of their blood *before* they ever entered a jail. Explaining what promoted such "scorbutic" constitutions, he listed an array of issues that blended moral actions with physical, environmental, and even emotional factors in an imprecise motley stew of disease causation: Fever "most commonly attacks Persons of weak Nerves, a lax Habit of Body, and poor thin Blood; those who have suffered great Evacuations, a long Dejection of Spirits, immoderate Watchings, Studies, Fatigue and the like; and also those who have used much crude unwholesome Food, vapid impure Drinks, or have been confined long in damp, foul air; that have broken the Vigor of their Constitutions by Salivations, too frequent Purging, immoderate venery &c." Obviously, the dietary and hygienic claims long ascribed to the poor in plague treatise were here represented. Prisoners and their ilk were presumed to have survived on low-grade food and drink in filthy homes. Of course, Huxham's reference to "poor thin Blood" demonstrates another echo of "depauperated blood" a century after that term entered medical use. William Grant's 1775 treatise on jail fever employed similar terminology. Grant identified jail fever as Sydenham's pestilential fever and declared the most predisposed bodies to be "those whose blood had been impoverished by bad living."[38] Impoverished people had impoverished blood, characterized by putridity, which rendered them predisposed to a disease bordering on plague. And their "bad living" had a lot to do with it.

Huxham's claims about sexuality also stand out. He raised two issues. On the one hand, he vaguely referenced the constitutional effects of too much sex. He nowhere explained the point, though his use of *et cetera* to punctuate the claim suggests that he did not feel clarification was necessary.

But he also clearly referenced venereal disease. When he mentioned a "broken constitution," he used a term that was common in popular texts and advertisements for VD care. The pox—also a putrid disease—was said to lurk, leaving its "taint" behind even after it had been cured, laying the seeds for future putrid diseases. Moreover, its treatment, mercurial salivation, was held to be deeply destructive to the constitution. Lind would later agree that patients who had undergone the operation were highly liable to putrid diseases. Thus those who survived mercury treatment were rarely believed to possess truly full health, whether because their constitutions were now so severely weakened as to be called "broken," or because remnants of the pox lurked in their blood and threatened to spark a new round of putrefaction at some later date. If putridity predisposed to fevers, then the debauched who had caught the "foul disease" were prime candidates.[39]

By Huxham's logic inmates entered jails with constitutions predisposed to fever from their previous years of poverty and sin. Layard made precisely this point early in his 1772 jail fever treatise. Describing the mixture of different kinds of bodies in a jail, and almost certainly referencing the plight of debtors, he lamented, "Prisons . . . are too frequently crouded, with the healthy, strong, vigorous, cleanly and decently habited, together with the infirm, weak, feeble, filthy and naked." Discussing the danger of the latter to the former, he made a key assertion. "Accustomed to every hardship, which the most abject poverty can suffer, the one are inured to misery, by the depravity of their minds; and vice rooted in their hearts, keeping them bound in the chains of wickedness, they are totally changed in constitution, as much as in principles; and both filth and disease are become as natural to them as cleanliness and health are to the virtuous and industrious." Few claims express the moral biology of the plebeian body as succinctly. By the tandem effects of poverty and vice, felons were "totally changed in constitution." Layard emphasized the preexisting state of prisoners' bodies, twice referencing "the share of health brought in with them" as one of the most important causes of jail fever. Although debtors, first-time offenders, or the wrongfully accused might "bring into their confinement, that share of health . . . which they have hitherto enjoyed," it provided little protection against the emissions from "the bold offender hardened in iniquity." The latter "rather finds an Asylum, in his prison, from cold and hunger; and in return, adds more poisonous, and baneful steams from his breath and body, to increase the stock of contagion, and destroy others. . . . Such a motley set of beings crouded together, breathing the same infectious air, which daily grows more pestilential as the healthy grow more corrupt, produce such an acrid, powerful and destructive change in it that no wonder the very walls are infected with the noxious vapours." The bodies of the virtuous were transformed by their proximity to the bodies of the wicked, taking on the latter's noxious quality. Layard thus implored authorities to heed the lesson that logically followed; bodies lay at the heart of the jail fever threat, thus bodies must command attention. This was not a crisis that could be solved by architecture alone. "The care and management of the prisoners in regard their health, require as much attention, as the building, or convenience of the prison." No edifice, however carefully constructed, could remain wholesome "while the effluvia of the jail distemper are continually rising from a croud of miserable wretches."[40] There would be a mania for ventilation later in the eighteenth century, as we will see, but this was only ever a strategy to manage the toxic by-products of rotten bodies.

The quality of bodies before they entered prison was thus a crucial element in discussions of jail fever, one often framed by moral assumptions. Few treatises made the point as thoroughly as John Mason Good's *Dissertation on the Diseases of Prisons and Poor Houses* (1795), written for the Medical Society of London's annual essay contest, which that year addressed the question: "What diseases are most frequent in workhouses, poorhouses and similar institutions; and what are the best means of preventing or curing them?" That Good won and saw his essay published shows just how much his ideas had impressed London's medical elite. (The contest's topic, of course, conveys how pressing the question remained even in the last years of the century.) Good broke institutional diseases into two categories: those generated inside workhouses and prisons, and those brought into such institutions, harbored within the bodies of the paupers who entered them: "In Poor-houses workhouses, and prisons, there are . . . diseases which are continually presenting themselves, though they do not originate in such places of public confinement, being solely introduced by those who enter, in consequence of prior vice, misfortune, or uncleanliness." Vice, filth, and poverty worked in tandem, as ever. Good reasoned that patients with three conditions flooded Britain's carceral institutions. The first were those with ulcers, which, as open sores on the skin, were construed as arising from inner putridity that the body pushed to the surface. Vice mattered in these cases. Workhouses, he argued, saw milder ulcers than prisons because parish paupers "have seldom had it in their power to enlarge the ulcer by their intemperance. But this . . . we frequently meet with in Bridewells, and other Prisons, on the first admission of patients." Vice played an even greater role in accounting for the other two diseases—itch and venereal disease—which "the idle, the unclean[], and the abandoned" carried with them into prisons.[41]

Of course, Good spent considerable time detailing the generation of jail fever, paying due attention to issues like ventilation and hygiene. However, of all the jail fever theorists he made one of the strongest cases for considering the importance of plebeian bodies' preexisting putridity, and reminded readers that wickedness helped forge the moral biology of the English lower class. "The poor are, in general, but little habituated to clean-liness; they are liable to a thousand accidents, and a thousand temptations, which every superior rank of life is free from; and they feel not, from want of education, the same happy exertion of delicacy, honor, and moral senti-ment, which every where else is to be met with. It is not surprising, therefore, that such diseases as the above should be frequent in almost every prison, and every poor-house, in the kingdom.[42] In theory, a collection of healthy bodies breathing each other's waste would eventually sicken if confined for long enough. But that was theory. In practice, epidemic fever was generated by the noxious congregation of particular kinds of bodies. The bodies Good describes—poor and wicked, harboring syphilis or visually rotting before doctors' eyes with ulcers and itch—emitted far more dangerous effluvia than did a respectable citizen. Who could doubt that it rendered the air poisonous in very short order?

Moreover, writing at the dawn of the nineteenth century Good demon-strates the profound longevity of the notion that poor bodies could intensify mild ailments into the worst diseases. He warned that drinking, idleness, and the "riot and debauch" found in poorly governed jails ensured that simple fevers descended into contagious and deadly typhus. However, when he made this point, he tellingly stressed poverty more than vice: "In bridewells this is more particularly true than in work-houses or any other kinds of prisons; for in bridewells we generally find the greatest poverty and want."[43] In other words, the power of bodies to intensify fevers—something doctors had warned about since the 1620s—was still contingent on class: the poorer a body, the greater its capacity to magnify disease. The seriousness of jail fever was never in doubt; Good shows that in 1795 doctors still held that it was essentially a weak form of plague. On plague he asserted: "I know not of any other phenomena that render it different from the typhus, excepting, perhaps, a greater activity in the virus."[44]

꙼

Jail fever captivated Britons for many reasons, not least because it was terrifying. Its ability to act as a vehicle for the medicalization of moral and policing discourses was profound. However, poverty was the real killer. Good gave a lengthy description of prisoners' descent into sickness and death that vividly reminded readers of how poverty transformed bodies with tragic results, a discussion largely free of the moral condemnations that characterized other sections of his book.

> Vagrants, and petty offenders, when they are first led into bridewells, have perhaps, scarcely a penny in their pockets at the time, and the cloaths that cover them are already rags. . . . In a fortnight's time it frequently happens that their rags are of little or no use to them. I have seen them in many prisons in this metropolis, as NEWGATE, CLERKENWELL BRIDEWELL, and the SAVOY PRISON, bare-footed, and bare-legged and nearly bare-breached, with only a jacket over their bodies, and that very much tattered, and without any shirt. And I have seen many women nearly as indifferently cloathed. Colds are caught as fever is introduced. If there be an infirmary, the patient is admitted into it; if not, a straw bed is procured for him, and he lies down in the common night room of the prison, subject to all the noise and outrage of his companions. If a good constitution, or the timely application of medicine, and other assistance, enable him to triumph over the disease, still has he to contend in a state dreadfully reduced and debilitated, with the same exposure to colds, the original cause of his disease, as before he was affected. And, if in the more full possession of vigor, he was unable to resist the powerful agency of such a cause, how may he now hope for success, and the recovery of former health. Such relapses, and from such fresh application of cause, I have known occur for three or four times successively, and often, at last terminate fatally.[45]

The fact that the body described here is incarcerated is almost a technicality. The prison merely acts as one more cause of its impoverishment. It is the descent into poverty that inevitably brings on disease—and not just a

single disease, but disease everlasting. Through poverty the body is debili-
tated so that even if it began with a "good constitution," it soon acquires
the pathogenic and weakened corporeal state attributed to paupers' bodies
for almost two hundred years. Indeed, the lethal poverty described above
began well before these hypothetical prisoners' incarceration; Good describes
them as penniless and in rags "when they are first led into bridewells." Here,
ventilation and architecture are neither the culprits nor the solutions.
Good's rhetoric depends on readers accepting the virtually inevitable link
between poverty and disease in its starkest form, portrayed here by the figure
of the pauper shivering in rags before he finally succumbs. By pathologizing
vice, jail fever texts undoubtedly advanced and supported disciplinary
rhetorics. Part of the fascination with the disease was surely its power to
wed the medical and the moral. The idle, drunk, and sexually abandoned
were dangerous, of course. But so, too, Good reminded his readers, were the
simply poor. As was the case with plague, medical claims never limited themselves to the disorderly poor but always stretched beyond to address the poor
more generally. Treatises on jail fever thus represented some of the most
fertile eighteenth-century vehicles for expressing the continued belief in the
pathology of the plebeian body.

However, it also bears repeating that jail fever was never just physicians' theoretical plaything, a debating point for medical hypotheses or
veiled social commentary. Notwithstanding the clear worry about jail-born
diseases earlier in the century, or the ways in which an event like the 1577
Oxford epidemic became historically embedded in national memory, the
crisis of 1750 brought altogether new focus to the dangers of prisons. It did
so because of the direct threat they posed to London's propertied classes.
What drove so many doctors to write about jail fever after 1750 was a
profound anxiety arising from the powerful belief that jails could provide the
epicenters for terrible new epidemics. It was not fantastic to imagine that the
horrors of 1665/6 could return and that such a crisis was more likely to start
in a jail than anywhere else. That anxiety would lie at the heart of numerous
strategies aimed at protecting the bodies of propertied men from poorer
ones. It will be my contention in the coming chapter that while the movement to reform prisons in the late eighteenth century had many goals, what
may have driven it more than anything else was sheer class self-preservation
in the most literal sense of that term. To make that case, we have to return to
the Old Bailey in May 1750.

5. Jail Fever and Prison Reform

London, 1750–1789

On May 26, 1750, the epidemic was still just two weeks old. London newspapers reported the funeral of Sir Daniel Lambert. Fellow aldermen acted as pallbearers and "a great Number of vessels in the River dropped their colours and fired Minute-Guns on the Occasion." Along with the tolling of funeral bells, these shots must have sent a somber sonic signal throughout the city about the current crisis. Action was needed. That same day newspapers reported the initial responses.

> In the first place, the jail of Newgate has been thoroughly cleansed, and all the Filth carried into the Fields: It was likewise this Day washed throughout with Vinegar, and the Prisoners are also to be washed with Vinegar, before they are brought to the Sessions House to take their Trials. Strict Orders have been likewise given that not more than Twelve, or at most Fifteen prisoners shall be brought down at a Time to the Sessions House to take their Trials, half of which to be arraigned at once; and that the said Prisoners shall be remanded back to Newgate one by one, after their Trials are over, and fresh Prisoners brought down in their room; so as the Number at the Sessions House shall not, at one Time, exceed Twelve or Fifteen. There is this farther Satisfaction to give the Public, that about Twenty prisoners for Debt (out of Fifty Debtors, or there abouts, in Newgate) were discharged this Day.

We later learn that a proposed strike by the magistrates helped spur such quick action: judges resolved "not to attend at the Old Bailey, till Measures were concerted which should secure them from a like catastrophe."[1] Each of the city's initial responses—and as we will see, its responses over the next four decades—reveals profound assumptions about bodies.

First, they cleansed. Drawing on practices inherited from plague times, aldermen deployed an old standby: vinegar. Accused felons would be doused in it before entering the courtroom in the hopes that the disinfectant would counteract the putridity they emitted. Proposals included the provision of linens and laundering facilities so that prisoners could attend trial in clean clothes, a recommendation driven by the long-held fear that pestilential effluvia could lodge in fabric. Through hygiene, therefore, officials hoped to engineer prisoners' rotten bodies. They also spent considerable energy cleansing spaces: the courtroom, the prison, and the passageway between them. More than just disinfecting them, they scraped the walls clean. The medical belief that human breath expelled excrement inspired fear that prisoners' effluvia had adhered to the walls, building up over years to form a pestilential layer of deadly filth that had to be carved off and carted away. It stood to reason that this material was poisonous, as was, of course, prisoners' actual excrement. We have already encountered the acute fears associated with plebeian waste. It is thus telling that one of the very first responses to the Old Bailey crisis was to ship cartload after cartload of Newgate's filth out of London and bury it ten feet underground. A city with more than half a million people hardly lacked for dunghills, but Newgate's waste was just too toxic to keep within city limits.[2]

Officials also moved to govern bodies spatially. For starters, as we have seen, they reduced the number of prisoners brought into court at one time, returning each to Newgate after his proceedings and bringing up new defendants in like number. By this strict and orderly process, officials sought to guarantee that only a handful occupied the court at any one time. This is again revealing, because most accounts of the outbreak emphasized the crowded gallery for Captain Clark's trial. Yet officials leave no evidence that they limited onlookers. If a room full of people breathing one another's exhalations was risky, one might expect a limit on spectators. However, such a policy would have necessarily required an assumption that bodies were created equally. The policing of polite bodies seems not to have occurred to authorities, whose policies show pretty clearly which bodies needed governance.

Aldermen demonstrated this point vividly with moves to protect polite bodies further still. As a later report explained, they changed the positioning of defendants: "A new Bar for arraigning the Prisoners, few at a Time, was erected just without the Court, partly in the open Air, instead of their being brought into Court to the trying Bar, as had been the practice; whereby the Hazard of catching Infection from the Prisoners was considerably abated." This arrangement was corroborated by a report describing the new bar as "within a Yard or two of the Door opening into the Court." Previously, prisoners were arraigned twenty at a time at the center of the courtroom, where "if there had been any infectious Disorder among them, the Court was in the greatest Danger of Catching it." Now the number of defendants arraigned was just nine, and "the *Effluvia* . . . could not dilate itself so far into the Court."[3] Note the small discrepancy between these accounts; the latter suggests that prisoners were arraigned just inside the courtroom, while the former (published sooner after the event and so perhaps more accurate) describes them situated *outside* the courtroom. In either case, aldermen moved to maximize the distance between the prisoners and the bench, a bench at which, we must remember, they often sat.

And of course they released debtors. Readers are excused their befuddlement at this development, considering the threat posed by bodies departing Newgate in the spring of 1750. But it makes sense in light of what we now know about the concerns for debtors since at least the time of Oglethorpe, demonstrated by so many Insolvency Acts. Thus on the same day that Londoners heard funeral bells for victims, they read about released debtors. And as early as May 22 papers reported deliberations about a new jail that could accommodate all of Newgate's debtors and an influx of donations to help discharge those confined for small debts. Such pleas represent some of the earliest and most passionate responses to the Old Bailey epidemic. A letter by "P.Q." employed the language of rot to describe conditions he considered "inhuman even to Criminals" but that much worse for debtors "rotting away with Vermin and . . . perishing of a Goal Distemper." A submission to *Old England* two weeks later deployed religious overtones to critique Newgate, where debtors' quarters were said to be as bad as felons'. Warning of an epidemic, the writer made one of the most self-aware claims regarding the class dynamic implicit in the Jail Fever Panic: "It is hop'd, as Reformation never begins till the Great and Wealthy become incommoded, it may produce a Jail-Reformation in favour of our miserable Fellow-Christians."[4] Like the reorganization of courtroom space, the releasing of debtors demonstrates a drive to cope with the crisis by distancing polite bodies from plebeian ones.

These moves notwithstanding, voices called for a more radical restructuring of prisons, especially Newgate. Newgate held a special place in the British psyche as easily the most notorious prison in the nation.[5] Commentators rarely tired of highlighting that it received prisoners from jails across southern England. The holding pen for everyone tried at the Old Bailey, Newgate was a kind of hodgepodge cauldron wherein was mixed the effluvia of some of the worst people southern England had to offer, each of them potentially carrying filth and disease from various bridewells, workhouses, and lockups. Given theories that fevers intensified into more dangerous ailments, it was easy to believe that the worst forms of jail fever necessarily hailed from Newgate. Many thus feared that vinegar baths were simply not up to the task.

Stephen Theodore Janssen, sheriff in 1750 and soon lord mayor, published a series of reports and proposals that aldermen received during the crisis, the first of which called for building a new jail. The author, a Mr. O'Conner, presented jail fever as inevitable in the current jail, "scarce possible to prevent." There were simply too many foul bodies and not enough space. He suggested that Newgate be torn down and built anew, modeled on York's county jail. While brief on detail, he stressed that it should allow firm separation between debtors and felons and have a large airing yard and substantial water supplies. Aldermen clearly took the suggestion seriously, for newspapers soon reported surveys conducted for the explicit purpose of enlarging Newgate, and Janssen wrote to York to request plans for its jail. He would later claim that the political will that summer would have easily swayed Parliament to support rebuilding the jail. Given the level of panic—and the clear motives of "Self Preservation" that he identified among city officials— he was confident on this point.[6] That the aldermen did not embark on building a new prison is largely down to one man, Stephen Hales.

A Breath of Fresh Air? Ventilating Newgate, 1750–1755

Hales may have been uniquely positioned to influence events. A minister in nearby Teddington, he was already a celebrated scientific figure by 1750. His experiments on plant and animal bodies laid the groundwork for pneumatic chemistry but also made him an authority on numerous issues central to theories of jail fever. His work on respiration, for example, led him to posit that breathing performed essential cleansing, with experiments exploring the materials that bodies consumed and excreted when they breathed. His 1733 work on "haemeostaticks" focused on the blood and touched on key medical ideas underpinning the plebeian body, including the effects on blood of fever and putrefaction, predisposition, and even how blood became "pestilential" or "depauperated." Civic activity connected him to the issue of prisons and fever, because he was heavily involved with Oglethorpe's project that immediately followed his work on jails: the foundation of Georgia as a colony for released debtors. Not content as a theoretician, Hales tried to address problems practically, as through numerous charities. In the case of fever he devised an invention to defeat it: a ventilator.[7]

Hales compared man-made structures to animals in their need to breathe to remain healthful. He thus devised ventilators as a kind of artificial lung, pumping clean air into buildings or ships and forcing foul air out. To him, ventilation was a technology of hygiene. Breath expressed waste, so ventilation acted like plumbing for the air. In 1741 Hales presented a paper to the Royal Society detailing ventilators for ships that he insisted could work in buildings, ideas that he developed in his 1743 *A Description of Ventilators*. "Can it therefore be an unreasonable proposal to furnish ships gaols, hospitals etc. in the same manner with the wholesome breath of life in exchange for the noxious air of confined places?" Hales had thus been thinking about jails and health for a decade by 1750. More than think about it, he had already affixed ventilation systems at both the Savoy Prison and Winchester County Gaol. Large windmills fashioned to their roofs drove bellows forcing air through a series of ducts, a contraption Robin Evans aptly described as "a gigantic and extremely inefficient lung" (Figure 5).[8]

Hales's ventilators must have been well known because city officials received multiple calls for them during the first days of the crisis. Economically, they had a major advantage over rebuilding the prison. Evidence supports A. E. Clark-Kennedy's opinion that aldermen divided over the choice. Ventilators had been ordered for Newgate by mid-August, yet a report by Hales a full year later confirmed a long delay: "Deliberations, whether Newgate should be pulled down and new built, have with good Reason delayed the fixing of Ventilators there." Clearly, some did not think

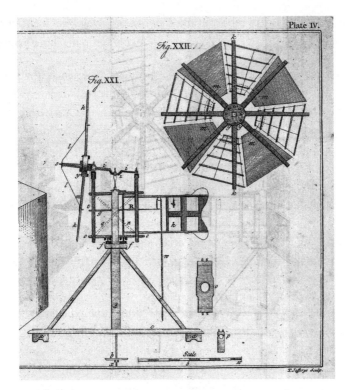

Figure 5. "Ventilation Apparatus Devised by Reverend Stephen Hales," from Stephen Hales, *A Treatise on Ventilators* (London: Richard Manby, 1758), n.p. Courtesy of Wellcome Library, London.

his contraption was up to the task. But his invention soon received endorsement from the leading medical authority on jail fever, John Pringle. The Court of Common Council requested that Pringle and Hales tour Newgate together and make recommendations, and they consulted on Newgate over the next several years. Sufficient aldermanic support was won by spring 1752, and the ventilators were erected in May. They remained controversial, however, because more than half of the workmen installing the machines allegedly caught jail fever and spread it to their families.[9] The workers' epidemic later assumed a key place in the lore constructed around the 1750 Black Assizes, as we will see. But for the moment these deaths only confirmed the pressing need for the ventilators.

Early reports trumpeted their success and show how extensively theories of the plebeian body informed this example of enlightenment technology. Hales's 1752 report in the *Gentleman's Magazine* focused mainly on technical details. However, he paused to explain the machine's purpose.

> It is well known, by long and too frequent experience, that the destructive goal distemper is occasioned by the bad air in prisons, which is filled with the great quantity of vapours that arise from the breath and perspiration of the prisoners . . . [which] by long stagnating is very apt to putrefy; and putrefaction being the most subtile and powerful dissolvent in nature, it dissolves the blood and humours of human bodies, and thereby produces that very infectious, pestilential disease, which is called the goal distemper. And such close-confined, damp, putrid air will not only dissolve human bodies, which are framed of materials strongly tending to putrefaction, but also even heart of oak, as is well known, by daily experience everywhere.

Here Hales references at least three ideas pertinent to medical theories on jail fever and putrid bodies. First, he underscores that air in a jail was rendered dangerous by the bodies incarcerated therein. This may be obvious, but it is vital to note because discussions of Hales's role in prison reform so often emphasize environmentalist assumptions about the air. The air was indeed the medium that conveyed disease, but prison reformers' focus on ventilation has drawn historians' attention toward ideas about air and architecture while occluding what these debates conveyed about *bodies*. Yet here Hales, the figure most closely associated with the notion that prisons needed clean air, makes clear that the body remained of primary, not secondary, importance in assumptions about the etiology of jail fever: prison air was poisoned by "vapours that arise from the breath and perspiration of the prisoners." Second, Hales clearly emphasized putrefaction. And finally, comments that prisoners' vapors were "*apt* to putrefy" and that their bodies comprised materials "*tending* to putrefaction" signal his reliance on predisposition. Given his close work with Pringle, who expressed all these ideas, this should hardly surprise us.[10]

By early 1753 Hales felt sufficiently satisfied to publish a report on his invention's success. In keeping with the period's fascination with quantification, he did so numerically. Fewer than two prisoners per month had died since his windmill was affixed, while more than sixteen prisoners per month had died previously. The Savoy showed similar success. Ventilators quickly cropped up at institutions like St. George's Hospital and the Middlesex Small Pox Hospital, and on more and more ships.[11] Enlightenment technology had saved the day.

The honeymoon was short-lived. For starters, not everyone was enamored of the ventilators, least of all people who lived near Newgate. For all the trappings of modern engineering and medical promise, it stood to reason that pumping pestilential filth out of Newgate presented a serious health risk to its neighbors. Reports from 1752 make clear that such concerns were registered right from the start. The *Public Advertiser* tried to reassure readers that "there will be no Danger, as some fearful People are apt to apprehend," arguing that ventilators flushed air out before it could putrefy. But the ventilators did not sustain their initial success. Deaths of Newgate prisoners typically went unreported in the popular press, though after the 1750 crisis they may have become more newsworthy. Clusters of prisoner deaths like those reported in May and June 1753 were probably unnerving. And then a spate of deaths in the winter of 1755 turned Londoners' opinion strongly against relying on ventilators to protect them. An anonymous contributor to the *Public Advertiser* invoked "the great number of strong-bodied Prisoners, who have died in Newgate of the Gaol Distemper, within these last weeks past" as the reason for recounting events dating back to the 1750 epidemic. He lauded Hales as ingenious, but the recent epidemic demonstrated that "Precautions of this sort are sometimes Ineffectual." He then reminded readers of the scuttled plans to rebuild Newgate. The time had come to revisit them—not merely, or even primarily, for the sake of the prisoners, but rather, as ever, for the security of respectable London. A new prison would "be a Security, under God, against various contagious Distempers, which may possibly happen to the Destruction of many thousands of his Majesty's healthy, able Subjects, in this trading City." The whiff of plague was hardly subtle. Hales defended his work the following week, noting, for example, that Newgate received prisoners from unventilated prisons and thus that this fever was probably imported. His comments confirm, however, that neighbors had indeed continued to complain that his ventilator threatened their health, a worry that the latest epidemic surely heightened. The crisis caused Janssen, now lord mayor, to seek the opinion of Hales's partner John Pringle, who grudgingly admitted that he had lost confidence in Hales's contraption. He politely pointed out that the machine often sat idle because no one adjusted the sails toward the wind. But then he came to the point:

"The truth is, I despair of getting thoroughly the better of the Distemper and Contagion without building a larger Prison, better aired."[12]

The ventilator experiment represents one of the more fascinating episodes in the history of eighteenth-century contagion anxieties, revealing prevailing wisdom about jails and bodies. However, it is also important to the chronology of prison reform because it helps explain the five-year lag between the 1750 epidemic and the decision to enlarge Newgate. That delay was peanuts. The new jail would not be completed for almost twenty-five years.

The Struggle to Rebuild Newgate

On June 12, 1755, the Court of Common Council established a committee to "inquire into the State and Condition of the Gaol of Newgate and to Consider how the same may be enlarged and rendered more healthy and commodious." At its first meeting Mayor Janssen presented the five-year-old report recommending building a larger jail and perhaps inadvertently revealed the core mission: "The Lives of many unhappy Objects may be preserved & the publick thereby rendered more safe from any dangerous Infection." Janssen's syntax lays bare that plebeian bodies in the jail were being saved expressly as a way of protecting the wider community from them.[13]

Newgate keeper Richard Akerman gave a report in which he, too, spoke in terms derived from medical parlance. He reminded the committee of the uniquely dangerous constitutions in his institution, lamenting that many prisoners died from "an ill habit of body." There were just too many such bodies in the space allotted, frequently more than thirty men to a room. And while he mentioned need for fresh air, he drew greater attention to inadequate water and toilet provisions: "the privies &c. are frequently stopt and overflows which may contribute to the Distemper." He here referenced the need to ship Newgate's filth out of the city, advocated for an Insolvency Act, and lamented that the navy was reluctant to accept men from prisons for fear of infection. However, medical ideas did not need to be refracted through lay commentators like Akerman, because Pringle addressed the committee directly. While only rough minutes for that meeting survive, the pride of place given to Pringle's published works stands out. The committee discussed his report in the *Philosophical Transactions* and his *Diseases of the Army*, a treatise in which we have seen Pringle expressly link poverty, putridity, and predisposition to fever. The clerk was ordered to copy passages from both texts into the official record and instructed to purchase the *Philosophical Transactions* for that purpose. We learn that Lord Mayor Janssen owned *Diseases of the Army*, because he lent the clerk his personal copy.[14] We thus need not doubt the centrality of medical theory to this committee's work.

The following week the committee heard from a very different kind of authority. On July 24, Newgate's neighbors assembled to have their say. Their comments reveal both the day-to-day anxieties experienced by common Londoners and the extent to which the medical theories underpinning constructions of the plebeian body had diffused throughout the general public. For example, a hosier named Holmes complained of the danger caused when prisoners cast dirty water or filth out the windows. He was especially concerned about foul smells, though his comments show that he perceived this not just as a matter of olfactory aesthetics but as a pressing health threat. "That he has frequently Smelt a Stench from the Prisoners, and that the same has likewise been smelt by other Persons going thro' the Postern nothing being more Common in Hot Weather than to see Persons holding their Noses as they go thro' Newgate. That in 1750 he was very much frighted. His Customers declaring they were afraid of coming to His Shop and that they came round by Saint Pauls Church Yardd, rather than come thro' Newgate. That he has frequently Observed the Smoke or Effluvia come out of the West Windows in several of the Rooms when the Ventilators were working." Other citizens expressed similar anxieties and, like Holmes's customers, some altered their routes to avoid areas that were now identified as biohazardous zones. For example, a neighbor named Mr. Say claimed that the stench prevented him from standing at his door and that for the sake of safety "he frequently goes round thro' the Market rather than the Postern." Newgate's neighbors had opposed the ventilators from the start, and the minutes of the Gaol Committee now revealed how such contagion anxieties influenced their daily lives, in this case changing traffic patterns to follow routes of perceived safety. Londoners who needed to move about near Newgate were literally led around by their noses, negotiating an imagined urban geography governed by smell. Unsurprisingly, they argued that the prison be moved: "Others were of Opinion that there was danger of Infection from the present condition of the Gaol and all argued that removing the Gaol to a place where more Room and a convenience for airing the Prisoners would be the most effectual Means to Remedy the Same." Two days later architect George Dance reported that the only plausible course of action was to demolish Newgate and build an entirely new jail. Revealing rough minutes capture the sense of pressing danger; Dance advised the committee "to Report Goal very dangerous & infectious State not only unhealthy but ~~Dangerous~~ unsecure in as strong Terms as can."[15]

The committee did just that in its report back to the Court of Common Council. An undated rough minutes entry includes a list entitled "Proofs," which accompanied the report to support the case for the expensive solution of building a new jail. These included the neighbors' depositions, Pringle's account of the deaths of the workers installing the ventilators, Dance's architectural report, details on the number of prisoners, and the account of the jail fever epidemic in the early months of 1755. The report itself crafted these themes into a historical survey that related the 1750 epidemic, the 1752 deaths of the workmen, and the 1755 epidemic, seasoned by references to inadequate privies, stench, frightened citizens, and alarming mortality figures, to make a powerful case that there were simply too many of the wrong kinds of bodies pent up together. As ever, wider public safety, rather than the lives of felons, punctuated the argument: "We apprehend the Lives of His Majesty's Subjects in general and of the Inhabitants of this Great City in particular, are in eminent danger from the present filthy and loathsome State of Newgate." Deliberations occurred against a backdrop of press reports about yet another respectable fever victim. In late August, Reverend John Grierson, imprisoned for marrying a couple in contravention of the recently passed Hardwicke's Marriage Act, was transferred to Newgate, where he caught "Gaol Distemper." The Court of Common Council approved the report, ordering the committee to proceed with the plan. But even now there were delays. City officials haggled with their counterparts from Middlesex County (with whom they shared responsibility for Newgate) over money, designs, and locations, and by February 1757 the committee was still only preparing a parliamentary petition to request funding. To no avail. The chancellor of the Exchequer soon informed the lord mayor that Parliament could not help.[16]

The records inexplicably then jump nine years, to February 1764. The committee's self-reflection helps us piece together the delay. A rough draft of a report probably from 1764 or 1765 explains what a crushing blow the failure to secure parliamentary support had been. Yet again recounting the history of events starting from 1750, it concluded: "It appearing . . . that the Government cou'd not then Assist the City in any supplies towards rebuilding the said Goal the Affair was dropt." Janssen later lamented losing the initiative. Invoking the £100,000 grant to victims of the 1755 Lisbon earthquake as an example of how a crisis could be seized, he complained: "No one will entertain a Doubt, in case an Application had been made the ensuing Session [in 1750], while the Terrors from the Jail Distemper were still fresh in people's Minds, but the Parliament would have granted liberally, towards rooting out so ignominiuous, and so dangerous a Nusaince, from the very Heart of the first City in Europe, whereby the whole of the Kingdom was in some degree liable to be affected." But aldermen had waited seven years to strike, and by then the iron was no longer hot. The reports and activities of 1755 demonstrate that "the Terrors of Jail Distemper" were indeed still fresh in the minds of Londoners. But seven years was long enough for the government to find other priorities.[17]

However, that apparent lack of activity on Newgate 1755–1764 should not suggest a waning of concern about prisons and health. In fact, it may be partially explained by the city's dealing with other prisons, notably those for debtors. When Parliament declined the City of London's petition for Newgate in 1757, it may have been because it had just funded the rebuilding of the King's Bench debtors' prison in 1754, a project completed in 1758. The aldermen then turned their attention to another decrepit debtors' prison, Ludgate. Much smaller than Newgate, Ludgate held only around forty prisoners, making its refurbishment much more affordable. In July 1760 newspapers reported the decision to pull down that prison and transfer its debtors to the London Workhouse in Aldersgate. It was not a small project, but transferring the prisoners to the city-owned workhouse was, in terms of costs, far more manageable than constructing a new jail. Thus, while Newgate languished in the late 1750s and early 1760s, the city went ahead with other prison-reform projects, privileging debtors, of course.[18]

Architectural historian Harold Kalman suggests that damage to Newgate from a 1762 fire provided the impetus to take up Newgate's cause once again. Outbreaks of jail fever at the Poultry Compter in 1762, the Savoy in 1763, and the county jail in Surrey in 1764, as well as reports of a significant epidemic in Paris jails the same year, surely helped fuel the opinion that crowded, unhealthy Newgate could not be ignored forever. Indeed, Newgate was the site in 1763 of yet another outbreak, with roughly twenty casualties. Aldermen revived the Newgate Committee in February 1765 and endowed it with more than £500 to submit another petition to Parliament. Debates highlight just how treacherous Newgate was now believed to be. City justices lamented that coroners refused to enter its cells, that they could not persuade a physician to tend to the sick, and that the apothecary "sayd he'd not endanger his life on any Accot. whatever." Sustained pressure resulted in a 1767 act providing £50,000 to rebuild the jail.[19]

The committee already had plans on hand, drawn up a decade earlier by George Dance the Elder and architect William Jones. As historians like Robin Evans have explored, the new Newgate, like virtually all prisons henceforth, was conceived with special attention to ventilation. Airy courtyards, windows, and high ceilings presented strategic opportunities to maximize airflow, design details Evans linked expressly to concerns about fever. However, one feature vividly reminds us that anxieties about Newgate fundamentally concerned bodies: the toilets. Dance and Jones's plan contained a remarkable number of privies: one for every two prisoners. Since at least the late seventeenth century prisoners' bodily waste was imagined to be toxic. In 1750 it was carted out of the city and buried. Newgate's planners now hoped to provide enough privies so that fully half the prisoners could relieve themselves at any one time. Moreover, their structure and placement stand out. The architects situated them in the buildings' corners inside independently ventilated silos, with air ducts inside the walls rising up to "nostrils" on the roof that whisked the vapors out of the building before they could seep into the prison itself. These privy silos were thus conceived as virtually separate buildings unto themselves, providing a specific form of quarantine for the putrid products of putrid bodies. Dance's son, George Dance the Younger, took over in 1768 and updated the existing plans. He had to sacrifice certain features because spatial limitations and security concerns precluded having as open and airy a prison as originally hoped. But the privy silos remained. They are visible as the semicircular structures in the many corners of Figure 6. Said Evans, "The only hint that the prison resulted from a fever scare were the ten semi-circular ventilation walls behind the still numerous privy closets."[20] Privy silos were texts, each one asserting a profound claim about the perceived danger of the plebeian body.

Yet delays continued. Agitation to secure funding and discussions about design—including a failed attempt to secure land farther removed from the heart of the city—drew yet more attention to the issue of jail fever. For example, former mayor Janssen pressed for action by publishing an open letter to the Newgate Committee with considerable detail about the 1750

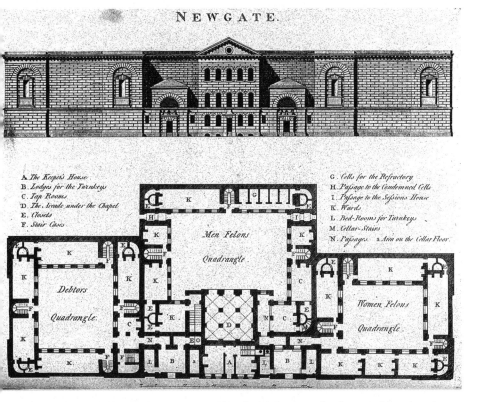

NEWGATE.

A. *The Keeper's House.*
B. *Lodges for the Turnkeys.*
C. *Tap Rooms.*
D. *The Arcade under the Chapel.*
E. *Closets.*
F. *Stair Cases.*

G. *Cells for the Refractory.*
H. *Passage to the Condemned Cells.*
I. *Passage to the Sessions House.*
K. *Wards.*
L. *Bed-Rooms for Turnkeys.*
M. *Cellar-Stairs.*
N. *Passages. a Area on the Cellar Floor.*

Men Felons

Quadrangle.

Debtors

Quadrangle.

Women Felons

Quadrangle.

Figure 6. George Dance II, Newgate Prison Plan, from John Howard, *The State of the Prisons in England and Wales* (London, 1792), plate 20. Courtesy of Wellcome Library, London.

crisis and the initial efforts to fight fever, a text that physician Layard in the previous chapter told us was "almost in the hand of every one." Readers had to have been struck that rebuilding Newgate had been one of the very first suggestions in May 1750, yet here they were still debating details seventeen years later, all while reports of jail fever deaths continued to dot the newspapers.[21]

Mundane details like agreements with contractors slowed the pace of work. But one obstacle is particularly noteworthy. The plan required the purchase of land from Newgate's neighbor, the Royal College of Physicians. That body's representatives addressed the committee in December 1768 to lodge protests. Its library, for example, would be darkened by the enormous shadow cast by the forty-five-foot-high prison. But that was hardly their main concern. Who but physicians could be more aware of the health threat posed by having a prison right next door? "The College of

Physicians cannot but look upon a Prison so near them as an infectious nuisance. The Foul Air from the Goal however will . . . be necessarily thrown upon that part of the College Building where the public Business must be done." That danger might even force them to move, which would be difficult due to the plunging real estate values triggered by widespread contagion anxieties about the neighborhood. "The College apprehend they cannot meet together in their house, without exposing themselves to great danger of catching a Distemper which generally proves mortal, some instances of which cannot yet be out of the memory of the City of London. The College therefore desire the Committee to consider whether the Law under which they act can admit of such a Construction, as to give them power of bringing a contagious and most dangerous distemper close to a Body of Men, who meet for no other than public purposes: and who must, if the design of the Committee take effect, in consequence of their apprehensions either think no more of any further Meetings, or dispose of their house, which *by reason of its neighbourhood to the Goal,* cannot be done but to great disadvantage." There may have been some hard bargaining here, for the Royal College eventually agreed upon a price, although not until a year had transpired, despite the city's pleas that "no further delay can be permitted."[22]

These delays meant that the first stone would not be laid until May 31, 1770, almost twenty years to the day after the Old Bailey epidemic. The College's remonstrance suggests strongly that that the 1750 event was indeed not "out of the memory of the City of London." To the contrary, decrepit Newgate stood as a frightening reminder to Londoners of the pestilential sword of Damocles perched above them. Men still died there, and prisoners continued to expose polite citizens to danger when they stood trial at the Old Bailey. Debtors still went in and out, and so did chaplains, doctors, parish officials, court officers, and visitors.[23] How long would it be, Londoners must have wondered, before the horrors of 1750 struck again? The answer, as it turns out, was not very long at all.

In the autumn of 1772, while the new jail was still a construction site, another epidemic claimed the lives of judges at the Old Bailey. The outpouring of fright and anger that met this incident reflects the powerful pent-up emotions of Londoners who had carried this precise worry for twenty-two years. Indeed, we will see that this outbreak was a major immediate catalyst for the spate of well-known activities of the 1770s that established penitentiary reform as a sustained national issue.

The Black Assizes Redux, 1772

It was not unusual for newspapers to report the transfer of prisoners to Newgate in advance of a new session at the Old Bailey. However, in September 1772 reporters noted great numbers filling the jail. Ninety were said to come from New Prison alone. "It is said that there are more prisoners to take their trials at the ensuing sessions at the Old Bailey, than at any general goal delivery for many years past." Then, like a recurring nightmare, the events of 1750 began to replay. The clerk for judge William Henry Ashurst died, and Ashurst took ill as well. As before there seems to have been a rush to judgment that they had caught their illness on the bench. The first report read: "Judge Ashurst is extremely ill of a disorder he caught by attending the last sessions of the Old-Bailey; his head Clerk is dead of the same distemper, and many apprehend that it will prove epidemical." Within days reports laid the crisis firmly at the feet of the Newgate Committee, citing its slow progress building the new jail. "The death of Judge Ashurst's Clerk, and the illness of his Lordship, from a disorder catched at the Sessions-house, are very alarming circumstances. 'Tis pity the building of the new goal is not carried on with more expedition." It is difficult to pinpoint how many died in the epidemic, but over the course of October and November newspapers reported the deaths of nine Newgate prisoners, one prison employee, one lawyer, one alderman, and four jurors. Another alderman was infected, and although Ashurst recovered, his sickness was followed closely in the papers. The *Middlesex Journal* now reported that like the judges who threatened to strike in 1750, "the counsellors of law . . . are afraid to attend at the Old Bailey." The sessions were adjourned until December. Just as Pringle had done in 1750, physician Daniel Peter Layard published a treatise on jail fever almost immediately after the start of the outbreak. He suggested that prisoners should attend court in special garments that closed tight at the wrists, ankles, and neck to trap their pestilential effluvia, and that screening should be used during interrogations to keep prisoners and magistrates safely apart. Such clothing was in use by late October. Some recommended ventilators for courtrooms, while others suggested a kind of a fire-heated dome situated over the bar to draw prisoners' effluvia up into a series of pipes that, like those of Newgate's privy silos, ran straight to the roof and out of the building. Still others proposed that judges should stuff rue or tobacco up their nostrils for prophylaxis.[24]

The presence of a sitting committee tasked to prevent precisely this crisis may explain why the 1772 epidemic became more overtly politicized than the 1750 one; for critiques of the city government were plentiful and fierce. Reports accused authorities of neglecting hygiene, or sheriffs of failing to conduct inspections.²⁵ But the bulk of critiques aimed squarely at the Newgate Committee for moving so slowly.

The Morning Chronicle, October 9

The late fatal fevers caught at the Old Bailey are the strongest reproach imaginable to the Committee which has the charge of erecting the new gaol. It is to be hoped therefore that some benevolent friend to mankind will take up the shameful inattention to that necessary business at the next Court of Common Council, and get put in better hands.

London Chronicle, October 8–10

It is the Complaint of every Citizen, and indeed all the metropolis, that the building of Newgate goes on most uncommonly slow. Surely, if any thing the late dreadful calamity of so many lives being lost by the jail pestilence at the old Bailey; will urge the Newgate Committee to insist upon expedition in the builders.

The Morning Chronicle, October 10

It has more than once urged in this Paper, how exceedingly important it was that the building of the New Prison . . . should be expedited. The shamefully negligent Surveyor, no doubt, thought the hints and reflections thrown out by us upon his scandalous inattention, equally impertinent and unnecessary; and the sleeping Jacks in office, who constituted what has been termed "The Committee for rebuilding Newgate," were probably of the same opinion. The matter is now unhappily come to the proof; the ravage the gaol distemper . . . has fatally evinced how absolutely a matter of public concern it was, that the new prison should be erected with all possible expedition. . . . As it is, however honest and worthy in other respects the surveyor of the New Prison now erecting may be, thousands are bound to curse both him and the negligent committee of the Common Council appointed to look after this business, for having entailed on them, their children, and their children's children, a measureless weight of misery, occasioned by the loss of those who lately died of the Putrid fever caught at the Old Bailey.

The Public Advertiser, October 14

It is now impossible to eradicate the Disease from the infected Walls of Newgate, and therefore the only Way is to pull down that loathsome Dungeon as soon as possible, which indeed cannot be done until the new one is built. I therefore take the Liberty of recommending to the Persons entrusted with the building of a new Newgate, that they set about that Business with Alacrity and Vigour, and not suffer that Affair to remain in its present languid and neglected State. . . . I would advise the Committee to call upon the Public for Assistance, and surely there can be no Doubt of their being able to borrow Money upon so good a Security. Let the aldermen themselves set an Example, by lending Money for this salutary purpose, which will shew their Patriotism in a much more amiable Light than their present absurd Contest for a Lord Mayor. . . . I hope that this Call upon the Committee will rouze them from their present torpid State.

That the crisis coincided with the mayoral election undoubtedly raised the stakes and elevated the epidemic to a topic of the widest interest. This was so because one of the candidates was a lightning rod for controversy, none other than John Wilkes. Already a celebrated, if notorious, national political figure, the famed champion of "Liberty" and master of rough politics was an alderman in 1772, with aspirations of becoming mayor. Important to our story is that he had been the sheriff of London and thus responsible (along with the Middlesex sheriff) for inspecting and maintaining Newgate. Wilkes's opponents were thus probably behind the criticisms that "the late sheriffs" had neglected the jail, claims that his supporters vehemently countered with claims of his diligence.[26]

In the mayoral contest Wilkes was outmaneuvered by former ally, James Townsend, whom Wilkes's supporters accused of betrayal. On Townsend's accession day Wilkes's supporters responded as they so often did, by assembling as mob. Five hundred men crowded around the Guildhall, shouting insults, setting fires, and trying to block entry. Townsend had the protesters arrested and locked up—where else but Newgate!—bringing the question of whether fever still raged in the prison straight into the political spotlight.

Wilkes demanded that they be incarcerated elsewhere, arguing that imprisonment in Newgate was a death sentence, even accusing Townsend of trying to kill his supporters. The Court of Common Council hotly debated the health of the jail and grilled Newgate's keeper and surgeon for the latest details of the epidemic—all of which played out in the press and intensified public anxiety.[27]

Representations of Wilkes's supporters in these debates carry intriguing implications for class. As is well known, Wilkite crowds included men of both mercantile and artisanal classes, and this mixed composition allowed for selective constructions of them as either respectable or lowly, based on one's politics. For example, Wilkite arguments presented them as polite, protesting that Newgate was "a place of confinement fit only for criminals." Townsend retorted that he had already afforded the rioters privileged status by separating them from the felons. Indeed, he challenged one of Wilkes's allies, Sheriff Watkin Lewes, reminding him that Newgate's debtors were situated between the Wilkites and the felons and thus lived in closer proximity to danger. He asked rhetorically how "Mr. Lewes' Heart should bleed for the innocent rioters, and feel nothing all this while for the unfortunate Debtors, who were the Sheriff's prisoners, were charged with no Crime, and yet had long been kept by Mr. Lewes in a Situation more dangerous." Moreover, an opponent of Wilkes blamed the epidemic on the presence of his supporters in the courtroom: "Several persons having caught contagious fevers at the Old Bailey, in consequence of the late admission of the lower classes of people into that court, by favour of the late patriotic Sheriffs." This critic drew on the idea that congregations of poor bodies perpetuated contagion, notably omitting reference to the infected prisoners on whom virtually all other commentators blamed the epidemic. Thus while Wilkes's supporters were elsewhere depicted according to the model of the polite debtor deserving of privileged treatment, they were here besmirched as pestilential in ways that carried forward links between contagion and the poor that had been forged more than a century earlier.[28]

Such use of jail fever as a rhetorical weapon undoubtedly increased news coverage of the epidemic and enhanced the levels of fear felt in late 1772. Numerous sources attest to heightened anxiety, especially on the part of those with cause to enter a courtroom. We saw that lawyers were afraid to attend court. An open letter similarly conveyed a distraught woman's terror when her husband was called to jury duty. In tears she expressed the "utmost anxiety" that he would inevitably be exposed to "Pestilence and Death." The writer implored the sheriffs not "to trifle with the lives of my Countrymen." Another paper commented on the grave risks that attended the position of alderman: "He must in course attend at the Old Bailey, and if he is elected Sheriff, his close attendance about the prisons may make him obnoxious to catching the gaol distemper."[29] The panic carried into early 1773 despite reports that fever in Newgate was abating.

The palpable worry in 1772/73 must also have resulted from the looming sense that an epidemic was bound to happen as long as Newgate remained unreformed. The framing of the 1772 epidemic was thus profoundly historical, as time and again the older epidemics—1577 in Oxford, 1730 in Taunton, and 1750 at the Old Bailey—were referenced to explain to Londoners the threat that they now faced.[30] These historical narratives contributed a sense of inevitability to jail fever. As long as the conditions associated with poverty—filth, hunger, inadequate clothing, spoiled food, and dirty water—were institutionalized in jails, the biological ramifications of those conditions would necessarily follow. It was a matter of science, which meant that another epidemic was merely a matter of time. History and the politics of memory thus became powerful tools in these debates. Consider how the *Morning Chronicle* threatened the Newgate Committee with the suggestion of a memorial to the dead.

> As an atonement for the fatal consequences . . . which have arisen from their [the surveyor's and the stone mason's] mutual neglect, they are now determined with their wonted expedition to erect at their own cost, a grand and extensive Mausoleum, or receptacle for the bodies of those who have fallen victim to the gaol distemper since May 1770, the period of time when they allow the public had a right to expect a new prison to have been completed. Open as we are to conviction, we cannot but allow that this, like a greasy dish-cloth, wipes off a part of the disgrace, and we recommend to their consideration the following inscription for this deadly repository: "Large as this Catacomb for those who fell sacrifice to the malignant gaol fever in the years 1770, 1771, 1772, 1773 and 1774, may appear, the architects have a double claim to the public admiration; they not only erected it at their own expence, in token of their having been favoured with the most convenient marks of inattention, from the committee appointed to inspect their building of the new prison, intended for the use of the old gaol of New-Gate was for many years put to, but they happily contrived, through their

own immediate care, that a sufficient number of proper subjects should be ready to closely cram every corner of it as soon as it was erected."[31]

Among the many fascinating elements of this passage is the inclusion of both past and future dates on the proposed plaque. It would not merely commemorate the dead of the present crisis but would look backward and forward commemorating deaths from years past as well as those that would inevitably come. Here was London's past. More frightening, here was London's future.

As the 1772 epidemic sent people scurrying to history for lessons, it is clear that many of those lessons concerned plague. It was no accident that critics of the Newgate Committee referred to the disease as the "jail pestilence." Medical theory, specifically the idea that the jail distemper represented a weakened form of plague that paupers could intensify, was now conveyed in the popular press. Writing in the *Public Advertiser* under a pseudonym, "Titus" compared prison reform to maritime quarantine. "It is of the highest national Consequence, and claims the Attention of Government equally with the Means of preventing the Plague being brought into this Country; for many learned Men think the Jail Fever a Species of the Plague.—Its Effects are as fatal—and should it once be carried from Newgate to some Parts of the Town by the wretched Inhabitants of both Places, and take deep Root there, it will be almost impossible to root it out, without a Conflagration of such a Quarter of the Town."[32] In citing "learned writers" he surely meant the works of physicians who had long linked fever and plague. But he clearly read beyond those passages because he also referred to the unique danger of the poor, demonstrating revealing slippage between prisoners specifically and the poor generally. The vectors responsible for intensifying and spreading plague would be the "wretched inhabitants" of Newgate *and* London's slums. The fear that a jail-born epidemic might not just kill a few judges but could explode into a repeat of 1666 remained firmly in Britons' minds in the autumn of 1772.

And so prison reform indeed became an issue of "national Consequence." Titus hadn't exaggerated. Wilkes's national profile played a role. But critics also set their sights beyond London authorities, demanding that Parliament act. If the Newgate Committee could not act, "some higher Powers" must. The *St. James's Chronicle* demanded that MPs "interfere to bring it [Newgate] to a Completion." A writer calling himself Benevolus similarly called for parliamentary action under direct threat of plague. "It is a national concern and ought therefore to no longer be delayed; or . . . we I fear shall be visited with a secondary plague." The eruption of epidemics in other parts of Britain during the London crisis, for example, a worrying fever outbreak in the Lewis Islands off the Scottish coast, could have only enhanced the sense that controlling the spread of fever truly represented a national issue.[33]

The 1772 Old Bailey epidemic thus marks an overlooked turning point in British history, because it provides crucial background for contextualizing the prison reform activity that immediately followed. John Howard is often presented as a singular visionary who set off to tour English prisons based on his personal experience as a sheriff in Bedfordshire, sparking prison reform seemingly by his own hand.[34] He tends to appear like a deus ex machina, who from an excessive capacity for sentiment set out in 1773 to tour prisons and shock Britons to action by forcing them to confront prison conditions in explicit detail. But these conditions were hardly a secret awaiting a hero to uncover them. To the contrary, prison conditions and their danger to wider public health had been a subject of concern for a very long time. Now in the autumn of 1772 the issue came to a head. It is thus hardly a coincidence that Howard embarked on his tour in 1773. He was less a singular voice in the forest than a self-appointed champion for a much wider movement.[35]

The Jail Fever Panic and the Age of Prison Reform: The 1770s and 1780s

The 1770s and 1780s represent a fundamental era for penitentiary reform. The spate of legislation and pace of activity were intense and unprecedented. After what appears to be a century of incidental, ad hoc, and periodic attention, prison reform efforts got serious, immediately after 1772. The key events and figures have been extensively studied and need not be itemized here.[36] Their importance here lies in demonstrating the depth of the contagion anxieties that had long existed in British culture but which now intensified to panic levels. Jail fever became nationally important. Throughout 1773 Howard inspected jails all over the country. And when in the spring of 1774 he stood in Parliament to report his shocking findings—namely, that jails throughout the land presented epidemic threats to their communities—he had the nation's ear. We will explore Howard in the next chapter, but in what remains of this one I want to demonstrate that issues of health and the dangers of the plebeian body were at the forefront of prison reform efforts every step of the way. Here lies an opportunity to support the claim made by both DeLacy and Porter that the fear of epidemics was a primary driver of penitentiary reform, an assertion that has not resonated as loudly as it should have done, although Philippa Hardman's recent study of Gloucestershire may signal that this is changing. But the point is not primarily to revise the historiography of penitentiary reform. Rather, the goal is more modest: to approach debates about prisons as a high-profile and wide-ranging discourse about bodies. When prison reform became a national debate, claims about the plebeian body sounded more widely than at any time since 1666.[37]

For all the prison building that was soon to come, and for all the lofty debates about how best to discipline the wicked, the development inaugurating this golden age of penitentiary reform was medical: 1774's "Act for Preserving the Health of Prisoners in Gaol, and preventing the Gaol Distemper." Howard's speech to Parliament, delivered with the support of his friend the Quaker physician John Fothergill, was instrumental to its passage. It is probably not coincidental that the bill was introduced by an MP from Taunton, where, as we saw, a 1730 jail fever epidemic became part of the disease's lore and a key feature of that town's history. The initial bill called for baths in jails so that prisoners could be washed before trial. The bill concentrated on plebeian bodies, omitting any reference to debtors' prisons and specifying that its regulations were meant for those jails "to which felons are usually committed." It said nothing about innovative architectural structures, making it clear that the processing of bodies was its primary aim. In the event, the act reached farther than the bill, empowering justices to enforce such health measures as paying prison surgeons from the poor rates; scrubbing, scraping and whitewashing walls; and providing infirmaries. The bill was initially two-pronged, with other provisions aimed at eradicating fees that allowed keepers to detain acquitted prisoners who still owed. These different provisions were unbundled and passed as separate acts, but their initial links support the reading that these measures also had health in mind, and, like Insolvency Acts for debtors, were aimed at facilitating the movement of bodies out of jails. If MPs needed a reminder of what was at stake, they got one in the midst of their deliberations. Two weeks after Howard addressed the House, and just two days after MPs agreed to split the bill into parts, newspapers reported that "Baron Adams is dead of gaol fever contracted at the Old Bailey." While MPs worked to pass the act, further rumors circulated of an outbreak in Hertford, while a writer calling himself "Anti-Pestlientia" published a lengthy call for action on "a national danger," warning that jail fever was actually plague. The "Health of Prisoners Act" received royal assent on June 2.[38]

A close look what transpired between the passage of that law and the Penitentiary Act (1779) spotlights how radically the situation intensified over the next few years. If crowded jails were dangerous, then the American Revolution was a public health disaster. The abrupt end of transportation in 1775 occasioned by the revolution brought an altogether new crisis. Relief that Britons may have felt in 1774 because their local jails now promised to be cleaner must have been short-lived, as those jails quickly filled to the brim with the bodies of felons who had been sentenced to sail away but now had nowhere to go. It may help to note what a significant role transportation played in the criminal justice system at this point. More than 60 percent of those found guilty at the Old Bailey in 1774 were transported. Now that option disappeared. Simon Devereaux has called the ensuing period "a crisis of overcrowding in English jails that had no equal before or since," while John Beattie asserted that in 1775 "the government was clearly willing to accept any expedient to clear the jails." Hitchcock and Shoemaker support this view, seeing the end of transportation as promoting a massive adminis-trative crisis.[39]

The immediate expedient was resort to the hulks. Parliament took quick action in 1776, ordering prisoners sentenced to transportation to serve hard labor on prison ships floating in the Thames. Never designed for the purpose, these decrepit vessels became quickly notorious as floating pits of disease, with even higher mortality than terrestrial prisons. It is notable, however, that even here we find antecedents. In the midst of the 1772 epidemic Londoners already considered this solution. The *Morning Chronicle* suggested prophetically, "Perhaps it might contribute much towards destroying infection in Newgate, if an old vessel was fitted up, to remain at anchor at a convenient distance down the River, on board of which those who were convicted for transportation might be put."[40]

Studies of prison reform often present debates in this period as contests between advocates of different policies, transportation on the one hand and imprisonment on the other. Beattie, for example, points to a decline in trans-portation sentences in the early 1770s as evidence of a desire to move beyond transportation even before the American war. He explores thinkers like Blackstone, Hanway, and Eden who pushed for the expansion of incarceration based on the workhouse model and lauded the social engineering promise of enlightened institutionalization. However, while penitentiary advocates eventually triumphed, it is notable that in the short term they lost. Devereaux has shown that only a small number of supporters of the Penitentiary Act actually sought to replace transportation with imprisonment and that efforts to bring in more sweeping measures jeopardized the act's passage. Moreover, the jails envisioned in the act were simply not built. Devereaux has usefully demonstrated the intellectual influences on these debates such as reformers' thoughts on deterrence, liberty, and humanitarianism.[41] However, viewing these debates against the backdrop of the jail fever crisis suggests a different motor of change.

For it was a crisis. Consider that Parliament was already debating the Hulks Bill by November 1775, just a few months after the outbreak of hostilities in America, and attempts to postpone debates were soundly defeated. The lord mayor had by then already ordered 140 Newgate convicts loaded onto ships because he feared an epidemic. Moreover, while debating the Hulks Bill, Parliament gathered information on prisoners scheduled for transportation for the express purpose of trying to arrange pardons, thereby using yet another mechanism to try to move bodies out of jails. After all, this is what transportation had done so effectively. The reason that "sentiment for transportation still ran so high" throughout the American Revolution was that transportation emptied prisons. Worries about crowded jails had been building for decades; little wonder that so many yearned for the resumption of a policy that took potentially pestilential bodies and simply sent them off to sea. When imploring Parliament to resume transportation, Edmund Burke was not speaking metaphorically when he called prisons "nests of pestilence."[42] By the 1770s transportation was as much a public health policy as a penal one.

The debates on how England's penal system should be reformed had many positions, of course, but in some ways they constituted different sides of the same coin. Reformers calling for new prisons sought to relieve overcrowding by providing more space, while advocates for transportation addressed the same problem by reducing the number of incarcerated bodies. Bodies in space: this was the issue that needed managing. Indeed, the unity of these seemingly different strategies can be detected in Blackstone's reformulation of the Hard Labour Bill (1778), the preamble of which made clear that the public's health was its primary aim. Famed as a champion of the penitentiary, Blackstone stressed four quite different strategies: resuming transportation, establishing new prisons for London, retaining the hulks, and enlarging county jails. It seems schizophrenic if viewed through the lens of adversarial policy stances: transportation *and* new prisons *and* the hulks *and* larger county jails. However, the bill makes sense when viewed against the backdrop of the jail fever crisis, because its various policies all combatted pestilence by reducing the deadly ratio between bodies and space. Each in its own way resulted in fewer bodies per square foot in Britain's jails, and this, according to generations of physicians, was vital to keep plague at bay. In the event, the hodgepodge represented in Blackstone's bill roughly predicted the course of events. No strategy was neglected as public fears drove authorities to use every tool at their disposal. The temporary hulks became permanent and then expanded as new prison ships came into use. Howard's hugely influential *The State of the Prisons in England and Wales* (1777) revealed how dire the situation was, sparking the well-documented spate of jail construction that saw as many as forty-five prisons rebuilt by 1790. And authorities continued to explore options to resume transportation.[43]

This was the case because anxieties ran high well into the 1780s. Consider the situation back in London. Builders finally completed Newgate in the spring of 1780, at long last enabling authorities to order the first prisoners transferred from the old jail on May 25. Unsurprisingly they moved debtors first and, ever conscious about class, ordered that their rooms "be fitted up for Prisoners of a Superior Rank." It turned out not to matter. Within a week the Gordon Riots erupted and burned the brand-new prison to the ground. From the point of view of propertied Londoners, there were many unsettling elements to these riots, not the least of which was that they significantly set back the city's strategy to protect them from jail-born pestilence, a campaign that had been waged—frustratingly in the case of Newgate—for thirty years. The prison would not be fully operational until 1784.[44]

What started as a religious protest exploded into a massive uprising targeting numerous institutions of authority, with particular venom for prisons. More than sixteen hundred inmates were freed as mobs moved from jail to jail. Hitchcock and Shoemaker see the riots as the culmination of anger toward a hardening criminal justice system that had percolated throughout the century and now reached a boiling point. Prison overcrowding of the late

1770s played a role by bringing together large numbers of plebeian Londoners for long periods in deplorable conditions, helping to create the conditions for larger-scale collective organization. While these scholars stress hatred of an unfair justice system, they also acknowledge that concerns about disease in prisons ran hot in the lead-up to the riot.[45] And it is hard to imagine that such concerns were a monopoly of the propertied. It stands to reason that poor Londoners resented that even petty transgressions could get them locked up for extended periods in toxic dungeons, a sentiment comprising equal parts anger and fear that could have only enhanced their hatred of prisons in the summer of 1780. Unfortunately, the parameters of the current study largely limit its ability to delve into plebeian experiences of epidemics. However, in their reflections on prison breaks as a form of agency, Hitchcock and Shoemaker offer a useful insight that allows us to take a momentary glance at how poor Britons may have incorporated discourses about disease into their survival tactics during the Jail Fever Panic.

Unsurprisingly, numerous men fled the pestilential hulks. George Morley explained his motivation to escape as the fear that if he stayed, "I should not live a month." William Bateman knew that he risked a death sentence when he ran away from the *Stanislaus*, the Woolwich hulk on which he was imprisoned for more than three years. But when a fellow inmate presented an opportunity to make a break, Bateman declared, "I did not care, I would as soon die as live." John Purdy was equally eager to join fellow prisoners who invited him to join their escape from the hulks at Langston Harbour. "I said I did, for it was a place of sad distress." None of these prisoners specified that he feared disease precisely. But George Barrington did. He spent five long years on the hulks before being pardoned on condition of banishment. However, he did not leave the country and subsequently stood at the Old Bailey. He pleaded for mercy, crafting a defense that not only highlighted illness but did so in ways that deployed references to fever and putridity, detailing how the hulks ruined his constitution: "Colds that I had repeatedly caught had ulcerated my lungs . . . and putrified air by night, had greatly reduced and wasted my frame. . . . My constitution is destroyed by those sufferings; I trust you will consider my behavior, and the state I am now in, laboring under a nervous fever and shortness of breath." He begged not to return to the hulks: "My Lord, my disease is of such a nature, it is not in the power of medicine to relieve me if I go down to that place; and certain death must be the consequence." Other trial defendants tried to use the delirium of prison-born fever to excuse their actions. And if some deployed words in the courtroom, others let their actions speak. Following the riots soldiers were stationed around prisons to prevent escapes. Two such soldiers ran afoul of the law and found themselves imprisoned for theft. In a disgusting turn of events, inmates terrorized them for having helped keep them locked up by submerging one of them in a tub of stale urine. They announced that "they would serve every soldier in like manner for preventing them getting out of Goal." Hitchcock and Shoemaker correctly point out the shaming nature of this ordeal, but we should not discount that the prisoners here tapped into the profound contagion anxieties long associated with plebeian waste and strategically used them to add an element of biohazardous threat to this act of violent resistance.[46]

Whatever the case, the Gordon Riots dealt a massive blow to London's carceral system. Prisons and jails bulged throughout the land. Demobilization at the end of the American war (1783) again ushered in a period of high unemployment and crime, and, as in the 1750s, anxiety about social disorder soared. Beyond public sentiment, this crime wave enhanced the sheer number of bodies that the overwhelmed justice system had to accommodate so that, according to Beattie, "The problem of crowded prisons was being felt all over the country by 1784 and 1785." Pressures were particularly acute in the capital. By 1786 aldermen petitioned the king to press for a resumption of transportation to deal with the more than four thousand felons who they felt should have been exported long ago. Newspapers did not mince words: "The King's Bench and Fleet Prison are at this time so full that a gaol fever is dreaded every hour—perhaps a plague may be the consequence." MPs finally discovered a solution in the form of Australia, with the first ships departing for Botany Bay in early 1787. Once transportation resumed, London banished felons at rates faster than anywhere else in the country.[47]

Further evidence supports viewing decisions about jails in this period as attempts to manage a crisis of plebeian bodies. Hitchcock has recently demonstrated that London's system for vagrancy underwent dramatic reform as a direct result of prison crowding. Vagrants were typically whipped and imprisoned in houses of correction before being "passed" back to their home parishes. However, the jails that usually housed vagrants and petty offenders filled up with felons once transportation halted, especially following the Gordon Riots. At that point "the system for holding prisoners in the capital was in meltdown." As a result, magistrates and justices began reducing the numbers of vagrants imprisoned by dramatically increasing the number that they simply loaded onto carts and shipped out of the city. Vagrant removals increased almost 400 percent between the mid-1770s and the mid-1780s. Moreover, the composition of vagrants changed, as many men who would have previously been charged as felons were now charged as vagrants so that they could be quickly removed. Unable to use the long-effective strategy of transportation across the ocean, London and Middlesex justices opted for a form of transportation over land, adjusting sentences to employ a different legal mechanism to resume shipping away thousands of poor men and women who came to stand before them. That vagrant removal was part of a health scheme is further supported by complaints of the contractor who transported them, that many vagrants were "dangerously ill, some of which have died in his Hands." In other words, not only were city officials now shipping plebeian bodies out of the city without bothering to administer their legal punishment, they may well have targeted the visibly unwell in order to export particularly worrying bodies. Indeed, the refusal of the contractor to remove the ill forced city authorities to hospitalize sick vagrants just to be able to send them packing. In vagrant removals we may witness the policy that comes closest to Defoe's utopian strategy six decades earlier: the forced exodus of poor bodies out of the city for the sake of preventing an epidemic. Although it bears repeating that banishing the homeless had been a mainstay of early modern plague orders for two centuries.[48]

ꙅ✕ꞓ

Throughout the period of penitentiary reform that followed the 1772 epidemic, doctors churned out treatises on jail fever like never before.[49] We have already seen how these works advanced theories of plebeian putridity until the end of the century. Such a flurry of publication helps signal the magnitude of concern during Jail Fever Panic. But more than that it reminds us that when confronted with the pressing dilemma of prison crowding, Britons robustly consumed medical literature, books that time and again warned them that poor constitutions were uniquely dangerous. Moreover, the prison reformers whose books occupied shelves alongside these medical treatises—John Howard's magnum opus in 1777, or those by Jacob Leroux in 1780, George Onesipherous Paul and Jonas Hanway in 1784, and Jeremy Bentham in 1791—were forever grounding their ideas in the works of physicians.[50] The crossover between these genres was significant, as evidenced by the fact that the prison reformer Paul published a treatise on the disease, while physician William Smith published one on jail conditions. Scottish and Irish publications reveal the same links.[51] In this way theories of the putrid plebeian body provided essential scientific evidence in a debate that was sustained at national levels and a fevered pitch throughout the last quarter of the century.

The men most committed to prison reform were often those who viewed themselves as particularly vulnerable. DeLacy has shown how frequently reformers came from the ranks of magistrates, justices of the peace, or sheriffs: propertied men whose civic responsibilities demanded that they regularly come face to face with paupers from jails. While lofty ideas about the social engineering potential of the Panopticon garner the lion's share of attention in penal histories, the 1785 comments of Lancashire prison reformer Thomas Butterworth Bayley make clear that more immediate concerns of personal safety often dominated their thinking: "Many of the judges, and the greater part of the Magistrates—have no other Object in view—than to prevent the Contagion of the Gaol fever; Fear, and the selfish ideas of personal Safety carry them so far; the other great points of Policy and Humanity in the plan of the Penitentiary house, Solitary Imprisonment, etc. have been treated as chimerical—and expensive Experiments."[52] Many issues informed late-eighteenth-century prison reform, perhaps none more than the naked survival instincts of the British ruling class. The evidence from London, where aldermen died, magistrates threatened to strike, and a mayor like Janssen crusaded against jail fever decades before penal reform became a national movement, goes a long way to support DeLacy's argument. And Howard, of course, famously first served as a sheriff. But whereas the intense emotional reaction to Howard is often framed in terms of late-eighteenth-century senti-mentality, evidence suggests that this response represents less the music of plucked heartstrings than an outpouring of relief born of real terror.[53] Howard, as we are about to see, was a hero because he was a savior. He offered a solu-tion to a most vexing problem. In the clean, spacious, well-ventilated, well-provisioned, and diligently inspected prison he offered respectable Britons the mechanism that promised to save them from a pestilential specter that terrified them throughout the second half of the century. Exploring in greater detail not Howard the man, but Howard the cultural phenomenon, offers us a unique way to take the pulse of wider British culture during the Jail Fever Panic.

6. Braving Contagion

John Howard and Ordinary Men

The story of John Howard is well known. A Bedfordshire sheriff who toured English and later European prisons decrying their conditions, he became a hero in his own time, lauded as one of the great humanitarians of his age. His 1790 martyrdom by fever in Russia transformed Howard from hero to legend. In this chapter I seek not to retell that story but to recontextualize it. The longer history of concerns about public health that this book has charted invites us to look with fresh eyes at the material left behind by and about Howard. Moreover, as I began to suggest in the last chapter, and as Roy Porter once argued, Howard should not be considered singular—as his hagiography often presents him—but rather as epitomizing a broader cultural phenomenon.[1] I seek to use Howard as a point of departure for a wider exploration of how the Jail Fever Panic was experienced by common Britons. When writers praised Howard, they said as much about themselves as they did about him. For example, it is widely known that Howard was praised for his sympathy for the downtrodden and superior Christian heart. However, less noticed have been portrayals of Howard as brave. It is axiomatic that bravery relies on danger; the former cannot exist without the latter. Commentary on bravery can be thus be mined for expressions of fear. Similarly revealing are the methods by which Howard protected himself when entering spaces that virtually everyone agreed were treacherous. Late-eighteenth-century Britons came to incorporate such strategies into their own lives. Thus Howard offers a point of entry for a broader exploration of how the Jail Fever Panic registered in wider British culture. Moreover, our investigation offers a chance to see how average citizens responded when faced with the prospect of following in their hero's footsteps. An analysis of common Londoners forced to serve as jurors investigating prison deaths gives us a unique glimpse of how men less extraordinary than Howard confronted jail fever. While Howard bravely entered prisons, fever be damned, London shopkeepers were not so bold. Finally, Howard's own work makes it apparent that while he battled jail fever, he also set his crusade against that older, deeper and ever more frightening monster, plague, a disease whose terror prevailed even at the dawn of the nineteenth century.

Howard Confronts the Prisons

If Londoners were uneasy walking *near* Newgate in the 1750s, how frightening must have been the prospect of actually entering a jail by the mid-1770s? Howard's own *State of the Prisons* suggested that prison conditions were bad precisely because many authorities were too afraid to supervise them properly. Supervisory visitation was standard practice at eighteenth-century institutions.[2] Yet when Howard met with wardens he heard stories of men too frightened to enter their own jails. "Many County-Gaolers excused themselves from going with me into the Felons Ward. In one County-Gaol the Felons told me once and again that the Gaoler had not been in their ward for months." And it was not just the jailers. The critique applied to sheriffs, magistrates, and JPs who were similarly "fearful of the consequence of looking into prisons." Gaolers commonly divulged that such fear was widespread among the country gentlemen who served in these positions. One confided, "None of those Gentlemen ever looked into the dungeons, or even the wards of my Gaol," while another exclaimed, "Those Gentlemen think that if they came into my Gaol, they should soon be in their graves."[3] In a later edition, Howard even suggested that keepers manipulated these fears to prevent inspections. "When a gentleman, particularly a magistrate, has come with an intention to visit the gaol, the keeper has pretended the utmost willingness to accompany him, but at the same time has artfully dropt a hint that he fears there may be some danger in it, as he is apprehensive that *the fever* has made its appearance among them. The visitor, alarmed, returns thanks for the kind caution, and instantly leaves the house." Medical men were not immune to these fears. The Health of Prisoners Act of 1774 mandated that all prisons provide doctors. Yet the surgeon contracted at the High Gaol in Exeter demanded a provision in his contract excusing him from visiting any dungeon in which the jail fever raged. The situation in Worcester was similar. The surgeon there had once caught fever and had "ever since been fearful of going into the dungeon: when any felon is sick there, he orders him to be brought out."[4]

The extent of such fears helps us understand the emotional reaction to Howard, who more than just volunteered to enter prisons, he insisted on it. His attention to detail made it clear to readers that he was physically present in even the dankest of English gaols. "I have described no prison but from my own examination. . . . I entered every room, cell, and dungeon with a memorandum-book in my hand, in which I noted particulars on the spot." And he did not enter them just once. He repeated his tours over three years, visiting many prisons, including the notorious Newgate, as many as four times and some even five. Polite readers must have been thus struck by the courage it took to expose his body again and again to spaces that would have sent them running.[5]

For indeed, the details were terrifying. No fewer than sixty jails were filthy, unwholesome, or "offensive," an adjective that referred to stench. Lack of sewers or sufficient water plagued even more. Howard critiqued seventy-two for these deficiencies, which would have been understood as serious hazards to anyone familiar with the long-standing connections between putrid diseases and human waste. Notwithstanding that the law now mandated infirmaries and doctors, Howard reported that thirty-seven jails lacked an infirmary or medical staff, or else had surgeons who neglected their duties. (Some of these were bridewells, whose keepers made the case that their institutions differed from "prisons" and thus were exempt from the act.) By all accounts Howard entered many frighteningly unhealthy buildings.[6]

Moreover, jail fever did not just lurk in the background of his text. Howard entered thirty jails that had been the sites of recent epidemics, and in some he encountered the disease directly. In 1776 he found almost forty ill men in the Savoy, "many of them sick of the Gaol-Distemper," and he entered the King's Bench Prison during a smallpox outbreak. Howard reported witnessing sick prisoners in fully twenty-one jails. His descriptions suggested to readers that he neither shied away from them nor based his reports on the keepers' notes. Rather, he came face to face with illness despite the obvious risks. When he described the "meagre sickly countenances" of ill prisoners in Chesterfield, or the woman "languishing on the floor in a consumption" in Shrewsbury, Howard made it clear that he saw these prisoners up close. Passages describing direct conversations with sick prisoners, detailing their skin tones, the sound of their cries, or the smell of their rooms, all conveyed the vivid picture that Howard was right there. The point of explaining that "upon examining two sick prisoners, I found they had no Irons" was that the Maidstone jail treated sick prisoners humanely. However, readers would have also taken from it that Howard had yet again examined the sick up close, something that they themselves were almost certainly too afraid to attempt. And there was every reason to feel such fear. The keepers and magistrates whom Howard criticized for neglecting to inspect prisons could reasonably defend their inaction by pointing out fully thirteen instances in Howard's own book in which keepers, surgeons, or other prison staff had caught jail fever, often fatally, and even spread it to their families.[7]

There were many lessons here. First, jail fever had left its morbid mark not just in London but in tiny jails and lockups all across the country: the Chelmsford Gaol in Essex, bridewells at Horsham, Usk, and Cowbridge, the Worcester Castle and the Knaresborough Prison, and county gaols at Hertford, Bedford, Warwick, Monmouth, Winchester, and Launceston. Casualties of nonprisoners in communities large and small surely helped convince Howard's readers that jail fever was indeed a "national concern."[8] But Howard's descriptions of jail fever's ravages also worked on another level, namely to convince readers that only a superior form of courage could enable someone to walk willingly into so many jails that had seen men die. Jail fever terrified late-eighteenth-century Britons, but John Howard stood up to it and looked it straight in the eye.

His friends worried about him. Surviving letters from physicians John Haygarth and John Coakley Lettsom, surgeon John Aikin, and minister Samuel Stennett all expressed concern for the danger they believed he faced. An anonymous writer from Georgia spoke for many when he heaped praise on Howard, not just for caring for the downtrodden, but for his manly courage "risk[ing] liberty and life." To this writer Howard was more than a friend to humanity; he was a "guardian angel" who, through "Herculean labor, patience and fortitude," "bid defiance to every species of contagion, and calmly confronted death in every horrid form." Of course, Howard was afraid too. Reports on particular jails offer glimpses. A dismal dungeon in Chester crowded men into cells with no windows and but a tiny aperture in

the door. It "brought to mind what I had heard of the *Black Hole* at Calcutta."
Howard was not above admitting his fear; "It was not, I own, without some
apprehensions of danger, when I first visited the prisons." However, he grew
more confident as his missions proceeded, in part because he believed that
gradual exposure to prisons slowly armored his system to pestilence.
Showing the influence of constitutional theories of the body, he noted that
his time in prisons "abated the force of noxious impressions upon me."[9]

Nevertheless, he protected himself, especially through prayer. Howard's
devotional writings demonstrate its ever-present role for a man who saw
himself as an unworthy instrument of God.[10] More intriguing than his devotional writings are his notebooks. He carried them to record prison conditions
and vividly described airing them before the fire each evening because he
feared their pages had absorbed pestilential effluvia from so many dank cells.
Inside one's front cover Howard inscribed, probably as the first entry, not so
much a prayer as a kind of oath that stressed courage. Given its position on the
inside cover, it may have even served as a kind of mantra to read at the start of
each day or right before entering a jail to strengthen himself for what lay
ahead. "A Traveller should have *Temperance Prudence,* and *Fortitude;* or firmness of mind, to bear sufferings or meet dangers undaunted. These are necessary for the active scenes of life and maintenance of the rights of others; for,
the truest pleasures arise from *extensive benevolence.* Dejection and Despair are
the consequences of Pusillanimity." The passage was clearly important to
him, for he transcribed it in another memorandum book and later expounded
on it in ways that further emphasized the masculine qualities of strength and
courage that he felt were necessary for his work. "To maintain the rights of
others requires strength & vigour of Constitution, wisdom in the conduct of
affairs, & the firmness which can baffle difficulties and dangers. Thus Temperance, Prudence and Fortitude are necessary to practice Justice."[11]

Howard's determination to stay courageous was probably also grounded
in medical theory. Since plague times doctors asserted that fear weakened the
constitution and predisposed it to infection. They drew on theories of the six
nonnaturals, but instead of stressing air or food, they charted the impact
of "the passions" upon physiology. For plague, powerful negative emotions
like grief or fear were most dangerous. Seventeenth-century doctors like
Willis advised readers to keep spirits up during epidemics, arguing that plague
took the "timorous" more than the "bold" and thus that "confidence [is]
a good Preservative." Yet another legacy that plague bequeathed to the

Enlightenment, this was standard advice throughout the eighteenth century and applied to fevers by such medical heavyweights as Lind and Cullen. The influence on Howard is made clear in the third edition of *The State of the Prisons* (1784), which included a new chapter on Gaol Fever arguing that the dejected emotions of prisoners impacted fever rates. Thus when Howard recited his passage about fortitude before entering a jail he almost certainly believed that it had physiological merit, strengthening his constitution against the pestilential effluvia he was about to confront. Cowardliness was deadly.[12]

Bravery Remembered

While Howard's writings are fascinating, it is through the writings of others *about* Howard that we can more clearly take the pulse of Britons living through the Jail Fever Panic. One of the most influential texts on Howard was the 1792 biography written right after his death by his friend the surgeon John Aikin, a book on which scholars agree virtually all subsequent biographies are based. Aikin consulted closely with Howard, and even helped write the *State of the Prisons* because Howard's prose was so poor. He exuded admiration for Howard and like so many believed that his achievements stemmed from a superior character. In keeping with the genre of biography he emphasized the moral foundation Howard displayed in youth that would ground him later in life. He thus spotlighted early examples of charity, devotion, discipline, and especially sympathy—the trait that so vividly colors sentimental depictions of him. However, bravery was every bit as important in Aikin's construction of his dead friend. Indeed, just three pages into the book Aikin may well have hit upon what rendered Howard a subject of such passionate hero worship, namely his singular combination of sympathy and bravery. He punctuated a list of accomplishments thus: "and to have done all this as a private unaided individual, struggling with toils, dangers, and difficulties, which might have appalled the most resolute; is surely a range of beneficience which scarcely ever before came within the compass of one man's exertions."[13] Danger made Howard's actions special.

After all, the eighteenth century did not lack philanthropists to celebrate. One merely need reflect on a figure like Thomas Guy, who singlehandedly funded a hospital for patients turned away from other hospitals, or perhaps more poignantly Thomas Coram, who devoted his life to Britain's youth, building the Foundling Hospital to save abandoned infants.[14] Howard founded no such institution and yet he received the moniker "*the* philanthropist."[15] This takes some explaining. In an age when sentimentality marks British culture so vividly, Howard's care for the neglected stands out. But this alone cannot explain why he was lionized even beyond a figure like Coram, who was just as easily constructed as the loving man of feeling, and indeed who saved victims who were far less complicated than the morally dodgy beneficiaries of Howard's goodwill. The difference lies in what they risked. Coram or Guy or any of the scores of institution-building reformers paled in comparison with Howard because all they gave was money. They were celebrated, of course, with good reason. But risk rendered Howard's actions an altogether different sort of activity. Howard's courage in braving contagion, in literally risking his life day after day, allowed for constructions of him to borrow simultaneously from sentimental depictions of so-called men of feeling and from masculine tropes that more commonly typified military heroes.[16] This one-two punch set Howard apart as a national saint.

Books like Aikin's thus afford considerable material for a gendered analysis of Howard as a masculine hero. Aikin offers hints in this direction, as when he described one of Howard's appeals for greater prison research as "forcible and manly." Moreover, he embeds bravery in Howard's essential character when describing early career developments like his acceptance of the post of sheriff. Non-Anglicans faced the severe penalties of the Test Act if they shirked the job's mandatory oath, an oath that a devoted nonconformist like Howard could not in conscience take. Of course, he opted to serve despite the risk; Aikin proclaimed, "It was perfectly suitable to Mr. Howard's character to make option of *the office with the hazard*," notably adding, "and as to personal hazard, *that* was never an obstacle in his way." Tessa West has shown that the risk was actually quite low. But it made a great story. Aikin demanded readers to consider what a loss it would have been had Howard neglected public service because he caved to "those apprehensions which would have operated upon most men." But Howard, Aikin was at pains to show, was not most men. He similarly stressed Howard's courage in braving repeated research trips to France even though his critiques of French prisons exposed him to arrest.[17]

But it was in regard to contagion that Howard represented "A Hercules who went about in order to contend with monsters." And when it came to disease, no monster was more terrifying than plague, the disease Howard graduated to confront in 1785. While prison reformers scrambled to apply his advice throughout Britain, Howard declared that he was leaving to study Europe's lazarettos. Aikin, who warned him about the trip, described Howard's resolute intent as "nothing less, than to plunge into the midst of those dangers which by other men are so anxiously avoided; to search out and confront the great foe of human life, for the sake of recognizing his features, and discovering the most efficacious barriers against his assaults. Who but must be struck with admiration of the firmness of courage, and the ardour of benevolence, which could prompt such a design!" Like any great martyr, Aikin's Howard knew that his life was at stake—he issued final farewells to friends before departing—yet he pressed on regardless. Aikin made sure to quote Howard's response to friends' warnings: "My medical acquaintance give me but little hope of escaping the plague in Turkey. I do not look back, but would readily encounter any dangers, to be an honour to my Christian profession." And when the inevitable fatal infection came during his later tour of prisons in Russia, Aikin described Howard's courage to the end, reporting that he proclaimed on his deathbed that "he all along expected [death] to take place; and he often said that he had no other wish for life than as it gave him the means of relieving his fellow-creatures."[18]

It is no stretch to say that Howard was framed as a martyr, because Aikin's concluding comments on Howard's character made the point explicitly, offering one of the clearest expressions of Howard as a masculine hero.

> His whole course of action was such a trial of intrepidity and forti-
> tude, that it may seem altogether superfluous to speak of his posses-
> sion of these qualities. He had them, indeed, both from nature and
> principle. His nerves were firm; and his conviction of marching in
> the path of duty made him fearless of consequences. Nor was it only
> on great occasions that this strength of mind was shown. It raised
> him above false shame, and that awe which makes a coward of many
> a brave man in the presence of a superior. No one ever less "feared
> the face of man" than he. No one hesitated less in speaking bold
> truth, or avowing obnoxious opinions. His courage was equally
> passive and active. He was prepared to make every sacrifice that a
> regard to strict veracity, or rigorous duty, could enjoin; and it cannot
> be doubted, that, had he lived in an age when asserting his civil and
> religious rights would have subjected him to martyrdom, not a more
> willing martyr would ever have ascended the scaffold, or embraced
> the stake.

No Briton reading these lines in 1792 could have mistaken the comparison to the heroes in *Foxe's Book of Martyrs*, the most commonly owned book after the *Book of Common Prayer*, and one of the most influential texts in the entirety of British history.[19] It is difficult to imagine rhetoric of higher praise at that moment in history.

Those reformation martyrs had died for Britain (at least, the Protestant version of it that eighteenth-century citizens held so dear), and in many ways so did Howard. Despite sentimental claims about his compassion, we must remember that what animated the commentary and eventual action on jail fever was the fear that it would strike *outside* the jail. Howard's most important work was not saving prisoners, despite what his biographers suggested. It was saving everyone else. His clean, well-ordered prisons promised to stop jail fever in its tracks. Doctors still believed that prison fever could morph into plague, and so Howard did so much more than just protect prisoners. He protected the nation, and he risked his life doing it. This is why Aikin could present Howard as "marching in the path of duty," a claim that evoked military action and rendered the dead Howard as a kind fallen soldier not unlike Wolfe or later Nelson, who gave their lives defending the nation.

Aikin's attempt to frame Howard according to ideals of masculinity, such as his emphases on self-denial, discipline, and even clothing, was even clearer when he curiously addressed his subject's attitudes toward women. Aikin's Howard is a courteous gentleman, of course, as when he gave up his berth on a crowded ship to a servant girl and slept on the floor. But in ways that call to mind Lisa Forman Cody's discussion of male midwives, Aikin's Howard also had a soft side that allowed him to converse easily with women. Aikin went as far as to call it feminine, but, tellingly, did so only within a sentence that immediately returned to the more traditional images of virility and action that he had taken pains to trace for two hundred pages: "Indeed, his soft tones of voice and gentleness of demeanour might be thought to approach somewhat to the effeminate, and would surprise those who had known him only by the energy of his exertions." To clarify the point Aikin quickly followed this claim with an anecdote about Howard pursuing an attractive young woman.[20] He might have a heart of gold, but make no mistake: John Howard was all man.

It is also useful to acknowledge that the emphasis on Howard's bravery was not a postmortem construction of a martyred hero; it was part of his living legend. William Hayley's 1780 saccharine *Ode to Howard* typifies the effusive praise. Howard, who hated such proclamations and who was down-right angry at the campaign to erect a statue to him, must have bristled when he read Hayley's letter accompanying the *Ode* proclaiming his work "the sublimest example of charity that was ever exhibited." Stanzas like this one give a taste of how masculine bravery and national protection colored the deification:

> That Hero's praise shall ever bloom,
> Who shielded our insulted coast;
> And launch'd his lightning to consume
> The proud Invader's routed host.
> Brave perils rais'd his noble name:
> But thou deriv'st thy matchless fame
> From scenes, where deadlier danger dwells;
> Where fierce Contagion, with affright, repels
> Valor's adventr'ous step from her malignant cells.

The *Critical Review* commented favorably on the poem, seizing on the theme of courage in its own commentary. "It is well known that this humane traveller visited every loathsome dungeon in this kingdom, fearless of the dreadful consequences which he might naturally have expected from such a dangerous enterprize; but the same Providence which saved and protected the good bishop of Marseilles extended its care over this equally bold and pious adventurer." By comparing Howard to Bishop Belsunce of Marseilles, famed for toiling among plague victims in the 1720s, the *Review* once again connected Howard to the much longer history of plague that was forever forcing its way into eighteenth-century discussions of fever.[21]

Howard's bravery even played out on the stage, during his lifetime. Elizabeth Inchbald's play *Such Things Are* (1787), a tale involving a prison inspector in the exotic locale of Sumatra, fashioned one of its characters after Howard and emphasized courage throughout.[22] The inspector, Mr. Haswell, is the only virtuous character in the play, and he does what one expects a Howard clone to do: feel sympathy for miserable prisoners, advocate for them, and generally act nobly. When inspecting the local jail, he is warned about the dungeon's "noxious vapours" and given the option of ending the tour. Of course, he resolutely demands to press on. However, danger, fear, and courage shine through as themes in the play in numerous other ways. Haswell's valor is constantly set against other men who lack it. Sir Luke

Tremor, as his name suggests, is a coward. Having acquitted himself poorly in battle, he lives in fear that his cowardice will be revealed and becomes comically agitated whenever conversation turns to military matters. When he cannot muster the nerve to confront a man who insults his wife, she complains: "Sir Luke, show yourself a man of courage but on this occasion."[23]

Elsewhere Howard's caricature inspires fear through righteous strength. Elvirus, a young man whose father languishes in prison, does not recognize Haswell and threatens him physically. The prison inspector replies undauntedly: "What am I to fear?" When Elvirus later realizes that he insulted the one man who could free his father, he yearns to apologize but laments, "I dare not—I feel the terror of his just reproach." When he later cannot meet Haswell's eye, the stage direction notably reads: "Haswell looks on him with a manly firmness, then walks on." Haswell later discovers the sultan's wife languishing in a dungeon, unbeknown to the sultan. Precisely because he neglected to do what Howard does—inspect the prisons—the sultan feels not just shame but fear at the thought of confronting her. His cowardice, like that of Elvirus and Tremor, is unveiled.

> SULTAN: Why do I tremble? . . .
> HASWELL: Yes, tremble, indeed!
> . . . .
> SULTAN: O! do not bring me to a trial which I have not courage to support.

Haswell/Howard thus towers over all other characters, thanks primarily to his bravery, a theme that swims throughout the entire play. Susan Staves is correct that its portrayal of Howard was profoundly sentimental.[24] Yet Howard's manly courage was no less important.

Such extensive commentary on Howard's bravery offers rich material for charting the Jail Fever Panic. *The State of the Prisons* is a rather ponderous book to have so captured the nation's imagination. And indeed it did not. Roy Porter once suggested that Howard's fame was rooted in the greatness of his tome.[25] But that misses the point. It was not so much that *The State of the Prisons* was considered a great book as that its author was considered a great man. Charting the outline of Howard's deification offers a way to trace the size and scope of the Jail Fever Panic. Howard's reputation and his culture's fear of fever were connected in an almost mathematical relationship. Had people feared the disease less, his reputation would have diminished proportionally. But in practice things pushed strongly in the opposite direction. The enormity of the phenomenon that was John Howard, perhaps more than any other piece of evidence, reflects the enormity of the panic about fever. The monster stood in direct proportion to the hero who battled it.

Ordinary Men Confront Jail Fever: Investigating Prison-Deaths in Westminster

But what of ordinary men? How heroic were they? Allow me to shift gears for a moment. The rhetoric by and about Howard trumpeted that entering jails was dangerous. But most of the time law-abiding people could choose whether or not to enter a jail. However, at least one occasion demanded that ordinary men enter a prison: jury duty for a coroner's inquest.[26] Every so often ordinary men found themselves called upon to emulate Howard by entering jails as part of an investigative process. How they responded can teach us a great deal about how the fever panic was experienced during the height of Howard's fame. But before we explore how they responded when called upon to enter a jail, we should first take a look at the inquests themselves, because they reveal a number of telling patterns about how prison deaths were explored and recorded during the period of most intense worry about jail fever.

English law required a coroner's inquest for all deaths occurring in prisons. Theoretically, jailers could face criminal charges if prisoners died from abuse. Middlesex coroner Edward Umfreville, who penned an authoritative guide to the office in 1761, described the obligations. "For Murder may happen in a Gaol, and this taking of an Inquisition 'super visum corporis' [upon sight of the body] of Persons dying in Gaol, is not an inconsiderable Labour or Pain; for the Inquisition must be taken, and the body viewed in Gaol; Prisoners must be on the Jury; Prisoners must give Evidence of the kind or severe Usage of the Gaoler; the Prison may be at a great distance from the Coroner's Abode; and from a Diversity of Seasons, or Care, may be unwholesome; and however long and painful the Inquiry may be, yet the Coroner at his own Charges, must go and attend his duty; and be all the while under the Lock and Key of the Keeper." The comment that coroners had to enter jails despite the places' being "unwholesome" indicates an awareness of health risks long before Howard's reform activities had begun. The

A CORONERS INQUEST.

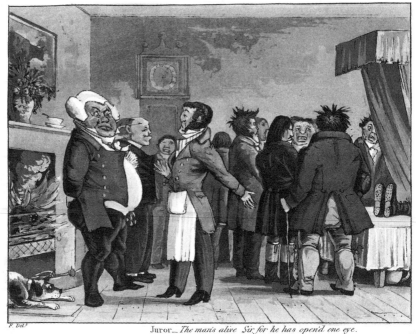

Juror— *The man's alive Sir; for he has open'd one eye.*
Coroner— *Sir; the doctor declar'd him Dead two hours since & he must remain Dead Sir; so I shall proceed with the Inquest.*

London, Published by Tho.' M.' Lean, 26, Haymarket, 1826.

Figure 7. Anon., *A Coroners Inquest* (London: Tho. McLean, 1826), Courtesy of Lewis Walpole Library, Yale University.

inquest had to occur inside the prison and in the presence of the body. Moreover, it was not just the coroner who would have to enter the prison but citizens as well. Jurors were expected "to inquire *upon the View of the Body* . . . how and in what Manner he came to his Death," a point nicely illustrated by the satirical cartoon in Figure 7. In cases of jail fever deaths, this meant that ordinary men had to follow in John Howard's footsteps, entering an unwholesome jail while contagion might still rage.[27]

We know that anxieties about Newgate ran high. So to test attitudes more broadly, I have examined a different, less notorious prison, Westminster's largest jail, the Tothill Fields Bridewell. This is possible because the Westminster coroner's inquests are unusually rich. Surviving for the period 1760–1799, they offer more robust witness depositions than are typical in surviving coroners' records for the period.[28] Those forty years nicely span the Jail Fever Panic, starting a decade before the 1772 Old Bailey epidemic and running for almost a decade after Howard's death. During that time the coroner investigated 106 deaths in the jail.

Tothill Fields housed a variety of inmates of both sexes. More than half the inquests identify the deceased's offense, offering a snapshot of the jail's population. These included ten thieves, three debtors, a forger, an accused sodomite, a man arrested for assault, and nine prisoners incarcerated for unnamed felonies and misdemeanors. More common were the sorts of lowly men and women typically associated with bridewells; three women had been arrested as "disorderly" (code for prostitute), and thirty-one men were vagrants.[29] Tothill Fields thus housed a large number of quite poor inmates, many of whom had probably been scooped off the streets as homeless. In 1776 physician William Smith described its population. "The prisoners in this gaol are a miserable set of objects; some of the very lowest order of abandoned women, covered with filth and vermin, eat up with the bad distemper [syphilis], and broke down by every species of intemperance. Debtors, felons, fines and disorderly people are all huddled together." But Howard gave Tothill Fields a more favorable review, stating that its rooms were "wholesome" and that prisoners washed every morning. It needed an infirmary, but considering Howard's reports on other prisons, Tothill Fields was hardly notorious. The inquests also give a sense of the kind of men who sat as jurors, frequently listing their occupations. The predominance of small shopkeepers and craftsmen suggests that juries deliberating on deaths in Tothill Fields typically comprised respectable merchants and artisans who were usually reputable householders and employers but hardly rich. The list of men summoned to inspect the body of prisoner George Hancock in August 1777 was typical: eight victuallers, four chandlers, two shoemakers, a cook, a pawn broker, a baker, a grocer, a haberdasher, a coach master, and a snuff salesman.[30]

Several features stand out about inquests at Tothill Fields. First, virtually all deaths in the prison were, at least officially, due to sickness. Only three deaths were attributed to other causes. Two prisoners committed suicide and in 1766 an intellectually disabled teenager was thought to have been murdered by the keeper, John Stevens, a charge of which he was acquitted. Second, as Umfreville noted, prisoners were supposed to sit on the jury. This occurred only once in forty years.[31] How the coroners, Thomas Prickard and later Anthony Gell, got away with routinely ignoring this law is unclear. (We did see that keepers of some bridewells shirked the stipulations of the Health of Prisoners Act by arguing that bridewells differed from prisons and thus that the act did not bear on them, so perhaps the Westminster coroners used the same semantic trick.) Third, prison inquests were perfunctory. For example, based on a sample comparison group, juries on deaths outside the prison heard testimony from nearly twice as many witnesses. Roughly three out of four prison inquests heard just a single witness. Moreover, testimony about nonprison deaths was typically much more detailed. Consider a simple word count. In 1768, to take a random year, juries for dead prisoners heard on average just 173 words of testimony, while other juries that year heard an average of 515 words. Thus juries on nonprisoners heard three times as much testimony from nearly twice as many witnesses as those investigating prison deaths. Thomas Forbes, Margaret DeLacy, Joe Sim, and Tony Ward have each noted the cursory nature of prison inquests in the early nineteenth century, and it certainly seems that this was already the case half a century earlier. Those scholars variously propose that such superficial investigation stemmed from communal indifference to the fate of prisoners combined with officials' attempts to avoid scrutiny.[32] We will see that contagion anxieties also played a significant role.

Testimony in inquests at Tothill Fields was not only short but formulaic. The 1776 inquest on prisoner Daniel Bradley is entirely typical and clearly geared toward exonerating the prison staff.

> Abraham Myam on his Oath saith That he hath been prisoner in Tothillfields Bridewell about three Months, That Daniel Bradley the Deced has been a Prisoner there above one Month, That the Deced appeared to be in good Health when he was brought to said prison[,] that he continued so until yesterday fortnight (January 13th.) when he was taken ill, and could not sleep at Night, Says that the Deced constantly had the Allowance in the Prison, being a Penny and a penny worth of Bread, that Deced ate the Bread and had some Watergruel for the Penny, and that the Governor ordered the Deced some Tea & Toast or Bread & Butter every Morning, That the Deced was Confined in the same ward with [this] Dept. [deponent] and in no Damp or improper place, That the Deced Grew worse and died Yesterday Morning Jany. 22d. in a natural way, and not by any ill Treatment from the Governor, or his Deputy or any of his Fellow Prisoners.[33]

This contains several components of typical witness statements about prison deaths. Fellow prisoners were usually deposed, often, as here, as the only witness. They typically identified roughly when the deceased entered the prison and noted his original state of health. Next, they pointed out when sickness began, usually with brief descriptions of vague symptoms. They then closed by assuring the jury that the deceased had been fed and not abused. In some cases this information was augmented. However, the format, indeed the order, of these components in inquest after inquest leaves little doubt that witnesses were coached, coerced, or led by questioning to hit key themes. Given that the legal purpose of prison inquests was to rule out abuse, this makes some sense. Although Bradley had been ill for nine days, there is no mention of medical care. This was also common, especially during the 1760s and 1770s, when all prison deaths but one were found to have been from sickness, yet barely a quarter of the inquests mentioned medical care, which was typically just a visit by an apothecary, who left medicines for fellow prisoners to administer. Finally, the verdict also stands out. Jurors ruled that Bradley "Departed this Life by the Visitation of God in a natural Way, to wit, of a Fever." How they reached that diagnosis is as baffling as it is revealing. The entirety of the medical information jurors heard was that Bradley was "ill" and had trouble sleeping. Such imprecise symptoms could suggest virtually any ailment. Moreover, this information came from a prisoner, not a doctor. Nevertheless, the coroner ruled that Bradley died of a specific disease: fever.

Fever verdicts abound in prison inquests during the 1760s and 1770s. Westminster juries attributed two-thirds of all prison deaths (20 of 30) to fever during these decades. Five inquests did not identify a sickness, merely noting that prisoners died "in a Natural Way." Leaving aside the aforementioned murder, there were only four other deaths, by dropsy and consumption.[34] Thus, in the 1760s and 1770s fever was practically a default diagnosis for sick prisoners, accounting for 83 percent of all verdicts that identify a specific disease (20 of 24). The lack of any mention in Bradley's inquest—or in so many like it—of any specific symptoms associated with fever suggests that Westminster jurors needed little convincing that a corpse in prison must have succumbed to fever.

This makes sense given what we now know about the atmosphere in London. The controversy over rebuilding Newgate gathered steam in the

1760s; the second Old Bailey epidemic flared in 1772; Howard launched his activities in 1773; transportation halted and the hulks appeared by 1776; and then a rash of reform activity built to the Penitentiary Act in 1779. Each development generated more commentary, broadcasting that prisons generated fever. Respectable Londoners were thus conditioned to presume that fever would explain nonviolent deaths in jail. That different collections of men sitting as jurors over twenty years reached the same conclusion again and again—often without any medical evidence to suggest it—speaks volumes about the silent assumptions framing their decisions. Moreover, because their neighbors shared those assumptions, such verdicts were unlikely to be questioned. A vagrant entered a jail, got fever, and died; that narrative was as powerful as it was mundane. Taking into account contemporary concerns about prison conditions, we should not presume that the public simply didn't care what happened in jails. Rather, Londoners had a ready-made and quite convincing explanation for why prisoners sickened and died. Holding an inquest to prove it must have seemed superfluous. Thus juries went about their business with minimal effort at due diligence: hearing a single witness provide formulaic testimony before reaching a verdict that confirmed what most Londoners already assumed about prisons and their inhabitants.

And yet things changed as the Jail Fever Panic intensified. With John Howard as the spokesman, with the hulks filling up, and with the predicament of prison crowding worsening once the Gordon rioters razed Newgate, the specter of epidemic catastrophe loomed ever larger by the early 1780s. Inquests reflect these developments. It is noteworthy, for example, that they begin to contain more mentions of medical care. Whereas previously three-quarters of dying prisoners received no medical attention, inquests in the 1780s show the reverse: fully 72 percent recorded that a surgeon or apothecary attended dying prisoners. Doctors had not become more immediately prevalent in Tothill Fields following passage of the Health of Prisoners Act (1774). However, Howard's book seems to have had a direct impact. It is probably telling, for example, that the first inquest to mention a sick ward was just the second held after publication of *The State of the Prisons,* a book that specifically critiqued the jail's lack of an infirmary.[35]

Local developments also spurred change. The prison suffered an epidemic in 1785. Deaths in Tothill Fields were relatively rare: up to 1784, it witnessed an average of just 1.65 deaths per year. In 1785 there were nearly ten times as many—fifteen deaths—including seven in March. Testimony in several inquests specifically mentioned fever, and a surgeon testified that Mary Fokes "had a Fever which . . . was a Putrid one." Jail fever was thereby officially recognized. What demands explanation is the sudden *hesitancy* to render fever verdicts. The official cause of death returned in seven of fifteen verdicts that year was merely "in a Natural Way." In three inquests witnesses used the word *fever* to describe the deceased's condition, but the jury merely recorded the nebulous verdict of "natural death."[36] Previous juries rendered fever verdicts without any symptoms to support the diagnosis; yet now jurors hearing that prisoners suffered from fever resisted reaching what should have been the obvious conclusion. After two decades of knee-jerk fever verdicts, juries confronting a named epidemic became suddenly vague.

This is not a coincidence. Thanks to the fanfare surrounding Howard, presiding over a jail that incubated fever in the 1780s was a serious problem. Hence when the body count mounts in 1785, we see attempts to play down rates of fever in the prison.[37] Westminster magistrates certainly would have been tempted to do so, given that they were responsible for administering the jail. Moreover, local merchants sitting as jurors would have had a stake in whether their neighborhood was declared home to an epidemic. Like the shopkeepers near Newgate whose commerce shriveled when anxieties about fever spiked in the 1750s, locals would have been motivated to resist proclaiming fever in the jail.

It is also significant that this epidemic took place against the backdrop of "alarming reports" circulating at the very same moment that plague—actual plague—had struck the Lock Hospital, killing six people that week in an institution that sat barely a mile away. Hospital authorities assured the public that it was merely putrid fever and that rumors of plague were exaggerated. Regardless, it is hard to imagine that this outbreak failed to influence affairs just a few blocks away. Moreover, it can hardly be coincidental that a Tothill Fields prisoner chose this precise moment to escape. Among the examples of prison breaks that Hitchcock and Shoemaker unearthed in their exploration of the phenomena was the March 8 attempt of Tothill Fields prisoner William Stewart, whose friend, William Gibbons, was caught smuggling him a rope. Surely it was Tothill Fields' fever epidemic, along with rumors of plague up the road, that persuaded Stewart to bolt at this very moment. He risked his life if he left, but he may have felt the risk was greater if he stayed.[38]

Ambiguous verdicts became even more pronounced in the 1790s. Only one of the twenty-two inquests from 1792 to 1799 attributed a Tothill Fields death to fever. The rate of fever verdicts had thus fallen from 66 percent in the 1760s and 1770s to just 4.5 percent at century's end. However, before we conclude that the prison was healthier, consider that mortality shot up almost 300 percent during the last fifteen years of the century. In place of the politically sensitive fever verdicts, more than two-thirds of inquests now recorded simply "Natural" death or a handy new diagnosis, "Decline"—which meant only that prisoners were healthy when they entered but then worsened and died. They declined.[39]

Westminster prison inquests changed in a potentially even more revealing way in the 1780s, and here we can begin to unpack the extent to which Londoners sought to emulate their hero John Howard. Inquests moved. Three components of coroners' inquests typically noted a location. First, the most formal document was the inquest itself, providing staple details like the names of the deceased and the jurymen, date, and cause of death. It began formulaically by stating where the inquest had been held. For example, the 1765 inquest on prisoner James McDaniel began by noting that the inquest was held at the jail. "An Inquisition Indented taken for our Sovereign Lord the King at the Gaol or Prison of Bridewell, in the Parish of St. Margaret within the Liberty of the Dean and Chapter of the Collegiate Church of St. Peter Westminster in the County of Middlesex . . ." Second, most surviving inquests include the jury summons. The parish constable summoned twenty-four men to appear at a specified time and place so that at least twelve could be sworn in. In the McDaniel inquest potential jurors were summoned to report to the jail. The coroner ordered the constable to "summon and warn twenty-four able and sufficient Men of your Liberty personally to be and appear before me . . . at Bridewell in the Parish of St. Margaret." Finally, the "Informations" section recorded testimony. Its formula similarly noted where testimony was given. Again, in the McDaniel case we learn that jurors heard depositions inside the jail: "Informations taken this Third day of January 1765 at Bridewell in the Parish of St Margaret . . . on an Inquisition taken on View of the Body of James Mc. Daniel a Prisoner there lying Dead." McDaniel's inquest follows the model of all those at Tothill Fields until 1783. Twenty-four men were summoned to the prison, where twelve or more became a jury to view the body in the jail, hear testimony in the jail, then deliberate and reach a verdict at the jail. For thirty-seven straight inquests the entire investigative process took place within the walls of the prison. As Umfreville noted, the coroner and jury should be "all the while under the Lock and Key of the Keeper."[40]

Then on September 12, 1783, an inquest on the death by fever of a debtor named Jane Smith recorded two locations. The inquest was said to have been held "at Tothill Fields Bridewell," and testimony taken there. But jurors were summoned not to the jail but rather to a coffeehouse, the Green Coat Boy, just up the street. While coroners commonly used public houses for inquests, this was a clear departure for Tothill Fields. The multiple locales listed make it difficult to know precisely where different elements of the process took place. This particular jury served double duty, also hearing the case of an infant who had been pulled from the Thames in an advanced state of decay. It is possible that the jury met in the coffeehouse to deliberate on the infant and moved to the prison to proceed on Jane Smith. Regardless, it started a trend. Until the end of the century, all remaining seventy-two inquests on dead prisoners were held, at least in part, at the Green Coat Boy coffeehouse.[41]

Several factors suggest that it was Londoners' anxiety about contagion that drove this relocation. First, both bodies that the above jury inspected, Jane Smith's dead of jail fever and the decaying infant, posed an infectious threat. Thus the coroner may have allowed the jury to remain safely in the coffeehouse rather than enter the potentially contagious space of the jail. This possibility is supported by an inquest on a man dead of putrid fever, not in the prison but in the parish workhouse, which reveals how fears of infection could influence these proceedings. The Westminster Infirmary turned away William Stephen because of the "great danger" his fever posed. He died hours later in the workhouse. His inquest includes a note from the parish apothecary warning that the coroner "Should have this Man buried, as Soon as possible, to prevent any infection spreading thro' the house, & likewise there is no Necessity for [the] Jury to sitt on him." The coroner routinely held inquests in the workhouse, but in this instance he held it in a pub.[42]

From 1783 to 1786 the coroner continued to summon jurors to the coffeehouse, even though depositions were still said to be taken at the prison. Perhaps jurors assembled at the coffeehouse, moved to the prison to see the body and hear testimony, and then deliberated back at the coffeehouse, thereby reducing time inside the jail. It is also possible that the coroner alone entered the prison to view the body and record statements to read to the jury in the safe confines of the coffeehouse, although this would have been in contravention to both custom and law. Regardless, we witness the beginning of a separation between the investigative process and the space of the prison. This separation was augmented in 1786, when a felon named Henry Young died of what was officially deemed just a "natural death" but which deponents identified as "gaol distemper." For the first time, not only were jurors summoned to the coffeehouse but testimony was recorded there as well.[43] Presumably the lone prisoner deposed was transported out of the jail, enabling jurors to remain safely at the coffeehouse. Where the body was, and whether jurors even inspected it, remains a mystery. The jail soon faced what looks like another epidemic in 1787 and 1788, with a spate of fever deaths, some identified as "violent fever" or "putrid fever."[44] Inquests again became conspicuously vague, this time about location. For the next four years, half of all prison inquests show jurors summoned to the coffeehouse but testimony heard merely (somewhere) "[in] the parish of Saint Margaret's Westminster." Then in August 1792 a new pattern was set; a vagrant named Andrew Farrell died in the jail, and the location listed on every element of his inquest was the Green Coat Boy Coffeehouse.[45] All twenty remaining inquests on dead prisoners listed the coffeehouse as the location on the formal inquest, the jury summons, and the witness statements, leaving no evidence that jurors set foot in Tothill Fields Bridewell for the remainder of the century. The same juries that rendered so many vague verdicts of "natural death" or "decline" did not even enter that prison. A final severing of the investigative process and the jail occurred in 1794, when, instead of prisoners testifying (a legal requirement), jurors heard only the testimony of a prison employee, the turnkey. The turnkey was the lone witness in all remaining inquests. Changes in procedures might be partially attributed to the new coroner, Anthony Gell, who assumed the post in January 1792. However, these shifts only bear out patterns that were already under way well before he took over. Thus, from the mid-1780s, coroners' juries demonstrated both a reluctance to proclaim fever verdicts and a strong aversion to entering a jail.

Howard called for Britons to look more deeply into their jails, yet in Westminster investigations moved decidedly in the opposite direction. The most likely explanation for this discrepancy lies in the reluctance of propertied Londoners to expose their own bodies to fever-ridden corpses in pestilential jails. By 1794 Londoners serving as jurors were shielded from the dangers of prison just about as much as they could possibly be. They did not enter it. They did not view the body. They did not even hear testimony from other prisoners. Indeed, this last development may have been less an effort to silence inmates than one more strategy to shield the public from infection. After all, citizens cannot have thought it wise to bring vagrants from a jail (in which someone had just died!) into a public house. Thus excluding prisoners from juries and then denying them opportunity to testify may each represent an attempt to distance respectable Londoners from potentially infectious plebeian bodies. Howard stood eye to eye with sick prisoners, but Westminster shopkeepers were a lot less willing to do so.

That contagion anxieties influenced these developments finds strong support in evidence regarding jury service. Put simply, the coroner had difficulty finding men willing to serve when the body lay in a jail. Almost all Westminster inquests include lists of potential jurors summoned. In the case of prison deaths, compared with other inquests, not only did fewer men serve, fewer showed up for jury duty. First, twelve was the minimum number required for a coroner's inquest, but Westminster juries routinely exceed that number. The average size of juries for nonprisoners was almost fourteen (13.8), while for prison inquests it was closer to the minimum (12.7). Much more telling is the fact that some men simply refused to answer the summons. Twenty-four men were summoned, but twenty-four did not always appear. It is usually unclear what happened, but there are hints. Occasionally potential jurors were noted as "excused" or "came too late," while others reportedly "refused to come." A turner named John Panton, summoned in December 1776, apparently told the constable that "absolutely he would not come." What is important for our purposes is that occasions on which fewer than twenty-four men appeared were 37 percent more common when inquests concerned prisoners. Men shirking jury duty faced the not inconsiderable fine of forty shillings for noncompliance, but some probably thought it money well spent. Moreover, the fine could be waived if a man was sick, meaning that that feigning illness may have offered a simple strategy to avoid serving on a prison jury.[46]

However, what transpired when juries were being formed is often unclear. Frequently the list of potential jurors *exceeded* twenty-four. These often appear to be instances when the coroner had such difficulty getting men to serve that he ordered the constable to summon additional men. The names of summoned men were often numbered 1 through 24, with extra names—unnumbered—often following, seemingly appended to the original list. The 1778 inquest on Margaret Lane, for example, notes that one of the men summoned, stable keeper Richard Shout, "refused to come" and then shows the name of the owner of the pub in which the inquest was held added and then sworn to the jury in Shout's place. As a result, the many instances when the

number of potential jurors for prison inquests exceeded twenty-four may indicate just how difficult it could be to fill such a jury. Prison inquests were twice
as likely to see the constable have to summon at least two extra potential jurors,
and more than three times as likely to have to call in four or more substitutes.
On seven occasions constables assembling jury pools for service in Tothill
Fields had to bring in thirty or more men just to find twelve willing to serve. It
is telling that all seven instances involved prisoners—usually vagrants—who
had died of fever, including ones identified as "putrid fever" and "gaol
distemper." Constables rarely had to go to such lengths for nonprison inquests,
but instances when they did may be revealing: a drowned vagrant whose body
was probably in a state of decay, and a pauper woman in the workhouse.[47]

More than anything, the 1785 epidemic demonstrates how difficult it
was to fill a jury under threat of jail fever. While it was not uncommon for a
few men facing the prospect of entering the jail to refuse the summons,
during the epidemic the coroner saw potential jury pools—which should
have been twenty-four—of just seventeen, fifteen, thirteen, and eleven.[48]
Moreover, the men who did appear strongly resisted serving. Perhaps they
paid the fine on site, or feigned sickness, or declared some kind of conflict of
interest. Whatever the case, something fishy occurred. Consider that for the
inquest on prisoner Sarah Rawlinson only seventeen men answered the
summons, and just five were actually sworn to the jury. Nineteen men who
had been summoned avoided duty either by talking their way out of it or by
just not showing up. The constable, Charles Carey, had to append the warrant
with a list of seven additional men whom he somehow pressed into duty,
including, notably, Thomas Pearce, the owner of the Green Coat Boy
Coffeehouse. In other words, when Tothill Fields faced a clear outbreak of
jail fever, this inquest could proceed only because the owner of the coffeehouse came out from behind the bar to fill out the jury. A closer look shows
how common this became. Pearce had to fill out fully ten of fifteen prison
juries that year, while Carey—the constable—had to sit on five. Thrice the
coroner needed both of them just to reach quorum. This was not at all usual;
neither Pearce nor Carey sat on any other jury that year. Yet the coroner
could fill only three prison juries that year without impressing one or the
other. And it was these same juries that seem to have pressured the coroner
to let them to stay in the coffeehouse. The very first inquest in which witness
depositions were recorded at the coffeehouse rather than the jail occurred on
March 10, when a paltry thirteen men answered the summons—just two days

after William Stewart risked his life trying to break out of the prison and while hot rumors of plague in the Lock Hospital still swirled.[49]

One has to imagine that these same men who shirked jury duty probably considered John Howard one of their greatest heroes. The positions seem contradictory: their hero bravely marched into prisons while they ran away. But they are intimately related. With each paean celebrating Howard's bravery, the act of entering a prison became more treacherous. The more anyone read about Howard the more fearful he must have grown at the prospect of following in his footsteps. Of course, a spate of reformers did follow Howard, men like George Onisipherous Paul and William Smith.[50] But who were these Westminster jurors? These were not great men waging a reform campaign with evangelical zeal. They were average Westminster haberdashers and chandlers, men who consumed tales about Howard the hero and internalized their lessons: be charitable, but avoid prisons like the plague.

John Howard and Plague

For even now it was indeed plague that still lurked behind the Jail Fever Panic. Howard made that clear in his less heralded but equally fascinating follow-up to *The State of the Prisons*, 1789's *An Account of the Principal Lazarettos of Europe, with various papers relative to the Plague*. Howard claimed an epiphany while touring jails: "It likewise struck me, that the establishments, effectual for the prevention of the most infectious of all diseases, must afford many useful hints for guarding against the propagation of contagious distempers in general." So in 1785 he set off on a tour of plague lazarettos, first in France and Italy and later in the eastern Mediterranean and Turkey. The resulting book was meant to teach Britons how to build and administer institutions to ensure effective quarantine. However, Howard also took the opportunity to clarify medical opinion on questions related to disease and the body, questions that were still unresolved. In so doing he demonstrates just how influential early modern theories of the plebeian body remained even at the end of the Enlightenment.[51]

Aikin, Howard's biographer and friend, shows that Howard had kept medical theory at the forefront of his mind when planning his lazaretto tour. Indeed, along with physician John Jebb, the surgeon Aikin helped formulate a list of questions for Howard to pose to lazaretto doctors.[52] The list is invaluable for investigating the issues about which British doctors remained unsure.

Aikin's own beliefs matter in this regard, not only because as a close confi-
dant his thoughts surely informed Howard's, but also because he helped edit
An Account of the Principal Lazarettos and probably influenced what appeared
in the book.

Aikin's ideas on contagious diseases can be apprehended from his 1771
treatise on hospitals, which demonstrates concern for many issues central to
prison reform: the management of space, hygiene, and ventilation for establishing healthy institutions. He was clearly a disciple of Pringle, who, we
should remember, wrote the first book on jail fever and updated seventeenth-
century plague theories by identifying putrid blood as the feature predisposing poor bodies to fever. Aikin concurred with Pringle's assumptions.
Accounting for fever in hospitals, he immediately homed in on class:
"Whoever has frequented the miserable habitations of the lowest class of
poor, and has seen disease aggravated by a total want of every comfort arising
from suitable diet, cleanliness and medicine, must be struck with pleasure at
the change on their admission to a Hospital." However, "the peculiarly
noisome effluvia" issuing forth from such lowly bodies rendered hospitals "a
dismal prison" where the sick poor "perish by mutual contagion." He then
lamented, presciently: "Every hospital, I fear, without exception, may in
some measure be considered as a Lazaretto, having its own peculiar disease
within it. That dreadful distemper, little less malignant than the plague itself,
distinguished by the title of the jail or hospital fever, has long been known
as the inbred pestilence of crowded receptacles of the sick." He then cited
Pringle directly, calling fever "the offspring of putridity" and identifying
hospital fevers as those "which tend to aggravate the putresency of the
fluids." Putridity everywhere colors his book, frequently as the core feature
of the "constitutional indisposition," "habit of body," or "putrid tendency"
that he said characterized plebeian bodies. It is even possible that it was
Aikin—who repeatedly compared fever to plague, who likened hospitals to
"Pest-houses" and even referred to fever as "hospital pestilence"—who
influenced Howard to consider lazarettos as a fruitful source of information
to enhance domestic health. Regardless, if Howard sought Aikin's medical
expertise (or Jebb's for that matter), as he almost certainly did, he would have
learned that the poor were predisposed to pestilential diseases because of
their essential putridity, just as Pringle had said decades earlier and English
physicians had been saying for over 150 years. Aikin's views also influenced
his editorial decisions, because we know that he omitted responses by lazaretto doctors that he considered unhelpful. Howard thanked him for having

"methodized and abridged" that section, and Aikin later admitted that "all the queries do not appear, some of them having been misapprehended, or imperfectly answered." He notably emphasized "particularly such as related to the discrimination of other fevers of the typhus genus from the plague."[53]

When Howard set sail, British doctors were more than a century removed from plague. So when they had an opportunity to query doctors with firsthand knowledge of the disease, what did they want to know? Jebb and Aikin sent Howard with eleven questions:

1) Is the Infection of the Plague frequently communicated by the Touch?

2) Does the Plague ever rise spontaneously?

3) To what distance is the Air round the patient infected? How far does actual contact—wearing infected clothes, or touching other things—produce the disease?

4) What are the seasons in which he Plague chiefly appears; and what is the interval between the Infection and the Disease?

5) What are the FIRST symptoms of the Plague—are they not frequently a swelling of the Glands of the Groin and Armpit?

6) Is it true that there are two different fevers with nearly the same symptoms, one of which is properly termed the Plague, and is communicated from a distance by air, and without contact; while the other, which is properly termed Contagion, is only communicated by the touch, or at least by near approach to infected persons or things?

7) What is the Method of Treatment in the first stage—what in the more advanced periods—what is known concerning Bark, Snake-root, Wine, Opium, pure Air, the application of cold Water?

8) When the Plague prevails, do the physicians prescribe to those who have the disorder a more generous, or a more abstemious diet; and do they prescribe any thing to the uninfected?

9) Are Convalescents subject to repeated attacks of the same infection?

10) What is the proportion of Deaths, and the usual length of the disease?

11) What are the means to prevent the Plague, to stop its contagion, and to purify infected places?

Howard returned with responses from eight lazaretto doctors.

The questions reveal that the relationship between jail fever and plague remained altogether vexing even this late in the century. Question 2, whether plague could arise spontaneously, essentially addressed whether conditions found in Britain (as in jails) could spark plague or whether it could only ever be imported (as Mead had suggested back in the 1720s). It was probably not heartening to find the doctors still split on the issue, with most arguing that it must be imported but others warning that it could arise spontaneously. Several doctors explaining symptoms (question 5) spoke further to this issue, warning that plague "disguises itself under the form of other diseases" and "often conceals itself under the form of an inflammatory, ardent or malignant fever." Question 6 then circled back to the same topic via the contagion-miasma debate, inquiring whether there were multiple related forms of fever, one being plague. The possibility for pestilential fever to mask plague thus still loomed.

The answers to almost all the questions confirmed long-standing ideas about the putrid plebeian body. For example, numerous responses addressed predisposition. Doctors were not unanimous about whether plague had to be communicated by touch (question 1), but almost all said that transmission depended on the constitution. A surgeon at Marseilles explained that the "temperament of body" allows some to escape, while the physician in Venice stressed that "predisposition in the receiving body is necessary" for infection to occur. Doctors detailing symptoms (questions 4 and 5) argued that "difference[s] in temperament" explained why "predisposed" patients showed signs fastest and that symptoms varied based on the "constitution . . . of the body seized." When explaining treatments (question 7) a physician named Giovanelli at Leghorn identified putridity as key to such predisposition, claiming that "plague caus[es] always a disposition to inflammation and putrefaction." Moreover, blood remained central, as evidenced by a doctor identified only as "the Jew Physician at Smyrna," who stipulated that treatment must vary depending on a patient's "state of the blood." It is therefore particularly revealing that this same doctor offered the most unambiguous claim that constitutions varied by class: "The degree of infection in the air about the sick depends upon the greater or less malignity of the disease, and other circumstances. The air about poor patients is more infectious than about the rich."[54] Putting the pieces together, Howard's lazaretto book informed readers that predisposition to plague varied according to class based on levels of putridity in the blood. How little had changed.

But readers needed not piece together the picture themselves, for Howard was explicit at a different point in the book, leaving no doubt about his opinion on class and physiology. He joined generations of doctors who asked that perennial question—the same one Bradwell had posed back in 1625—why did only certain people sicken in an epidemic? "Why, of a number of persons equally exposed to the infection of the small-pox, or of gaol-fever, some will not take it? Perhaps physicians themselves are not capable of explaining this sufficiently. It is, however, evident in general, that it must be owing to something in the state of the blood and the constitutions of such persons which renders them not easily susceptible of infection.— The rich are less liable to the plague than the poor, both because they are more careful to avoid infection, and have larger and more airy apartments, and because they are more cleanly and live on better food and plenty of vegetables."[55] Something in the state of the blood rendered the poor more liable than the rich. So said Britain's hero. Howard braved contagion in its wickedest form to secure information from doctors on the front lines battling the worst disease of them all. And the project merely cemented the notion that poor bodies were different and dangerous.

Vinegar Sniffing, Lazaretto Lessons, and the Quest for Safety

But Howard was a practical man, not a theoretician. Hence he drew other lessons from lazarettos and offered other strategies for protection, many that had quite old roots. These strategies were eagerly adopted by ordinary Britons, and thus they offer further opportunities to knit together Howard's story with those of everyday people.

For example, on his jail tours Howard never entered a prison without his trusty bottle of vinegar: "I guarded myself by smelling to vinegar, while I was in those places, and changing my apparel afterwards." He aired his notebook by the fire each evening because he believed deadly effluvia lodged in its pages, and he refreshed his vinegar regularly because the pestilential air of even just a few prisons rendered it "intolerably disagreeable" and ineffective. His lazaretto tour then reinforced his trust in the virtues of vinegar and similar antiseptic agents that he found in use across Europe. At Marseilles, for example, officers received documents from incoming ships with tongs so that the papers could be "dipped in a bucket of vinegar standing ready for that purpose." Officials at Venice similarly used a stick to receive letters from those serving quarantine, promptly fumigating them before sending them on. The physicians at Malta and Trieste recommended vinegar, topically and internally, as the best preservative against plague and described various fumigation practices with it. Substances like lime, plants like wormwood, gentian, and zedoary, and the trusted antipestilential agent sulfur all had places in the medicinal arsenals at continental lazarettos.[56] Such practices were far from new, but Howard's books certainly lent them a strong endorsement to a wide readership.

Vinegar sniffing proved highly influential. Recall the 1772 Old Bailey outbreak. Physicians like Lind advised judges to protect themselves by stuffing their nostrils with lint dipped in vinegar as prophylaxis. But why only judges? In October, while newspapers were flush with reports of casualties, critiques of the Newgate Committee, and Wilkite politics, the *Morning Chronicle* published this advertisement disguised as a news item.

> The JAIL DISTEMPER, of which some people have lately died, shews the necessity of a preservative against contagion; this is to be found in the VINEGAR OF THE FOUR THIEVES, so called from having been used with success by FOUR THIEVES, who, during a pestilence in former time, preserved themselves from contagion, and carried on their robberies. It was adopted by those generous physicians who attended the sick in the plague at Marseilles, in the year 1720. Of upwards of Twenty that were sent to Provence from Paris and Montpellier, not one of them died by the distemper. This VINEGAR, so salutary in the plague, is still more effectual in preserving those whose profession or benevolence engages them, often at the hazard of their lives, to visit the infected in all other kinds of epidemical distempers. It is also the best corrective of the air, which is often malignant, and always too thick, where there are a number of people, as in churches, courts of justice, prisons, hospitals, ships and places of amusement, &c. &c.
>
> Sold by G. Arnaud, M.D. and Surgeon, in Church street, St. Ann's Soho, Price 3s. a vial, with proper directions for the use of it.

The ad conveys much of the legend about so-called Thieves Vinegar, one of the most popular pocket medicines of the late eighteenth century. In some versions the thieves received pardons from execution for disclosing their secret formula, in others they conveyed the recipe to their confessor as their final words. As with claims about the poor or prisoners who became habituated through long exposure to putrid effluvia, hawkers of Thieves Vinegar relied on the trope that denizens of the underworld could navigate epidemics in ways that respectable persons could never do.[57]

In some ways that sales pitch took the opposite approach of traditional ads boasting that elite doctors had concocted an elixir after years of high-brow study. Dr. James' Fever Powders represents the most successful example of such medicines for fever in the period.[58] But whereas James' Fever Powders were designed to treat the sick, Thieves Vinegar was a prophylactic that bourgeois consumers were encouraged to keep on hand and sniff whenever danger loomed. Although medicinal use of vinegar was quite old, and while this particular concoction may have dated to the Marseilles epidemic, discussions of Thieves Vinegar in the popular press indicate that it burst on the scene right as the paranoia about jail fever fulminated in the 1770s. Indeed, the chronology of references to Thieves Vinegar suggests that Howard may have had direct influence bringing the practice of protective vinegar sniffing into vogue. Searches of the *Eighteenth Century Collections Online*, for example, reveal barely any texts mentioning a medicine of that name before 1772. A similar search of newspapers reveals no references predating 1770, with more than 90 percent appearing after Howard endorsed vinegar sniffing in *The State of the Prisons* (1777).[59] Published recipes instructed those hoping to protect themselves to infuse a gallon of vinegar with aromatic substances like rue, sage, wormwood, lavender, mint, and rosemary, and then adding camphor after eight days. "Rub the temples and loins with this preparation before going out in a morning, wash the mouth, and snuff up some in the nostrils, and carry a piece of spunge, that has been dipped in it, in order to smell it pretty often." Polite Britons were thus encouraged to apply the medicine to their persons and clothing as part of their morning toilet routines so that its fumes would float around their bodies to neutralize any effluvia they might encounter. However, such perfuming might not be sufficient alone. Thus a bottle, or in this case a sponge, kept on hand for emergency sniffing provided an important tool for bourgeois self-preservation. This author similarly noted that a bag of camphor provided similar protection and specified the sorts of men he hoped to protect: "The recipe will be certainly useful to hospitals and workhouses. The Clergy may avail themselves of it in their attendance upon the sick; and, perhaps, the gentlemen of the medical profession may not think it entirely unworthy of their regard." It made sense that attendants of the sick might use such prophylaxis. However, when the author included workhouses, he subtly slid from the specifically sick to the simply poor. The vinegar could be worn and sniffed, or sprinkled about to disinfect rooms. While some critiqued Thieves Vinegar as a worthless quack elixir, it found its way into mainstream pharmacopeia and was sold by merchants beyond doctors and chemists. For example, perfumers commonly advertised it, emphasizing its "antipestilential" qualities. Such advertisements often played on genteel fears, emphasizing that the vinegar was "highly necessary for families in the summer," or calling the medicine a "most necessary article" in ads addressed to "the Nobility, Gentry and Connoisseurs."[60]

And people indeed carried these preventatives with them. A baroness remarked that when asked by peasant women for medical assistance, she "distribut[ed] some thieves vinegar which I had in my pocket." A governess responded to the crisis of a convulsing pupil: "I made her inhale some four thieves vinegar." A Newcastle man reacted almost comically to discovering that he had entered a hospital that housed fever cases: "His coulour instantly changed, he trembled, drew a camphor bag from his bosom and ran the length of Northumberland-street without halting." It is difficult to know what reveals more, the man's terror, or that he just happened to have a camphor bag with him. When he arrived home his family "also became alarmed; in consequence, a tea party was thrown into disorder, and abruptly dismissed." A 1778 newspaper account not intended to sell anything advised families to protect themselves from putrid sore throat by wearing camphor bags and sprinkling their homes. Travel writer Joshua Lucock Wilkinson visited Valenciennes after a siege had toppled the city in 1793. Walking among its sickly defeated citizens he proclaimed: "I had taken precaution of herbs, and also wore a silken bag of camphire, which I was advised to carry with me, to preserve my health from the infectious air of the town." If Britons wanted assurance that such medicines were scientifically grounded, they would have found it in William Falconer's experiments measuring levels of putrefaction in the blood after adding various antiseptic substances, proving that "camphor appears to have considerable power in preventing putrefaction in animal substances." The demand for medicines like "Rymers Antiseptic Elixir," "Imrac's Tincture," or the "Volatile Salt of Vinegar"— the last of which was advertised as "the best kind of smelling bottle"—points to just how common such practices were during the last quarter of the century.[61]

Fiction supports this picture. Samuel Pratt's novel *Family Secrets* (1797), for example, contains a scene in which characters have Thieves Vinegar on hand to assist victims when a street melee erupts. More evocative is a scene from *Barnaby Rudge,* Charles Dickens's novel about the Gordon Riots. Of course, he wrote it decades later, but when he sought to capture the London of 1780, camphor sniffing provided an evocative detail. The relevant scene depicts a locksmith named Gabriel Varden visiting Sir John Esquire. Varden informs him, "I am just now come from Newgate," prompting a nervous response:

> "Good Gad!" cried Sir John, hastily sitting up in bed; "from Newgate, Mr Varden! How could you be so very imprudent as to come from Newgate! Newgate, where there are jail-fevers, and ragged people, and bare-footed men and women, and a thousand horrors! Peak, bring the camphor, quick! Heaven and earth, Mr Varden, my dear, good soul, how could you come from Newgate?"
>
> Gabriel returned no answer, but looked on in silence while Peak (who had entered with the hot chocolate) ran to a drawer, and returning with a bottle, sprinkled his master's dressing-gown and the bedding; and besides moistening the locksmith himself, plentifully, described a circle round about him on the carpet . . . .
>
> "You will forgive me, Mr Varden . . . for being at first a little sensitive both on your account and my own. I confess I was startled. . . . Might I ask you to do me the favour not to approach any nearer?"

The scene plays out as they converse from a safe distance, each of them drenched in camphor and Varden confined to his tiny circle of the medicine on the carpet. Dickens was clearly writing for effect. Nevertheless, when he tried to capture the atmosphere of 1780, even if to spoof it, the paranoia about fever and its pocket prophylactics provided provocative details, ones that nonfiction sources from the period strongly support.[62]

And while these are more difficult for historians to chart, Britons fearing infection also probably controlled such minuscule personal actions as breathing and swallowing. Howard remarked that the most common query he received was how to protect oneself from fever. Predictably, trust in God was his response, but one to which he quickly appended: "I fear no evil— However, I seldom enter a hospital or prison before breakfast; in an offensive room I avoid drawing my breath too deeply; and on my return, sometimes wash my mouth and hands." Aylesbury physician Peter Kennedy similarly advised readers entering sickrooms or questionable crowds to "avoid swallowing the saliva or mucus secreted in the nostrils." Lind warned against attending the sick or potentially infectious on an empty stomach and advised chewing something like lemon peel to occasion frequent spitting. If, as with vinegar sniffing, Londoners took the advice and engaged in such actions of microprotection, they were probably unaware that they were following suggestions Mead had laid out the 1720s.[63]

A final element from Howard's lazaretto book offers one last way to gauge how the fever panic was felt on the ground in places like London. Howard paid great attention to the control of space and movement, especially architectural innovations that segregated potentially infected bodies (and goods) from the bodies of lazaretto officers. He was fascinated by the use of gates, fences, and windows that allowed for interrogation between participants kept safely apart. For example, ship captains arriving in Marseilles came ashore at a designated point cordoned by an iron gate through which they could be questioned. Travelers serving quarantine there could converse with visitors, but only at a distance, thanks to more gates, railings, and wire lattice. At Malta, posts, rails, and palisades served the same function. The space for interrogating ship captains in Venice was "an enclosed entry for that purpose, adjoining to the office, where his report is taken by a clerk, from a window at due distance." Here, a chamber connected to the office via a window so that potentially infectious newcomers could be questioned by officers seated in a separate room. Howard was explicit in the opening of his book that he intended his research on lazarettos to help render domestic institutions healthier.[64] As it happened, one need not wait long to see examples of the careful management of traffic patterns via architecture—with the specific aim of disease prevention—inspired directly by Howard.

In 1796 vestrymen in the London parish of St. Sepulchre invited architects to submit plans for a new workhouse. The successful plan survives. The unknown architect emphasized health concerns and cited two thinkers directly: Howard and physician John Coakley Lettsom, specifically the latter's thoughts on fevers in poorhouses. Lettsom, a friend of Howard's, was a key member of an influential circle of dissenting physicians in London, noted among other things for launching the dispensary movement as a model for health care that avoided the health hazards associated with institutionalizing the poor in hospitals. He founded the Medical Society, which had just a year earlier sponsored the essay contest on the topic of jail and workhouse fevers, won by John Mason Good's treatise that we explored in Chapter 4 and which was probably known to the architect, as it was published with fanfare just a year earlier. Good himself repeatedly cited Howard's lazaretto book and suggested that architectural details that Howard cited from lazarettos in Trieste and Malta should be applied to domestic workhouses and jails.[65] Howard's lazaretto book thus likely had a direct influence on the St. Sepulchre architect, who designed the workhouse with prominent features of the lazaretto.

For starters, it had a "Quarantine Room, where the poor on their first entrance are placed, and remain until they are certified to be free from any disorder." This space was not for the separation of the sick, but rather for *all* incoming inmates whose potential infection was assumed as a matter of course. The plan then addressed contagion anxieties by ensuring free circulation of air with high ceilings and many windows. This was typical stuff. However, a more telling innovation was the workhouse's committee room. This space held weekly meetings for parish officials to dispense poor relief. Week after week, in parishes all over England, local gentlemen sitting as vestrymen and overseers of the poor came face to face with paupers who lined up to tell stories of woe in the hopes of wringing a few shillings from the parish coffers. Although they still had to meet in person, St. Sepulchre's vestrymen and paupers now no longer occupied the same room. Drawing directly on continental lazarettos, the architect designed the committee room with an adjacent room for "inspection & Examination," the two rooms communicating by a window. Paupers waited in a separate room until one at a time they moved into the examination room where they sat by themselves and gave details through the window. Lest there be any doubt about the reason for this design, the architect was clear: "this Room is intended as a Separation to prevent the liability of infection being communicated to the Committee." Contagion anxiety was built into the very structure of a key local edifice, the one in which, perhaps more than any other, the respectable and the poor mingled with regularity. The building itself now pronounced the contagious threat of the poor to everyone who came to conduct parish business. The lazaretto had thus come to London.[66] Notwithstanding its design, one wonders how many vestrymen attended meetings with vials of vinegar in their pockets.

Like their neighbors who shirked jury duty when it meant entering a prison, St. Sepulchre's vestrymen took a rather unexpected lesson from the stream of eulogies to John Howard. Howard's greatness was fundamentally bound up in Britons' fear of fever, and fever was still hopelessly bound up in plague. Howard's move from prisons to lazarettos was thus no departure. Eighteenth-century logic about poverty and contagion determined that the one led to the other. In this way jail fever was always only ever the tip of a much larger iceberg. Particular events, like the Newgate epidemics of 1750 and 1772, gave fears a specific focus; in their wake hygiene in jails became a national issue and its reformer a national hero. But Howard's shift to plague signals that there was much beyond prisons that needed addressing. Indeed, the restructuring of St. Sepulchre's workhouse makes the point vividly, because the bodies segregated in its inspection room were not Newgate prisoners. Nor were they sick patients in a hospital. They were not even workhouse *inmates*, who might have understandably been similarly categorized by virtue of residing in an unhealthy institution. These were simply poor relief applicants. The respectable gentlemen of St. Sepulchre felt the need to protect themselves from even just poor neighbors, people who now found themselves treated literally like potential plague carriers. This point is surprising only until we remember that this is precisely how doctors had framed them for almost two hundred years.

Fear of infection thus colored late-eighteenth-century British culture powerfully and in ways that we have only begun to explore. The scope of hero worship for Howard offers a crude way to measure those fears. Moreover, that rhetoric conveyed as many practical strategies as moral lessons. Ordinary men and women longed to emulate the *spirit* of Howard's goodness, but many were clearly too frightened to follow in his actual footsteps. And so respectable Britons strapped on their camphor bags and rubbed themselves with vinegar as they prepared for their day. They navigated safe routes to avoid places like Newgate. They may have even controlled their breathing and swallowing while in the presence of the poor. And if a friend or loved one got locked up for debt, they assuredly thought long and hard about whether to visit. However, as tales of vinegar and workhouses have begun to suggest, there were many dangers beyond prisons, as we shall now see.

7. Typhus Ever After

In 1756 fever struck the Midlands weaving town of Kidderminster. Little about the epidemic is remarkable except that it had nothing to do with a jail. Physician James Johnstone described the outbreak. "It chiefly prevailed in poor families, where numbers lodged in mean houses, not always clean, but sordid and damp. It seemed to affect poor families most, where there was reason to think a sufficiency of the necessaries of life, on account of the dearth, had for some time been scantily supplied; yet the other poor persons, given to intemperate use of malt liquors, and ardent distilled spirits, were observed to be very much liable to its influence." Johnstone drew in features common to theories about plebeian pathogenesis such as diet and immorality; the poor's "acrimony of the blood," "bad juices," or "cachectic habit of body" predisposed them, and the seeds of disease "had been for some time lurking in the[ir] constitution." Predictably, fever then spread across class lines to strike "persons in easy circumstances." While Londoners scrambled in the aftermath of the first Old Bailey outbreak, doctors much further afield offered potent reminders that it was poverty, not incarceration, that bred fever. Of course, this had always been the case. The belief that slums bred plague was more than a century old. Jail fever drew considerable attention to prisons after 1750, but prisoners were hardly the only danger.[1]

Creighton's landmark *History of Epidemics in Britain* (1891) identifies outbreaks like Kidderminster's dotted across the British landscape throughout the late eighteenth century. Neither prisons nor London monopolized pestilential fever. In the last third of the century epidemics independent of jails struck cities like Liverpool, Newcastle, Chester, Carlisle, Leeds, Manchester,

Warrington, Lancaster, Hull, Worcester, Oxford, and Birmingham, as well as smaller communities and towns across Scotland. Jail fever certainly heightened anxieties about dangerous congregations of poor bodies. But if jails were dangerous because they crowded poor bodies in filth, then so were slums. Writing about his experiences visiting the London poor, army surgeon and anatomist John Hunter warned of malignant fever. "The disease, as it appears in jails and hospitals, has been well described by Sir John Pringle; and other authors have given accounts of it on board of ships, especially crowded transports and prison-ships, but I do not find that its originating in the families of the poor in great cities during the winter has been taken notice of." Hunter worried that slum-born fever demanded greater attention. It was about to receive it.[2]

In this final chapter I explore initiatives at the end of the century that set their focus beyond jails and squarely on poor neighborhoods, plebeian homes, and factories. The story of late-eighteenth-century fever has received excellent coverage from historians exploring the convergence of medicine, politics, and early industrial labor. The goal here is not to tell these stories anew but to set select developments within the longer history that this book charts and to argue for the continued centrality of quite traditional ideas about class, bodies, and disease as the nineteenth century dawned. This matters historiographically because the possible eighteenth-century roots of nineteenth-century public health has been a topic of considerable debate. Brian Keith-Lucas argued for seeing the origins of Victorian practices in initiatives such as those explored in this chapter, while E. P. Hennock replied with the cogent criticism that the scale of these enterprises paled in comparison to what transpired fifty years later, as did their tangible health outcomes. James Riley and Roy Porter each offered correctives to reductionist histories of nineteenth-century public health by arguing for the Enlightenment invention of the concept, at least inasmuch as eighteenth-century medical writers applied strategies like hygiene to populations, with prison populations notably central to these early programs. And although the thrust of much of John Pickstone's work on fever sought to recontextualize the sanitarians— and hence to explore the *distinctions* between them and their late-eighteenth-century predecessors—he offers important reminders of how much continuity there was between roughly 1790 and 1840. Drawing on the work of Margaret Pelling, he asserted, "We may at least conclude that most [mid-nineteenth-century] doctors *could* have maintained the elements of late eighteenth-century theory. And from my own research on Manchester it is clear that major medical figures did indeed do so." Indeed, Pickstone called for further research on fever that would span the traditional preindustrial and industrial divide and predicted that such scholarship "would probably underline both continuity and breadth in medical and popular views of the causes of fever."³ I hope to accomplish something along these lines. For by building *to* the 1790s—rather than starting from them, as so many Victorian histories have done—we can see not only that such continuities were indeed profound but that they themselves grew out of much older bodies of thought. Moreover, rethinking the modernist orientation of the prevailing scholarship on late-eighteenth-century fever affords me the opportunity to conclude this chapter with a Coda that explores how we might connect this book's findings to the more well-known history of nineteenth-century British public health.

Typhus Ubiquitous

Scottish physician William Buchan was among the most widely read doctors of the eighteenth century. His best-selling *Domestic Medicine* shows how easily the principles of jail fever could be extended beyond prisons. Here his jump from jail to plebeian home is seamless. "Wherever air stagnates long it becomes unwholesome. Hence the unhappy persons confined in jails not only contract malignant fevers themselves, but often communicate them to others. Nor are many of the holes, for we cannot call them houses, possessed by the poor in great towns much better than jails. These low dirty habitations are the very lurking places of bad air and contagious diseases. Such as live in them seldom enjoy good health; and their children commonly die young." On the surface physician John Heysham's *An Account of the Jail Fever* (1782) appeared to be yet another treatise on prisons. Its opening words revealed that this was not the case. "Altho' this Fever neither arose in a Jail, nor a Hospital, yet it so exactly resembles the Jail Fever . . . that I have not scrupled to treat it under that name." He instead identified the poor of Carlisle as the source of that city's 1781 epidemic, and, like Buchan, quickly implicated their homes. "This fever, chiefly, I may almost say entirely, raged amongst the common and lower ranks of people; and more especially amongst those who lived in narrow, close confined lanes, and in small crowded apartments." We know that "hospital," "jail," or "workhouse" fever were common names by the 1780s, but in 1784 Jeremiah Fitzpatrick enhanced the nomenclature tellingly: "I imagine a distinction unnecessary between the gaol, the hospital, or poor man's cabbin fever."[4]

And it was indeed still the same set of causes believed to generate fever among the poor. Fitzpatrick again: "There are but few physicians who visit the poor in city or country, who do not often find several narrow confined rooms, in the same bed, inspiring the air which another had that instant discharged, perhaps from putrid lungs; add to those annoyances, the exhalations from their excrements and perspiration; in apartments rendered damp by the discharges, and warm from the crouded sick, than which no other causes are more capable of promoting putrefaction." The poor still oozed putridity, contaminating the air with their breath, sweat, and waste. Just as prisoners poisoned prisons, paupers were believed to foul (and to be fouled by) their domestic environments in a pathological reciprocal relationship that had changed little over the preceding century. In 1788 physician John Alderson of Hull was still quoting Pringle and Mead to explain that fever was produced not only in jails but in "every Place ill-aired and kept dirty; that is filled with Animal Steams from foul or diseased Bodies." In a revealing relation Heysham initially lamented that he could not identify where the local epidemic had begun. Nevertheless, he confidently asserted that its cause must have been "human effluvia . . . generated in some little dirty confined place, of which there are great numbers in Carlisle, and every other large manufacturing town," places he called "scenes of poverty, of filth and nastiness." He then quickly bragged that further detective work revealed the source. Eureka! "It was in a house in Richard-Gate, which contains about a half dozen very poor families; the rooms are exceeding small, and in order to diminish the window tax, every window that even poverty could dispense with was shut up, hence stagnation of air, which was rendered still more noxious by the filth and uncleanliness of the people." Given his initial speculation, confirmation bias may well have influenced this "discovery." Regardless, we again see that, as in jails, it was not simply that stagnant air became poisonous but that it was rendered so by the filthy emissions from putrid bodies.[5] Thus, as I detailed at great length in Chapter 4, the putrid physiology of the poor remained medical orthodoxy throughout the late eighteenth century. It would have crucial ramifications for plebeian homes, neighborhoods, and workplaces.

One text is particularly revealing in this regard: when David Campbell's *Observations on the Typhus, or Low Contagious Fever* (1785) addressed plebeian homes, it presented a potentially even more frightening way of conceptualizing the threat. Campbell studied in Leyden and Edinburgh, undoubtedly hearing Cullen's lectures at the latter school before becoming physician to the Lancaster Infirmary. Adhering to his teacher's nosology, he identified jail/putrid fever as Cullen's "Typhus gravior." His influences were a mix of new and old, citing the likes of Cullen and his contemporary Francis Milman, but also drawing heavily on such stalwarts as Pringle, Mead, Lind, and even Sydenham. Like Cullen and Milman, he focused more attention on the solids than the fluids, but, also as for them, this did not preclude a central role for putridity: fevers damaged the fibers, causing their "tendency to ooze" fluids, which then rotted. Fever patients had "a tendency to, if not the actual presence of putrefaction," and therefore treatments should address the "disposition to putrefaction." On class Campbell did not mince words: typhus was generated almost exclusively by "the poor and laboring classes." Quoting Lind, he called it "the produce of filth, rags, poverty and polluted air." His main advice for readers was to "keep at a respectable distance" (note the class implications of that adjective), though he also advocated prophylactic practices à la Howard: vinegar sniffing, chewing tobacco or ginger when among the sick or the poor (but not swallowing the spittle), and blowing one's nose upon leaving. The vulnerability of polite homes was conveyed powerfully in a case that somewhat adumbrates *The Velveteen Rabbit*, whereby fever allegedly infected a respectable home when effluvia lurked in a child's stuffed animal.[6]

Much of Campbell's treatise is thus typical. However, in certain claims we can begin to chart in new ways the magnitude of the perceived threat of the plebeian home. Although physicians often spoke of outbreaks or epidemics—what appear on first glance to be periodic flashpoints—they frequently conveyed that these were merely eruptions of a constant threat. A single jail could be cleaned. But what could be done if the same kind of concentrated poverty characterized house after house, in slum after slum, in city after city throughout Britain? Fever thus approached both inevitability and ubiquity in the writings of doctors like Campbell. For example, after suggesting prophylaxis, he lamented how feeble such actions likely were given the magnitude of the threat.

But it is still to be feared, that notwithstanding every precaution, which may be enjoined the poorer classes of people; yet while their wants necessitate them to the modes of life that generally obtain amongst them, the spreading of a contagious disease, once intro-duced into a family, or even a community seems almost unavoid-able. Crowded together, in a small, and frequently dark, or damp rooms; those in health often sleeping in the same bed with the sick, from a want of any other resting place; without that change of linen which contributes, at once to the luxury and health of those in more affluent circumstances: we must whilst we deplore our inability to apply the same successful modes of prevention to them, as to those in other situations, be content to endeavor by charitable and medical assistance, to alleviate those ills, the existence of which is inevitable; and will probably be rendered still more severe, by the continued application of the causes, which either give rise to, or increase the malignity of the disease.

Fever among the poor was literally "inevitable," its spread throughout the community "almost unavoidable." Campbell's treatise discussed fever in Lancaster during the years 1782–1784. However, he repeatedly made the case that it was never absent from the city during that time, claiming that "it has continued to rage with more or less frequency and fatality."[7]

Medical theory about plebeian physiology mattered greatly in this regard, because the tendency for poor bodies to, in Campbell's words, "increase the malignity of the disease" played a powerful role in these depic-tions of fever's inevitability. Peter Kennedy conveyed the same point. Like so many doctors before him, Kennedy argued that a constitution must be disposed to receive infection. He offered a hypothetical scenario in which a hundred people were exposed to the causes of fever but none with a suitably predisposed constitution: all would remain healthy. However, just one putrid constitution made all the difference. "But if on the other hand, there should happen to be even one individual among the number, of a constitution disposed to receive the impression, he will not only fall ill of the disease himself, but will likewise communicate it." Because that one dangerous body could strengthen the disease, ninety-nine previously safe bodies became "new and distinct sources of infection" who (to use the language of inevita-bility) "*must necessarily* spread it more and more."[8] This factor helps explain why doctors' claims about moral causes of disease like intemperance or sex have played a peripheral role in this book, despite being clearly conveyed by some doctors. Transgressions aside, *all* paupers were potential vectors of disease. Even the most diligent, sober, and hygienic workers inhabited a world of filth and disease. Their constitutions may have been slightly better armored than those of profligate neighbors, but that protection was fleeting as fever quickly intensified all around them. There was simply no escaping the effluvia in their air, clothing, furniture, and walls, toxins that authorities from Sydenham to Cullen declared grew daily more poisonous. All paupers were potential incubators of disease.

Campbell was thus hardly alone in conveying fever as a fixed feature of plebeian life. A contemporary in Liverpool, James Currie, was on the front lines as physician at the city's dispensary. When it came to fever, Currie must have thought the town's jail paled in comparison to the threat posed by its slums. He quantified the scope of the problem. "Of the inhabitants of Liverpool, it is ascertained that about 7,000 live in cellars under ground, and nearly 9,000 in back houses, which have an imperfect ventilation, especially in the new streets on the south side of town, where a pernicious practice has lately been introduced of building houses to let to labourers, in small confined courts, which have a communication with the street by a narrow aperture, but no passage of air through them. Among the inhabitants of the cellars and of these back houses the typhus is constantly present." The living conditions later made infamous by the likes of Engels in the nineteenth century were already starting to take form in places like Currie's Liverpool, as industrialization took off and industrial centers absorbed a steady stream of migrant workers who crushed into rapidly growing slums. Currie clearly included the working poor—not just abject paupers—in his figures, referring to laborers in the above passage, and elsewhere to "the laboring poor." Liverpool had about sixty-three thousand residents at the time, meaning that sixteen thousand, or roughly one in four, lived where typhus was "constantly present." Data from Currie's dispensary bolstered this depiction. When readers learned that it treated more than thirteen thousand working-class patients per year, not a few would have drawn the frightening conclusion that that nearly all of the sixteen thousand souls Currie described in Liverpool's slums took ill each and every year. Currie included charts giving month-by-month figures for fever patients over seventeen years (Figure 8). Frighteningly, they showed no clear seasonal pattern. Polite Liverpudlians hoping for a respite at some point in the year must have been disappointed—and not a little worried—to learn that "the prevalence of fever is greater, and the influence of seasons upon it less, than might have been expected." Typhus

A TABLE,

Shewing the number of Fevers admitted on the books of the Liverpool Dispensary from the first of January 1780, to the last of Dec. 1796, inclusive ; distinguishing the numbers admitted every year, and each month of every year.

Year	Jan.	Feb.	Mch.	Apr.	May	June	July	Aug.	Sept.	Oct.	Nov.	Dec.	Total.
1780	150	125	179	173	168	183	191	150	129	186	150	133	1917
1781	130	146	180	200	187	154	157	127	167	234	208	223	2113
1782	268	265	231	292	148	159	120	140	143	182	150	158	2256
1783	210	158	184	207	222	212	286	227	265	316	257	273	2817
1784	170	194	245	247	232	225	270	230	266	247	369	297	2992
1785	285	268	296	294	219	187	173	180	186	250	244	182	2764
1786	191	166	216	244	202	155	159	188	169	211	167	197	2265
1787	256	209	301	234	313	356	255	192	218	234	283	326	3177
1788	236	174	213	255	253	245	271	311	258	341	315	295	3167
1789	319	176	338	323	391	205	184	162	212	214	204	208	2936
1790	176	248	337	294	281	247	343	270	310	340	355	269	3470
1791	253	247	277	230	233	240	266	248	300	344	335	371	3344
1792	359	361	269	278	261	237	236	223	211	330	212	174	3151
1793	174	209	221	259	237	334	199	197	338	305	224	228	2925
1794	157	230	383	280	337	305	291	245	303	290	258	326	3405
1795	152	265	546	204	234	230	248	159	196	239	317	180	2970
1796	197	161	266	242	288	176	203	182	254	329	153	247	2698
	3683	3602	4682	4256	4206	3850	3852	3431	4025	4592	4201	4047	48367

(210)

Figure 8. Fever Patients at the Liverpool Dispensary, 1780–1796, from James Currie, *Medical Reports on the Effects of Water, Cold and Warm, as a Remedy in Fever, and Febrile Diseases* (Liverpool: James M'Creerry, 1797), 210. Courtesy of Wellcome Library, London.

in Currie's charts is relentless. "For the last ten years there have been, on an average, 119 patients ill of fever constantly on the books of the Dispensary." In some months there were more than 350 fever patients, and there was never a moment in seventeen years when there were fewer than 120 feverish paupers.[9]

These patients in turn raised a series of frightening questions: how many more stood behind them, connected to them, from whom or to whom fever had been transferred, who harbored a feverish disposition in their blood about to worsen, or who carried the effluvia of these patients lodged in their ragged clothing? If in any given month there were 120 to 350 fever patients registered at the dispensary, medical theory suggested that there had to be many, many more disease carriers silently walking about the city. It was impossible to fix a number or to know who they were, but that only made the situation more terrifying. The dispensary had treated 48,367 paupers for typhus between 1780 and 1796, or an average of 2,845 per year. Readers able to do basic math would have been struck that nearly a fifth of Liverpool's estimated slum population—nearly 3,000 of 16,000—had full-blown typhus every single year. Typhus was here to stay. Currie meant every word when he warned: "It is constantly present among the poor."[10]

It may therefore be proper to speak of typhus as being conceived of as *endemic,* rather than *epidemic,* among the urban poor. Epidemics flared up from time to time, but endemic disease settled in for the long haul. Indeed, there is evidence to support the claim that assumptions about class were woven into the very definitions of these terms in the eighteenth century. Surgeon John Aitken (not to be confused with the Howard biographer of a similar name) defined epidemic disease numerically and temporally: "Disease prevailing generally, or seizing many individuals at the same time or season." By contrast, he defined endemic disease geographically: "Disease limited in its attacks to the inhabitants of a particular region." Here the issue was not how many people sickened or died, but where. Of course, nearly two centuries of commentary on epidemics had influenced epidemiological understandings of urban geography, meaning that when it came to cities attention to geography immediately brought with it attention to class. Such focus on geography followed from Hippocrates and influenced numerous writers of scientific dictionaries who defined "endemic" diseases as those common to particular nations. Robert Hooper's *Compendious Medical Dictionary* bore this influence. However, when he explained the term he put class squarely at the heart of his definition. "ENDEMIC. A disease is so termed that is peculiar to a certain class of persons, or to a nation." To take another example, the five-volume *Cyclopedia, or Universal Dictionary of Arts and Sciences* defined epidemic diseases somewhat as Aitken did—numerically and temporally, as diseases affecting many people in a short time—but also as did Hooper, according to what *kinds* of people were struck. Class was a key variable. "EPIDEMIC, denotes a general, or spreading disorder, as a plague, arising from some corruption or malignity of the air, which seizes great numbers of people in a little time . . . such diseases running among all kinds of people, of whatever age, sex, quality, &c. as arising from a common or general cause." Here the term *quality* can be understood to signify social rank, as connoted by the term *persons of quality*. According to these definitions, diseases would not be considered epidemic if they limited their violence to persons of the same class, regardless of the numbers affected. They only became epidemic when they struck beyond these victims and infected persons "of whatever . . . quality." It may be important that the *Cyclopedia* also set the term *epidemic* in opposition to what it called "Sporadic" diseases, the definition of which again highlighted class and invoked the language of bodily constitution. "SPORADIC . . . in medicine, an epithet given to such diseases as have some special or particular cause, and are dispersed here and there, affecting only particular constitutions, ages, &c. . . . *Sporadic* stand in opposition to *epidemic* diseases, which are those arising from a general cause, and that are common to all kinds of persons, of what complexion and quality soever." That this understanding was settling in as an influential mode of thought going forward may be suggested by commentary in an early-nineteenth-century Parliamentary report on contagious fever in London: "Epidemical sickness is an evil that threatens indiscriminately every class of the community." What was the evidence to support this claim? "The unhappy prevalence of Contagious Fever for the last two years, not merely amongst our poor and destitute, but amongst those [of] opulence."[11]

Campbell's and Currie's commentary on typhus helps make sense of what seem like alien definitions from a bygone age. The constant referencing by doctors to zones where typhus was "inevitable" or "constantly present" encouraged a kind of sociogeographic thinking whereby a city could be understood according to class, disease, and risk. In this thinking typhus became endemic to slums, its natural habitat, where it was expected to be found at all times. And as so many narratives about outbreaks conveyed, epidemics were frequently proclaimed only once the disease stretched beyond these zones to strike more affluent citizens. However, there were still other worrying contexts beyond plebeian homes.

Factory Fever

Campbell's opening lines pointed to one context that would command significant attention both from contemporaries and historians. He noted that for the past three years "a contagious fever has prevailed . . . at some neighbouring cotton works." He here referenced an outbreak that numerous historians have suggested was a key development in the history of late-eighteenth-century fever, namely an epidemic attributed to the cotton mill in the town of Radcliffe. Taking place about eight miles north of Manchester, the outbreak acted as a focusing moment for that city not unlike the 1750 and 1772 Old Bailey epidemics for London. Pickstone, Charles Webster, and Susan Carla Patterson all point to the outbreak as generating concern about the salubriousness of factories and initiating a series of reforms, including the formation of the Manchester Board of Health, the establishment of Britain's first fever hospital, and the passage of the first legislation to address working conditions in the Industrial Revolution: the Health and Morals of Apprentices Act, also known as the Factory Act (1802). Fever struck in 1782, and by

1784 worries about the health of mill workers and the threat that they might pose to greater Manchester reached a boiling point. Pickstone has expertly detailed the local political situation that provided the backdrop to its public health reforms, especially the role of Manchester radicalism animating key actors. However, it is useful to revisit these developments to set them in their longer context, because—progressive politics notwithstanding—they were powerfully influenced by quite old ideas about the plebeian body and its social threat.[12]

The latter point was demonstrated by one of the earliest documents from the crisis. In October the *Manchester Mercury* reported the call for action issued by Lord Grey De Wilton and "a great number of the most respected inhabitants" of Radcliffe and the county. They suspected that the epidemic originated in the factory, and they called on Manchester's leading physician, Thomas Percival, to lead an inquiry. The stated purpose of the inquiry is telling. The doctors were called not to save dying workers or distribute medicines but rather to "ascertain the Causes to which it was owing; and the most proper Methods to be used, to prevent the further spreading of the Contagion."[13] Checking the spread of infection—keeping it endemic rather than epidemic, we might say—was paramount.

The question of whether the mill sparked the illness was a political hot potato. Percival and his fellow doctors remained judiciously uncertain. Wherever it started, fever clearly had raged among the working class and its pattern seemed clear: "The Disorder has been supported, diffused and aggravated, by the ready Communication of Contagion to Numbers crowded together; by the Accession to its Virulence from putrid Effluvia." Their recommendations for the factory mirrored those for jails, a similarity noted by DeLacy, who points out that Lancashire men like Thomas Butterworth Bayley worked on behalf of prison reform and municipal health simultaneously. Unsurprisingly, the doctors called for better ventilation and fumigation. Rancid machine oil as one source of such "offensive Vapours" signaled that there might be health issues unique to a factory setting. However, Percival and his colleagues stressed that the most dangerous font of effluvia remained workers' bodies, a point made clear by calls for immediate attention to the privies. Not only should they be washed daily, but, as at Newgate, they should be separately ventilated so that their fumes never entered the workrooms. Percival's lengthy discussion of hygiene, special handling of workers' clothing, and instructions to wrap the corpses of dead workers in pitched cloth and bury them quickly all further convey the centrality of the body to Percival's recommendations.[14]

Campbell admired their report. He quoted it, showing that he concurred with Percival about who typically bred fever; speaking of cotton mills, he asserted that "the class of people who are employed in them, are most subject to the ravages of this fever." His choice of words matters. Percival did not claim that factory workers were most prone to the fever. The warning was broader. The *class* of people who work in factories was most prone to it. Percival here subtly exonerated the factory by immediately looking beyond it. This was probably due to the political clout of the mill's owner Robert Peel and his fellow industrialists, but that is not immediately important. Of course a factory could generate fever: like a jail, workhouse, ship, or hospital, it was a structure into which plebeian bodies crowded. Mines were dangerous by the same logic.[15] However, when Percival and his fellow reformers addressed the crisis sparked by the Radcliffe epidemic, we will see that they circled quickly back to the looming danger of the plebeian home.

That does not mean that industrialists were off the hook. As historians have shown, the health concerns surrounding factories became bound up in the larger apprehensions generated by early industrialization. And while this is not the place to analyze the complex politics and social impact of early factory work, it is worth looking briefly at medical discussion of factories because it allows for further reflection on the larger impact of epidemic disease in late-eighteenth-century British culture. In earlier chapters I demonstrated that when it came to prison reform, the drive to secure wider public safety from epidemics was not peripheral, as has sometimes been presumed, but rather a central force motivating political action. It was not coincidental that the very first piece of legislation during Howard's era of prison reform was the Health of Prisoners Act. Reforming prisons to reduce their contagious threat was neither an afterthought nor the by-product of other concerns. It was the very first thing reformers did. A parallel development occurred for factory legislation.

This is a fairly easy case to make, thanks to comments by Manchester's physicians and its nascent Board of Health. A list of proposals by Percival in January 1796 reveals the board's intention to pursue factory legislation as one of its very first actions. "We are therefore warranted by experience, and are assured we shall have the support of the liberal proprietors of these factories, in proposing an application for parliamentary aid, (if other methods appear not likely to effect the purpose) to establish a general system of laws, for the wise, humane, and equal government of all such works." The board reiterated the intention a few months later when it addressed child workers, the issue that came to dominate discussions of health in factories for several years. Overwork of children became a key medical concern, with doctors arguing that it "destroy[ed] the vital stamina" and predisposed them to fevers. Medically speaking, children's predisposition was framed much more around debility than putridity. Hygiene and ventilation remained important, but limiting children's hours became a goal to protect their constitutions, preventing the exhaustion that currently rendered them easy prey for fever. The board's efforts bore fruit six years later with the passage of the Factory Act of 1802, seen by many as Britain's first piece of legislation to address industrial working conditions. Like the Health of Prisoners Act, its full name reveals the centrality of health: The Health and Morals of Apprentices Act. It limited the work of children at night, but also mandated that factories be ventilated and cleaned with quicklime twice a year, meaning that hygiene practices developed at prisons and lazarettos now crept into factories as well. Joanna Innes is correct to situate its passage within the political debates about industrialization and changing ideas about the child. However, her study is invaluable for reminding readers of the pressing health concerns that initiated the push for legislation in the first place.[16] Nevertheless, as Percival suggested, when it came to fever, authorities believed that they had much bigger problems on their hands.

The Coming of Fever Hospitals: The Manchester Model

The Radcliffe epidemic made Manchester a center for medical activity on fever. Percival, and especially his younger colleague the physician John Ferriar, spearheaded research on fever throughout the 1780s and provided the medical leadership behind the drive to establish Manchester's Board of Health and its groundbreaking fever hospital, the House of Recovery. Pickstone has shown that Ferriar and his colleagues, who included numerous progressive Dissenters, were influenced by reformist politics, as evidenced by their work on behalf of sister causes like poor relief and abolition. Ferriar, physician at the Manchester Infirmary, conducted a study of a 1788–1789 outbreak and published a series of papers highlighting the danger of slums. His publications, as well as the considerable surviving material related to the establishment of the Board of

Health and House of Recovery, demonstrate the centrality of the putrid plebeian body and class terror to these developments that would establish the working-class home as the primary target for public health action and which provided a model for cities all over Britain. Scholarship on the establishment of the fever hospital often emphasizes conflict, whether political—because Ferriar and fellow reformers faced opposition from Anglican Tories—or in terms of medical paradigms, as in DeLacy's attempts to plot developments according to a contagionist/anticontagionist schema.[17] However, these conflicts again demonstrate how underlying assumptions about the plebeian body frequently spanned political or ideological spectrums. For we will see that advocates and opponents of the hospital deployed similar rhetoric based on a shared vision of plebeian physiology.

As has been noted, Ferriar was not above leveraging propertied citizens' fears in calls for reform. His "Origins of Contagious and New Diseases" repeatedly highlighted the threat of cross-class infection. Many schemes had been proposed to help the poor, he opened, but "it has not been sufficiently explained to the public, that their present situation is extremely dangerous, and often destructive of health and life, to the middle and higher ranks of society." Drawing attention back to plague times and using quasi-racialized language then current in stadial thinking (a body of thought we will explore in the Conclusion), he warned, "The poor still labour under those hardships which appear to have occasioned the frequency of pestilential diseases, in earlier states of society." Following John Hunter, he argued that "new poisons are now produced among the poor of great cities," but he warned that these toxins did not remain there for long. "The poor are indeed the first sufferers, but the mischief does not always rest with them. By secret avenues it reaches the most opulent, and severely revenges their neglect, or insensibility to the wretchedness surrounding them." He referenced the banishing of beggars in plague times as a useful if unfortunate measure and pointed both to the inevitability of poor homes producing such poisons as well as the corresponding impossibility of rich ones doing so. "That the poor perpetuate animal poisons cannot be doubted. When a fever either arises, or is introduced into the house of a poor person, every circumstance favours its progress. . . . Thus their dwellings and persons continually breathe contagion; and where this is the situation, not of one family only but a very great number, it is hardly possible to prevent the communication of the disease to the families of the rich, among whom it would never have been produced."

Yet again the body, not the building, was the font of pathogenesis. Ferriar broke no ground when he cited the poor's inadequate food, alcohol abuse, and filthy, meager wardrobes as readying their bodies for fever, and, predictably, he taught that "the essence of the disease, was putridity." And, as in the case of prison reform, calls to address putrid poisons in cities appear fueled by a drive for bourgeois self-preservation. Indeed, Ferriar used this exact term: "Thus it appears, that the safety of the rich is intimately connected with the welfare of the poor, and that a minute and constant attention to their want is not less an act of self-preservation than of virtue. For we are not only exposed now, to the ravages of disorders, the poisons of which are perpetuated in the abodes of misery, but we are threatened with the rise of new contagions."[18]

Such warnings must have seemed prescient when subsequent epidemics struck in 1792 and 1794 amid a backdrop of famine and economic crisis. These outbreaks occasioned Ferriar's follow-up essay "Of the Prevention of Fevers in Great Towns" and, he argued, led directly to the formation of the city's Board of Health, not because of humanitarianism among members of Manchester's political class, but because of their raw fear. "While the ravages of contagion are confined to the more unprotected class of the poor, the opulent and the busy, far removed from the sight of misery, little suspect the horrors with which they are surrounded. Their attention, when at length roused, by the approach of danger to their own threshold, often proves prejudicial at first, because it rises to alarm and panic." Here Ferriar nicely conveys that fever seemed naturally endemic to poor neighborhoods but caused panic when it crept beyond. Fever had ravaged the poor throughout the previous decade, but inspiration for action came only in 1794, when the "usual" fever among the poor appeared to intensify and began to "rage[] among all ranks of people." Domestic servants who moved between his readership's genteel homes and their own friends' and families' meaner ones were a particularly worrying vector.[19]

Perhaps more than any other late-eighteenth-century doctor, Ferriar placed the focus squarely on the plebeian home. Addressing the Manchester Committee of Police in 1792, he warned of the contagious threat of "cellars and lodging-houses." Cheap lodgings like those on Blakeley Street "threaten to become a nursery of diseases," he predicted ominously. He published an essay on the intensification of weaker diseases into stronger ones, and by the same Sydenhamian logic that still clearly mattered as 1800 approached described the inevitability of diseases strengthening to become permanently rooted in poor communities. Fever "became universal" in one neighborhood and "constantly subsists" in others. It is important that this address made only passing mention of factories. Surely overwork weakened workers' constitutions, and factories might crowd filthy bodies together in hot rooms. But the real problem was that workers brought deadly effluvia *into* them from their homes, returning to work while still contagious or unknowingly carrying poisons within their clothing. This assertion parallels John Mason Good's important claim—written at the same time and explored in Chapter 4—that the central challenge for jails was that prisoners brought their predisposed bodies into them. It went without saying that Britain needed clean jails and ventilated factories. But those reforms were hopeless unless something was done about the true nurseries of disease. Manchester's House of Recovery would offer a model for tackling this problem, one that would be replicated throughout Britain.[20]

Manchester itself drew on the pioneering work of Chester physician John Haygarth. Haygarth believed, following Cullen, that diseases like fever and smallpox were contagious but only over a short distance. He thus argued that patients could be safely segregated in specialized wards. Institutionalizing fever patients faced criticism, since the disease was so often held to be institutional to begin with. Indeed, it was the fear that fevers would intensify and run rampant in institutional settings that inspired the exclusion of fever patients at most eighteenth-century hospitals, a decision that in turn drove two further developments. First, the infirmaries of workhouses frequently became de facto fever hospitals, because febrile paupers often had nowhere to turn and workhouses' obligations under the poor law prohibited them from refusing legally settled paupers in need. Second, as scholars like Irving Loudon, Robert Kilpatrick, and Bronwyn Coxson have explored, the dispensary quickly became a popular charitable model in the 1770s—right when the Jail Fever Panic took off—precisely because it offered a way to treat contagious patients without institutionalizing them. Quaker physician John Coakley Lettsom is recognized as the prime mover of this movement, and his writings demonstrate the clear influence of theories of the putrid body on his thought. The appeal of dispensaries lay in preventing dangerous congregations of poor fever patients, who, we now know, were believed able to intensify fevers into plague. A major limitation, however, was that they left contagious patients in their homes and neighborhoods, an obvious danger.[21]

Haygarth, a traditionalist when it came to plebeian bodies and fever,[22] initially proposed hospitalization in 1774, to little support. Once again an episode of cross-class infection was to drive a key development, for there was a change of heart six years later, "when the inhabitants of Chester were alarmed by the progress of an infectious Fever, which was fatal to some of our most respectable fellow-citizens." With the support of propertied townsmen Haygarth now established fever wards in the well-ventilated attic of his Chester Infirmary. As at the plague hospitals that stand as clear antecedents, the policy for segregation was explicitly class-based. There was never any intention of hospitalizing middling or wealthy fever patients in the infirmary, an institution explicitly for the poor. Haygarth's reports suggested success in quickly separating fever patients from their families—and thereby protecting the home—without contaminating the rest of the hospital.[23]

It was to Haygarth that Manchester turned, his advice recorded as one of the first documents in the Board of Health's minutes. Haygarth promised that fever wards could be safe if well ventilated, though he immediately implicated plebeian homes, using typical language about "putrid Miasms" and "poison" arising from the "the breath, perspiration, faeces &c." in the "dirty & small rooms of the Poor." The key to success was speedy removal: "By taking out of a House the first person who sickens of a fever, we preserve the rest of the family from Infection together with an indefinite number of their Neighbours, who would otherwise catch the Infection." Haygarth's letter was dated January 6, 1796, and the body that became the Manchester Board of Health held its first meeting the next day. "At a meeting held this day at the Bridgewater Arms, which was very numerous and respectable, to consider of proper means to secure the general Health of the Town & Neighbourhood of Manchester, from the Contagion of an infectious Fever, which has long prevailed amongst the Manufacturing Poor." If we take them at their word, a group of Manchester's elite met with the explicit purpose of protecting the town *from* the contagion of the working class. The board was not to survey the health of the town generally but specifically to "superintend the Health of the Poor." Said committee would consist of magistrates, medical men, poor law officials, and members of the Methodist charitable organization the Strangers Friend Society, as well as a list of notable citizens that included ministers and industrialists like Robert Owen.[24]

The resolutions they reached demonstrate that a sense of panic had indeed invaded the town. The committee felt the need to reassure citizens that the situation, while bad, was not as dire as some warned. "Understanding that exaggerated accounts have been circulated," the committee resolved to have published "an accurate statement of the Number of the Deaths that have been occasioned by the Fever, and . . . that the Fever is at present abating." But public fears persisted and posed nagging problems for the board, especially concerning the fever hospital. Even six months later the board continued to face threats of legal action by citizens who sought either to prevent its establishment or else to force its relocation farther away. For example, the board had to commission a lawyer's report on what constituted a "nuisance" to defend the fever hospital's legality, despite what they acknowledged were "well-grounded fears." Nevertheless, citizens continued to voice strenuous opposition to the House of Recovery and its location. As evidence that plague still powerfully framed typhus in the 1790s, consider that critics literally characterized the hospital as a lazaretto. "We the undersigned, owners of lands and occupiers of houses in the neighbourhood near the place you have fixed upon to erect a lazar-house, with the most benevolent intention of checking the progress of fever in the town of Manchester, feel it a duty we owe to ourselves, our families, and the public in general, to offer to your consideration our sentiments upon the subject."[25] These complainants then lengthily deconstructed the board's own reports, a text worth exploring in detail because it conveys both the information the board distributed and how laymen digested and understood such advice.

Much like Newgate's neighbors who opposed the prison's ventilators, these Mancunians were ill at ease at the prospect of a fever hospital near them. Consider their remonstrance:

> In the report of the committee of the 17th of February, you state "the object of the first *magnitude* and *urgency*" to be, "to meet the existing evil in its present circumstances, and to provide an immediate remedy for impending *calamity* and *danger*." An epidemic fever is thus without doubt most properly described. You proceed to say, "there are not less than one hundred and seventy-eight persons at present under the care of the physicians of the infirmary, as home-patients afflicted with fever, and the number is increasing daily." But however *alarming* this statement may be, you "hope to check the future ravages." It is candid to allow that such an accumulation of infectious disease is *alarming,* and you say *"who can tell how soon* contagion may enter into those dwellings which seem furthest from the reach of danger and best protected against it?"

. . . You next introduce the report of your medical committee, and state, "Some degree of alarm may also be excited among those who reside in the neighbourhood of the houses to be so appropriated." The medical committee have very candidly *admitted* that some degree of *alarm* may be excited in the neighbourhood;—to do away which they report, that "there will be no access to, or communication with, patients in the wards;"—we presume that neither caution to persuade against, nor bars to resist, the approach of wards thus inhabited will be necessary to restrain those from visiting whose duty does not immediately call them thereto. But is it the intention of the committee that the public shall take this quoted passage literally as expressed; that "*no access*" shall be permitted? if so, patient adieu!

If, that the access shall be only for the nurses, and domestics of the house, will the medical committee be so good as to inform us that they can prevent those domestics from a communication with the neighbourhood, full charged through their whole dress with the effluvia of a fever-ward? We are next informed, that "their linen, beds, and clothes will be washed and aired in places *completely separated* from the neighbourhood."

The place thus *separated* from the neighbourhood, is separated from the public street only by a wall. The adjacent lands are covered with buildings, and if it be a fact that the linen, beds, and clothes, of an epidemic fever-ward can be washed and aired in a small yard, containing perhaps fifty or sixty superficial square yards so situated, without making the air unwholesome, it is a circumstance we believe only known to a learned few.

To this point, petitioners demonstrate clearly that laymen had taken on board long-circulating warnings about disease traveling silently in clothing and that they worried greatly about the range of actors who could become vectors. I have compared these petitioners with those living near Newgate, but they themselves made this precise comparison, quoting physician John Fothergill that it was a "known fact" that residents near Newgate were frequently infected.[26]

They then challenged the board's reliance on medical opinions such as Haygarth's, opinions that included even those of a figure who must have otherwise seemed like the ultimate authority on the matter: the recently martyred John Howard. Notwithstanding Howard's greatness, there was an even higher authority, the Law. When the petitioners invoked it, they conveyed just how powerfully plague still framed popular thought about plebeian fever.

> The services and labours of Dr. Russell [who wrote a 1791 treatise on plague and lazarettos] and Mr. Howard will always be remembered with gratitude and respect; but if Dr. Russell and Mr. Howard were both here, we presume they would not say that their opinions were to be taken in preference to, and in direct opposition of, the legislature of these realms in solemn assembly with paternal care watching over and protecting the safety of the people. This opinion of the legislature may be taken from the 29th of G. II. C. 8 which enacts "That all vessels being to the northward of Cape Finisterre having plague on board, were by the act of the 26th of G. II. To repair to the harbor of New Grimsby, in Scilly; but it now appears that the harbor of New Grimsby is an *improper* and *dangerous* place for the reception of ships or vessels infected with the plague, *by reason* that the same lies between the islands of Tresco and Bryers, both *fully inhabited*."

They thus took the stipulation that ships had to serve quarantine near uninhabited islands as legal precedent to prevent situating a fever hospital in a city—meaning that to these propertied Mancunians the febrile poor were perfectly analogous with plague victims. Moreover, if we needed proof that laypersons had absorbed medical advice about plebeian bodies' power to intensify diseases, the petitioners offer it in their worry that the fever hospital would be "so crowded as to render the disease fatally malignant."[27]

They then proposed what they believed to be a suitable alternative: the workhouse. Could there be a clearer signal of how class affected conceptions of citizenship? Just moments after arguing that the almighty Law prohibited situating infectious patients near citizens, the petitioners argued that it was perfectly fine to house them among paupers. The sense that fever was natural to such people—that they were practically fever patients anyway—powerfully underpinned, and therefore obscured, this otherwise glaring hypocrisy. Did it not make sense, they asked: "The poor house is situated on airy ground, distant from the town, well situated, and if fever-wards are there built, why not extend the plan and make them commodious for the whole poor? For without question this present intended house of recovery, can only be supposed for the use of the poor, for those who are able to remain in their own houses, and procure relief if afflicted with this terrible disease, will not quit their comfortable habitations for a lazar house."[28] There was never any question of placing respectable residents in the fever hospital, so why not just situate the fever wards in the workhouse and be done with it? The workhouse was already, and purposely, situated in an airy, distant locale so as to protect the town from its vapors. Thus the proposal made perfect eighteenth-century middle-class sense, notwithstanding pesky impediments like statutes.

Yet the petitioners were not alone in comparing the poor to plague carriers, for the Board of Health did the very same thing in its response. (And here we can see how opponents in a debate could once again draw upon the same physiological model.) The board reminded the petitioners just how pressing was the need for the House of Recovery by pointing straight back to the biohazard of plebeian housing. "Every lodging-house in the neighbourhood of the house of recovery, may be truly called a lazar-house, from which persons are daily issuing into the streets, whose clothes are loaded with contagious effluvia, because no pains are taken by the inhabitants to purify themselves, or their houses." The board reminded complainants that had it not appropriated the buildings slated to become the hospital, "they would have been let to poor families, among whom the common causes of fever would, in all probability, have soon introduced that disease, with much more danger to the vicinity." And these, Pickstone and DeLacy remind us, were among the most socially progressive men of the day. A 1796 letter from Currie to Percival shows similar opposition to attempts to establish fever wards in Liverpool driving a compromise there to locate them in the one location everyone could agree upon: the workhouse.[29]

As is well known, the Board of Health persevered and, in spite of opposition that would persist for years, established the House of Recovery on Portland Street. It could soon boast of success in reducing fever rates similar to that reported by Haygarth in Chester. However, that success hinged not merely on quarantine. Rather, the board took seriously its mandate to "superintend the Health of the poor" and developed a multipronged strategy to bring the plebeian home and workplace into the crosshairs of public health. Indeed, Percival's comments that begin the records of the Board of Health point immediately to surveillance of poor homes as a principal strategy. The surveillance of factories followed from there. The Board of Health, said Percival, had three objects:

I. To obviate the generation of Diseases

II. To prevent the spreading of them by Contagion

III. To shorten the duration of existing Diseases and to mitigate their evils, by affording the necessary aids and comforts to those who labour under them.

Under the first head are comprehended—the inspection & improvement of the general accommodations of the Poor;—the prohibition of such habitations as are so close, noisome, or damp, as to be incapable of rendering tolerable salubrious:—The removal of privies placed in improper situations:—Provision for Whitewashing, & cleansing the houses of the Poor, twice every year:—Attention to their ventilation, by windows with open casements &c—The inspection of Cotton Mills, or other Factories, at stated seasons with regular returns of the condition, as to the health, clothing, appearance, and behaviour of the persons employed in them; of the time allowed for their refreshment at Breakfast, and Dinner.

In order to stop the generation of fevers (objective I), or at least contain them within their natural ambit (objective II), it was necessary to inspect and purify plebeian homes and monitor factories. Manchester public health strategy thus hinged—from the very start—on active intervention in the plebeian home. While a pauper was quarantined in the fever hospital, Board of Health officials were to set upon his or her home to enact "subsequent cleansing and ventilation of their chambers, bedding & apparel."[30]

As a result, before the board could formulate plans to build the House of Recovery, let alone address concerns about its location, it had to address the legalities of its own policing power. Percival's opening comments went straight to this point, charging the committee to research how best to acquire the legal power necessary for such inspection and intervention. He gave the board three tasks:

I. Enquire into the power of the Committee of Police, and whether they be not competent both to originate & to effectuate the proposed reforms.

II. Or whether a Board of Health might not with more propriety, because with more legal authority be appointed by the Committee of Police, to act under their Auspices, and to hold from time to time communication with them?

III. Or might not a Board of Health be nominated by the Magistrates of the Quarter Sessions, and act under their Auspices in
connection with the Committee of Police?

Ferriar backed up his senior colleague, asserting that "the circumstances
which produce and propagate this disease"—by which we know from his
own writings he meant poor homes—"seem to require more immediately
the interference of a public body." That body should be empowered to
remove paupers from their homes—fever patients, but also family
members—so that the house could be whitewashed or scrubbed with quicklime. And it should possess the additional power to license rooming houses
in order to govern the hygiene of these abodes of the very poor. Moreover,
Ferriar explicitly pointed to moral policing as a component of the board's
mandate, although he surmised that this would probably require application
to Parliament, a petition he was eager to support.[31]

Rhetorical strategies that will be familiar to readers supported these
arguments. For example, a letter from Campbell to the board in March 1796
emphasized the threat to respectable citizens. Removing paupers and fumigating their homes provided benefits "not only to the lower orders of
society" but to their betters, who remained "liable to the contagion of fevers,
propagated from the usual sources by indirect, and little suspected means."
Targeting plebeian homes, said Campbell, "render[s] important services to
every rank of society." He then switched tack to deploy the language of inevitability, claiming that "remov[ing] all the sources of disease, to which the
habitations of the lower orders in large manufacturing towns are subject, *will
I fear be impossible*." It is difficult to know how poor families felt about these
measures, but Campbell offers a rare claim that officials should pursue them
without "injuring the feelings of the parties employed." In 1799 the board
boasted of the "cheerful acquiescence with which the poor have yielded" to
their interventions. Whether such cheer was real, feigned, or fictional must
await further investigation.[32]

Targeted hygiene and surveillance did not remain chimerical. The board
unanimously adopted proposals tabled by Percival offering cash rewards for
the reporting of fever cases. Once alerted to a case, the board empowered
physicians to "form the necessary medical regulations for the domestic
governance" of the entire family. Perhaps because the board lacked authority
to issue meaningful punishments, it ran with the idea of implementing its plan

by way of carrots rather than sticks. It offered rewards to heads of households who implemented hygiene regimens and instituted district inspectors to monitor poor homes. Case reports record such rewards being paid as early as May 1796. For example, Jeremiah Bowcock was removed from his home on Newton-lane, where he lived with eleven adults and three children. He appears to have been infected by his brother, whom he had taken in after he was turned into the streets with typhus. The board's physician reported that while Jeremiah was quarantined in the hospital, his apartment was washed and fumigated, his family's bedding and clothing purified, and that "a reward was promised to the heads of the family, provided their endeavors to extinguish contagion were attended with success." In 1801 the board distributed two thousand pamphlets offering health advice to the poor, reiterating the promise of rewards for anyone reporting fever in poor homes. Moreover, a pamphlet by Sir William Clerke, rector for nearby Bury, suggests that the withholding of poor relief may have functioned as a punitive device in that town to enforce ostensibly the same rules.[33]

Clerke's pamphlet is revealing, not least for demonstrating that similar initiatives were under way in smaller communities. However, Clerke further demonstrates how far health policing could bleed into moral policing. Bury stood just four miles from Radcliffe, and in the wake of the epidemic at the cotton works it incorporated a plan sketched by Percival. Clerke, brother-in-law to Robert Peel, tried to shield industrialists from responsibility, again stressing that disease prevention hinged not on attention to factories but on "a regard to the general state of the whole body of the poor." Mill owners could never know the state of their workers' homes, and it was from these that "epidemic fevers are introduced" to mills. Indeed, this may be why Bury's plan called for a public register of fever patients and the Manchester Board of Health published patients' names in the newspapers. In any event, in Bury we have an example of how the long-standing tendency to fuse moral concerns with medical ones could be institutionalized. Clerke hoped that the poor would come to appreciate the benefits of hygiene. But he lamented that regulations needed to be enforced upon "so numerous a class of people, who are, for the most part improvident and careless of their own health." By carelessness Clerke included that bugbear of eighteenth- and nineteenth-century reformers, "intemperance," a point he stressed repeatedly. Clerke's list of regulations nicely shows how Bury officials used the withholding of poor relief to enforce their plan and how the behavior of the poor was now supervised under the auspices of health. "Temperance and cleanliness to the whole body of the poor are here particularly recommended. And the Committee painful as it will be to them, will be obliged to withdraw their support from families who disregard the forgoing resolutions." Clerke, who chaired the committee to draw up and implement these regulations, thus encouraged inspectors to evaluate the poor's behavior, especially their alcohol consumption, even after fever had passed. The committee's ledgers included columns to record such factors as parish settlement and places of employment, but also one labeled "Rules observed or transgressed." Families named Smith and Dodd followed the rules and presumably received cash relief in addition to the bedding and linens recorded. By contrast, shoemaker Thomas May and his son, printer John May, "transgressed." Their transgression may have been hygienic, in not keeping their home clean in the weeks after their care. "House dirty" is all that is recorded. Regardless, a new form of political agency was necessary, Clerke argued, to effect what amounted to a civilizing mission.

> To accomplish purposes which the provision of public charities cannot reach, and the usual mode of parochial relief is incompetent, it certainly deserves to be considered whether a numerous class of people, the most liable to epidemic disorders, improvident and thoughtless to the greatest degree, should be left ignorantly to disseminate, to harbor, and fall prey to epidemic fevers, or whether it does not become those, the increase of whose property and opulence arises from their industry, to point out wherein they expose themselves to hazard, to assist them in regulations which . . . will conduce to diffuse general good will, to improve the morals, civilize the manners, and strengthen the general interests of society, by a more lasting influence than the warmth of zeal, by reflections arising from a becoming sense of our duty, and the knowledge of the necessity of mutual dependence.

The improvident and thoughtless poor, not unlike indigenous colonial subjects, one might say, needed moral education imposed upon them for their own good. Protection of the respectable required that the working class be "civilized." One wonders whether Clerke betrays his deeper worries when he orders the apparent dangers: namely that the poor would "disseminate, . . . harbor, and fall prey" to epidemic fevers. Clerke lists paupers dying from fever last, giving semantic precedence to their roles as vectors spreading fevers and as vessels secretly "harboring" them for later attacks.[34]

Regardless, Clerke's treatise is useful in one final way because it further documents the influence of Howard's lazaretto study on this crucial moment in early British public health. The teetotaler Howard wrote extensively about intemperance and probably influenced Clerke's thinking in that regard. But it was on the issue of whitewashing and fumigation that Clerke quoted Howard's lazaretto book directly. As at lazarettos, the movements of Bury's fever patients and their family members had to be strictly monitored—even outside institutional settings and in their own homes. For example, family members of the infected were prohibited from entering neighbors' homes and were to be sequestered in separate rooms within their own. Neither could they receive visitors. Homes were to be fumigated with lime according to Howard's specific instructions and clothing purified. Doctors administered prophylactic medicines—in this case mustard seed—to family members of the infected to reduce their levels of predisposition. And attention to bodily waste was paramount. Bedpans should contain water so that feces could be treated as toxins, kept submerged, and immediately removed from the dwelling. Inspiration for this practice was probably the similar use of buckets of water or vinegar that Howard described at continental lazarettos for the quick submersion of suspect linens or letters. Soiled bedding should not even be cleaned but simply burned. Percival's advice to Clerke similarly outlined strict quarantine procedures that clearly drew on the lazaretto model and folded moral admonition into the process. "The medical gentlemen . . . should give directions concerning regimen and clothing of the sick; the ventilation, temperance and cleanliness of their apartments; the precautions relative to their foul linen; their separation, as far as may be practicable, from the rest of the family; and the total exclusion of all visitors."[35]

Manchester's own policies also demonstrate the lazaretto's influence there. The House of Recovery strictly controlled the movements of both patients and staff and prohibited contact by friends of patients or even of nurses. As in the St. Sepulchre workhouse, the Board of Health utilized architectural innovations to enforce quarantine, in this case of nurses who had to leave the confines of the fever hospital and travel to the infirmary to obtain medicines. The board thus designated a special room at the infirmary for dispensing medicines to them, which relieved them of having to enter the main building. The board also developed specialized processes and spaces for washing patients' bodies, laundering clothing, and handling corpses, and it ordered constant fumigation of the house with quicklime, one of the most common purification agents that Howard had documented at lazarettos. Staff at the fever hospital were to keep buckets of the stuff on hand for patients' linens, which, like patients' feces in Bury or suspect materials at continental lazarettos, could be quickly submerged and transported away. Howard had died by the time Manchester's fever hospital opened; but in Manchester, Bury, and a growing number of British cities, his vision was coming to fruition, as the urban poor found themselves increasingly forced to confront the logic of the lazaretto, even in their own homes.[36]

By the 1790s, then, the attention to prisons had been superseded by a much wider focus on plebeian homes and neighborhoods as the most pressing threats to public health. Of course, worries about prisons continued, as did concerns about fever in the army, on ships, and in the colonies. Discussions still wandered back and forth between these topics, which is why reformers like Bayley can be found promoting causes like prison reform, factory reform, and the establishment of fever hospitals almost simultaneously. Yet for those looking backward from 1800, so little appeared new. The plans hatched in Manchester were portents of things to come, but what did they really do but advocate quarantine and fumigation, measures that had been deployed against plague for centuries?[37] The plebeian body was still thought prone to fever because it was putrid and feared because it could intensify weaker fevers into deadly ones. The causes of such fevers remained connected to the filth so long associated with poverty. Moreover, the debt to plague was not obscure, shadowy, or indirect. Doctors and reformers openly drew on much older medical writers, with Britain's great humanitarian hero pointing the way. Howard called upon his countrymen to look to the lazaretto as a model for domestic safety, and they listened eagerly. But even in their efforts to look beyond prisons, doctors and reformers of the 1780s and 1790s were not groundbreaking. Rather they merely *refocused* attention to where it had traditionally been. Poor neighborhoods had always been blamed for epidemics, and the Jail Fever Panic never displaced these fears. This wider scope, which looked beyond the subgroup of prisoners and apprehended the health risks posed by "the poor" generally—men and women, adults and children, idle paupers and diligent workers—had significant implications for the notion that class had a physiological component. Although they were rooted in quite old practices, the calls for action at the close of the eighteenth century would be amplified in coming decades and contribute to watershed developments in British public health.

Coda: Looking Backward, Looking Forward

We declare that Infectious, Malignant Fever is at all times prevalent among the Poor of the Metropolis, in whose habitations it has a constant tendency to difuse itself widely; that it often extends from them to the higher orders; that it derives its origin principally from neglect to cleanliness and ventilation; and that its communication from the person first attacked, to the other Members of a Family, is an almost necessary consequence of the crowded state of the dwellings of the poor.

These are the first words recorded in the minutes of the London Fever Hospital, written in 1801 by fifteen physicians calling for the capital to fight fever in its slums. The sense of fever's ubiquity among the poor, its inevitability in their homes, the emphasis on filth, and the danger posed by poor citizens to propertied ones: so many traditional themes find expression in the very first paragraph of the hospital's records. The authors recommended familiar techniques: removing infected paupers to a segregated institution and disinfecting homes. Failing this, "the infection of others is inevitable." They identified Manchester as the model to follow, and signatories like Robert Willan, one of the hospital's inaugural physicians, highlighted their debt to Manchester doctors like Ferriar. "We may hope a similar plan will soon be adopted in every conceivable town through the British empire."[38]

While Bynum has described its foundation, the records of the London Fever Hospital are rich and remain relatively underutilized for its early period.[39] However, many of its practices echo what we just learned about Manchester. Even the procedure to establish the hospital mimicked Manchester. Governors fielded opposition to various locations and had to call upon famed barrister William Garrow when threatened with a lawsuit based on the same legal principle (nuisance) that Manchester residents had used to try to block the fever hospital there. And on policy, London governors ran Manchester's playbook: strict segregation of patients, fumigation and whitewashing of homes, disinfection of clothing, and cash rewards for families that adhered to hygiene and ventilation regimens. Hospital authorities set up a system of surveillance, monitoring the condition of plebeian homes through visitation, and established a special committee for whitewashing poor homes with hot lime. The model that took form in the Midlands in the 1790s linking surveillance, segregation, and the disinfection of homes—the central strategies of modern British public health—had arrived in London, as it was soon to do straight across Britain.[40]

Of course, the state was not yet the player it would become, obviously a key development for any understanding of what we usually term modern public health. For now, fever hospitals remained local affairs, frequently modeled on eighteenth-century forms of voluntary charity. Much remained to be done, most important the passage of legislation, beginning with the 1848 Public Health Act associated with Edwin Chadwick. However, the sorts of actions called for and implemented in the late eighteenth century were clear precursors, albeit on a tiny scale and in a different statutory universe, of the actions that Graham Mooney and Peter Baldwin have shown authorities institutionalized throughout the Victorian age. Moreover, the medical debates surrounding Chadwick's famous reforms would continue to orbit the same constellation of concerns that had vexed doctors writing about infectious disease for two centuries. Hamlin has shown that in the 1830s and 1840s doctors like Thomas Southwood Smith worked to undermine the argument that poverty in and of itself predisposed bodies to disease, emphasizing filth alone as the primary cause of fever. This argument freed Chadwick and the sanitarians from having to address thorny issues like wages and allowed them to mount a public health campaign rooted in the belief that cleaning slums— without fighting hunger or poverty itself—would save the day.[41]

However, there remained a live debate, and throughout the first four decades of the nineteenth century leading doctors continued to debate putridity, predisposition, and the danger that poor bodies posed to their social betters, as Hamlin has shown. Michael Brown is among those who have cast the developments of the 1830s as far too stark a break from what preceded them. To hear him tell it, in the 1830s we witness "a move away from an eighteenth-century concern with climate and toward a nineteenth-century emphasis upon filth." This invites the obvious question: at what point in the seventeenth or eighteenth century was filth *not* emphasized as a major cause of plague or fever? Climate certainly played a role in theories about fever, as we have seen. But for the sorts of epidemics that concerned the sanitarians—infectious diseases among the urban poor—filth had always been a central concern, as Porter noted long ago. Moreover, what has not been appreciated, and what I have shown in this book, is that throughout the seventeenth and eighteenth centuries the bodies of the poor were *themselves* considered forms of filth. They were quite literally living forms of rotting meat, slowly turning putrid and endangering everyone around them. Here Pickstone is among those contributing to the now commonly accepted belief that sanitarian physicians like Smith were novel for thinking along these lines. Moreover, the forms of filth that most concerned the sanitarians, exhaled effluvia and fecal waste, were themselves merely by-products of these rotten bodies. Hamlin has shown that Chadwick succeeded in re-arranging the relationship between poverty, filth, and fever. But this should not be read to suggest that filth somehow burst onto the scene as an explana-tory factor in the nineteenth century. When historians like Brown suggest that 1825 brought a "significant shift" in medical thinking, which only *now* saw epidemic disease as caused by putrefying matter, we can appreciate just how much a closer look at early modern ideas can offer our understanding of nineteenth-century developments.[42]

Consider how reliant upon traditional thought was a mid-nineteenth-century doctor like George Leith Roupell. Roupell, a physician at St. Bartholomew's Hospital with publications on the related topics of poisons and epidemics, was a contagionist who held that typhus arose from a specific poison and thus would have found himself on the other side of debates from the sanitarians. His 1840 treatise on typhus did not merely bear the stamp of thinkers like Percival or Ferriar but recycled ideas from the seventeenth century. Consider, for example, his thoughts on blood from a section entitled "Putrid Symptoms." He attributed such symptoms to a "diathesis or state of the system, commonly denominated putrid"—in other words, a constitu-tion. "A proneness to become putrid appears natural in many constitutions," he claimed, arising from either climate or habits. He considered it unneces-sary to dwell on climate because "more decided causes and more palpable effects are to be found in certain habits of life." His very next sentence pointed to class: "Passing at once to the condition of that class in which a disposition to putridity is most especially shown in disease, we meet with it amongst those compelled to live in dark, ill-ventilated, and crowded apart-ments."[43] It was 1840, but what of this was new?

Roupell claimed that paupers' lifestyles were deleterious to sanguifica-tion (the production of healthy blood), the very same process that we saw seventeenth-century doctors implicate in theories of depauperated blood. Roupell drew on a leading thinker, French pathologist Gabriel Andral, who wrote extensively on the chemistry of blood and is often viewed as helping found the field of hematology. He emphasized coagulability and described impoverished blood as deficient in fibrin, the material thought responsible for clotting. In this he parallels seventeenth-century doctors like Willis who presented depauperated blood as similarly deficient in a key resource. They merely stressed different resources: for Andral fibrin, and for Stuart physicians nutrients, spirits, or chemicals such as sulfur. Roupell drew on these ideas when he moved from the quotation above implicating the poor to an explanation of their putrid constitutions and impoverished blood. In a passage with stunning early modern parallels he even described such blood in terms of its position along a continuum toward death.

> M. Andral . . . observes in his pathological anatomy, that there are certain morbid conditions in which before life has ceased the laws which regulate all matter overcome the resistance of vitality, and while consciousness remains and life still lingers, the system loses its power of generating heat, chemical affinities begin to exert themselves, and putrid symptoms result; these he refers to as depression of nervous energy, and then goes on to notice the different modifications of external influences, which more or less are in constant operation upon our frames, such as exclusion of the sun's rays, living constantly in a damp situation, and imperfect nutrition of the body: occupancy of unhealthy places, or deficient alimentation, at once strike at the function of the lungs and skin, the direct and indirect organs of sanguification; wasting ensues, *the circulating fluids are impoverished*, the blood becomes thin, watery, deficient in fibrin, and palpably disordered.

In 1659 Willis had called depauperated blood "lifeless" and "a poor thin juice," and here was Roupell, nearly two centuries later, saying rather the same thing. The blood of the working class was still thought weak, deficient in a vital resource and therefore literally "impoverished." In turn, this impoverishment explained the putrid constitutions "natural" to them and responsible for their special susceptibility to typhus fever.[44]

Changes were coming, of course. Hamlin demonstrated just how important was the shift in thinking on the relationship between poverty and fever. Deemphasized would be factors like meager diets as predisposing causes, issues that had allowed progressive voices to call for higher wages and against which Chadwick had to maneuver. In terms of political economy that change was small but mighty. But it bears repeating just how small it was. Rather than look at a contagionist like Roupell, we can look at the very medical architect of Chadwick's program, Thomas Southwood Smith, who himself made numerous claims about fever that readers of this book will recognize as deeply derivative of early modern thought. We can take as representative one of the texts Hamlin identifies as "the medical foundation of Chadwickian sanitarianism," Smith's "Report on the Physical Causes of Sickness and Mortality to Which the Poor Are Particularly Exposed" (1838).[45] Charting just how traditional were so many of Smith's ideas can help showcase the remarkable longevity of the ideas explored in this book, not among fringe thinkers but among the most influential and historically important British physicians of the day.

Putrefaction remained central to Smith's epidemiology. This makes sense. As the sanitarians came to focus heavily on filth as a cause of disease, they unsurprisingly emphasized putrefaction, as many scholars have shown. Neither is it surprising that Smith, like virtually all commentators on urban epidemics, focused on the poor. "Among the gravest [evils] . . . is the exposure to certain noxious agents generated and accumulated in the localities in which the poor are obliged to take up their abode." He considered it common knowledge—"known to everyone"—that the poisonous matter responsible for fevers consisted of animal or vegetable matter "in a high state of putrescency." Moreover, when such matter was inhaled it went straight to the blood. "When this poison is . . . transported to the lungs in the inspired air, it enters directly into the blood, and produces various diseases." Smith's understanding of respiration remained fairly traditional; it cleansed the blood, but filthy air in crowded spaces was ineffective at "depurating" it. Corrupt blood thus still had a role to play for Smith, just as we saw it did for Roupell, and indeed as Pelling has shown, for Victorian medical thought generally. While poisons from putrefying vegetation yielded intermittent fevers and agues, animal poisons from filthy bodies produced typhus, a disease that even now Smith continued to explain by referencing jails, ships, hospitals, and slums.

> The exhalations which accumulate in close, ill-ventilated, and
> crowded apartments in the confined situations of densely populated

cities, where no attention is paid to the removal of putrefying and excrementitious substances, consist chiefly of animal matter: such exhalations contain a poison which produces continued fever of the typhoid variety. There are situations, as has been stated, in which the poison generated is so intense and deadly, that a single inspiration of it is capable of producing instantaneous death. . . . There are others, again, as in dirty and neglected ships, in damp, crowded and filthy gaols; in the crowded wards of ill-ventilated hospitals, filled with persons laboring under malignant surgical diseases, and some forms of typhus fever; in the crowded, filthy, close, unventilated, damp, undrained habitations of the poor, in which the poison generated, although not so immediately fatal, is still too potent to be breathed long, even by the most healthy and robust, without producing fever of a highly dangerous and mortal character.

If at this point readers have become weary of what seem like so many versions of the same argument—one they have encountered in virtually every chapter of this book—perhaps their fatigue can be counted as evidence for the remarkable consistency in theories on urban epidemics over a very long time. The standard claim about Smith is that he differed from his peers in his singular focus on filth as the lone cause of fever, in contrast to multicausal schemata in which filth was one factor among many. That may be the case. And in the history of disease specificity it is quite important.[46] However, when Smith seized on his singular cause, it is clear that he chose an explanation that had stood the test of an enormous amount of time.

Hamlin also shows that the sanitarians deemphasized the role of predisposition. Yet this point shouldn't be taken too far, for as he and Pelling both note, the concept continued to influence medical thought, even that of Smith himself. According to Smith, animal poisons did not always convey disease immediately. In less intense concentrations such a poison "weaken[s] the general system . . . [and] acts as a powerful predisposing cause of some of the most common fatal maladies."[47] Smith's 1856 *Epidemics* offered an even more glaringly early modern explanation of the concept. Reiterating the standard view that causes of diseases could be split between predisposing and exciting ones, he asked the same question that Bradwell had asked about plague in 1625: namely, why did only certain people take ill during an epidemic? Smith's answer? They had corrupted blood:

The primary cause [of disease] cannot take effect unless the system be in a state of susceptibility to its action; that there is in the body an innate power of resistance to all noxious agents of this kind, rendering it, when in full vigour invulnerable to them; that there are certain circumstances which weaken or destroy this resisting power. . . . The predisposing causes of epidemics may be divided into two classes—External and Internal. The external are those which vitiate the atmosphere; the internal are those which immediately vitiate the blood.

The vitiators of the atmosphere include overcrowding, filth, putrescent animal and vegetable matters of all kinds. . . . The causes which more immediately act from within are those which either directly introduce pernicious matters into the interior of the body, in the shape of foul water or putrescent food; or which indirectly accumulate noxious matters within the system, by impairing the action of the excretory or depurating organs whose office it is to maintain the blood in a state of purity, but removing out of the system substances which having served their purpose have become useless and pernicious.

Even the attention to diet, long held as a primary predisposing cause of putridity in paupers, finds expression here, notwithstanding the contention that Smith sidelined it in favor of a singular attention on filth alone.[48] Plague doctors had long ago warned that consuming rotten meat brought systemic putridity, and here was the great nineteenth-century sanitarian reiterating the same idea.

Smith advanced other familiar rhetorics. For example, like his medical forefathers, he deployed the language of ubiquity. Notwithstanding seasonal variations, fever was "never absent" from poor neighborhoods; "the poison of fever is constantly generated" in places like Whitechapel, Bethnal Green, or Battersea, where the worst forms of fever "always abound." Moreover, like so many doctors before him, he argued that diseases intensified in such neighborhoods before breaking loose to strike wealthier bodies. If left too long, "the poison acquires a virulence"—what he later called an "aggravated character"—enabling it to spread "even among people above the rank of paupers, among the people of the middle class, and in numerous instances, even in the families of the wealthy."[49] To support this claim Smith advanced the idea that had logically followed for two centuries: namely that differently classed constitutions had different levels of predisposed vulnerability. Describing the slums in east London he asserted:

> It is not possible for any language to convey an adequate conception of the poisonous condition in which large portions of both these districts always remain, winter and summer, in dry and in rainy seasons, from the masses of putrefying matter which are allowed to accumulate. There is no strength of constitution, no conservative power in wealth, capable of resisting constant exposure to the exhalations which are always arising from these collections of filth. But the people who are obliged evermore to breathe the largest doses of this poison are, for the most part in a very wretched condition. In Bethnal Green they are almost universally hand-loom weavers, with the enfeebled constitutions of this class of people; not that if they had the constitutions of Grosvenor-square, they could permanently resist the malaria which they must breathe night and day. Were they in robust health, and had they, in every other respect, the best means of continuing so, they must inevitably, sooner or later, by their mere residence in these places, either fall into fever or suffer from some or other of the diseases indirectly produced by febrile poison; but under the wretched circumstances in which these people are actually placed, of course they become the victims of these maladies more easily and more generally.

Here was Smith, Chadwick's medical right-hand man, affirming an idea that doctors had advanced since plague times. Class *did* mold the human constitution, with the specific effect of establishing different levels of predisposition— rooted in either the purity or putridity of the blood—which in turn determined that poor bodies succumb to diseases more easily than rich ones. Of course, in order to support Chadwick's calls for action, Smith needed to highlight the danger that febrile paupers posed to wider society. So he portrayed the privileged eventually yielding to fever, too. Hamlin reads this point as suggesting that constitutional predisposition had become effectively irrelevant, since both rich and poor die if exposed for long enough. However, Smith clearly still differentiated between the "robust" constitutions from Grosvenor Square and the "enfeebled" ones from Bethnal Green, with the former holding out much longer when exposed to malarial poisons but the latter succumbing "more easily and more generally."[50]

We can push the point further. Smith perpetuated the old belief that simply living among the poor transformed the constitution because one's air was invariably tainted by the poisonous by-products of their filthy neighbors. Temporality is crucial here. Smith conveyed that fever's poison worked slowly over time. "Sooner or later," paupers who inhaled one another's effluvia "day and night" found their bodies changed, in spite of who they may have been and whatever lifestyles they had led. It was inevitable. Even those who escaped fever still carried the biological effects in their systems, both in the form of their predisposition and in the other diseases that were "indirectly produced by the febrile poison." Moreover, in his *Treatise on Fevers* (1830) Smith made it clear that the consequences of living in a poor neighborhood were inscribed on the blood. To support the claim he offered fascinating experimental data. Baltimore physician Nathaniel Potter had compared the blood of three groups: fever patients, healthy people from neighborhoods with high fever rates, and others hailing from healthy neighborhoods in a different city altogether. What had Potter found? He claimed that the blood (especially the separated serum) of fever patients and the apparently healthy inhabitants of feverish neighborhoods was indistinguishable. Both samples displayed the same yellow or deep orange discoloration, while serum from inhabitants of healthy neighborhoods bore no such signs. Smith saw in this powerful proof that the blood of slum dwellers—all of them, not just the sick—was transformed merely by living where they lived. Simply living in environments that produced fever—and we must remember that he believed fever was "never absent" from entire sections of London— meant that one's blood took on the qualities of diseased blood. Whether they showed signs of fever or not, paupers had tainted blood. This very idea had been advanced by plague doctors since the time of the great London epidemic: paupers' blood shared qualities with plague-infested blood. The remarkable durability of some of these ideas helps explain why a nineteenth-century doctor like Potter would cite both the 1750 Old Bailey outbreak and the 1577 Oxford epidemic to frame his experiments.[51] Even in the mid-nineteenth century and across the ocean the infamous jail fever epidemics remained valuable scientific examples.

Smith would have approved of such medical historicism, because he was quite open about the traditional roots of his own thought. He casually called his belief that typhus was a weakened form of plague simply "an old truth." Indeed, he bragged about relying on old thinkers. As Pelling has noted of him, he abhorred rigid adherence to systems and was especially irked by the blind following of Cullen. Admonishing his medical colleagues, he blamed their shortcomings on their ignorance of what came *before* Cullen! "Were it not that the professional reading of an age, is bounded by as strict a line as that which divides century from century; were it not that no one reads back beyond the authority which happens to give to the day its prevailing doctrines; were it not that the great repository of facts treasured up in the volumes of the close observers, though sometimes the bad reasoners of former days, thus becomes neglected for the dogmas of some modern writer." Thus it was, he lamented, that valuable insights about fever had been forgotten. We thus need not struggle to draw "parallels" between Smith and early modern thinkers. The links were clear, direct, and openly acknowledged. Like a Renaissance humanist calling for a return to the classics, Smith implored Victorian doctors to look past the faulty doctrines of Cullen and recapture the lost truths of great thinkers. Who were in his pantheon? Mead and Pringle. "To cite the ancient and the more modern authorities who have observed and recorded the influence of animal malaria in the product of plague, would be to enumerate every distinguished writer, from Pliny and Diodorus Sicculus, down to Galen, from Galen to Mead, and from Mead to Pringle." It was good rhetoric to cast his opponents as narrow-minded, but as a description of the state of current knowledge it was silly. The ideas of Mead and Pringle hadn't disappeared down some memory hole; they were alive and well in spite of Cullen's ascent, as we have seen. For our purposes the claim is especially helpful, because it showcases the intellectual debt that doctors like Smith owed to the thinkers explored in this book. If needed, we could get more specific still. From the above claim Smith moved directly to acclaim specific ideas: Mead's theory on the generation of plague in Cairo (which, as we saw in Chapter 2, he attributed to the city's filthy poor) and Pringle's theory of jail fever (explored in Chapter 4). And these points then led him straight into a subsequent claim about poverty and disease. "Penury and ignorance can thus at any time, and in any place, create a mortal plague. And of this no one has ever doubted."[52] Smith may have tried to rearrange the relationship between poverty and disease, but he in no way meant to sever it.

None of this is to deny vital developments in nineteenth-century medical thought but simply to point out that when Victorians debated plebeian bodies and fever, they took part in a centuries-old conversation to a much greater extent than scholars typically acknowledge. It bears stressing that the current discussion is not meant as an empty flanking maneuver on nineteenth-century specialists—an early modernist pointing out precursors for the sake of it. Hamlin's erudite history of fevers has explored robustly the genesis of theories of fever dating all the way back to the Greeks.[53] Instead, highlighting the continued strong presence into the mid-nineteenth century of so many of the core ideas underpinning belief in plebeian constitutional putridity adds considerably to what I hope will be one of the central contributions of this book: namely, that seventeenth- and eighteenth-century links between poor bodies and disease provide us a way to connect the ages of plague and cholera. Scholars who take the classed body as their focus can move in a relatively straight line from doctors like Thomas Willis to those like Thomas Southwood Smith. Sometimes continuity can be as dramatic as change.

The sense that poor bodies were physiologically distinct remained buried in Smith, however. You really have to know to look for it. Notwithstanding traces of the idea, we know that Chadwick argued strenuously in the opposite direction, as Hamlin has adroitly shown. And while work remains to be done to chart more fully ideas about the plebeian body in the nineteenth century, it is important to consider that Chadwickian politics may have been influential not just on policy, but for the history of the body as well. The shift described by Hamlin, in which poverty came under attack as a cause of fever, may be one factor that helps explain the complex and still understudied question of why class never achieved quite the kind of hard essentialism that nineteenth-century science would confer on race and gender, despite two centuries of medical thought suggesting that it had a strong biological component.[54] It may well be that the politics of early industrial capitalism forced debate on an issue that had until then been taken largely for granted.

I have encountered not a single seventeenth- or eighteenth-century medical text that pushed back against the notion of plebeian putridity. Of course, some doctors stressed other factors. It has never been my contention that plebeian putridity singly explained eighteenth-century epidemics. Fever was a complex disease, and plenty of writers chose to emphasize factors like climatic causes over social ones. But even those doctors never bothered to argue *against* the notion that congregations of putrid paupers were dangerous. The multicausal nature of eighteenth-century disease, and the dizzying varieties of fever itself, left ample room for different explanations to sit aside one another comfortably. With the nineteenth century, by contrast, would come direct conflict on the very question of poverty's role in pathogenesis.

However, early modern scholars must confront the *lack* of such a debate anywhere in the period. Seventeenth- and eighteenth-century doctors were a quarrelsome bunch, forever debating physiological models, treatment strategies, and such controversial policies as inoculation or quarantine. But without the political impulse of the great "Condition of England" question, there was little reason to argue about ideas that seemed so obvious to so many for so long: poverty *did* make people susceptible to illness, and poor bodies *were* dangerous. Although Hamlin rightly presents nineteenth-century medical debates as political, he also demonstrates that the sanitarians met with pushback in terms of medical theory. After all, by trying to deemphasize poverty as a cause of fever, the sanitarians were challenging a two hundred–year–old medical orthodoxy. Be that as it may, the lack of a corresponding debate in the seventeenth and eighteenth centuries offers powerful evidence for this book's argument. There was broad belief throughout the seventeenth and eighteenth centuries that the poor were physiologically distinct, and treatises on infectious disease were the most important mechanisms for the formulation and expression of that idea.

Conclusion

Plebeian and Other Bodies

We can summarize the central findings of this book succinctly. From the latter days of plague British doctors presented the bodies of the poor as uniquely apt to generate, intensify, and spread infectious disease. Plague deserves a prominent place in the history of poverty, alongside events like the Reformation and the Price Revolution, for dramatically changing how people thought about the poor. Sometime after the Marseilles epidemic, pestilential fever took the baton from plague and became the principal disease on which anxieties about impoverished bodies were hung. But plague remained a powerful ghost animating discussions of poverty and disease throughout the Enlightenment and beyond.

A litany of developments in medical theory altered how doctors explained disease. Humoural theory made room for iatrochemistry, animalculism, iatromechanism, and nervous vitalism; yet—whether emphasizing miasma or contagion—for almost two centuries one concept sailed through these changes and provided the critical mechanism for linking infectious fevers to poor bodies: putridity. For all their differences, doctors at the dawn of the nineteenth century still spoke a surprisingly similar language to that of their medical great-great-grandfathers. Poor bodies were prone to putridity, and putrid bodies generated fevers. Such was medical orthodoxy for two centuries. Enlightenment doctors debated many things. This wasn't one of them.

In part, this was because the period's flexible medical systems took so many factors into account. Corporeal putridity could be acquired because of a dirty environment, bad diet, or the remnants of a previous disease, by breathing the poisonous emissions of one's filthy neighbors, ruining the constitution through intemperance, or failing to sweat out impurities because of idleness. Doctors selected from a smorgasbord of causation to inscribe assumptions about the poor onto their bodies, and this moral biology lent the support of enlightenment science to contemporary policing agendas. However, this medicine was never simply a policing discourse, a convenient way to harness science to reform. When doctors warned about plebeian bodies generating fever, they gave voice to profound anxieties about epidemics in and of themselves. The return of plague, or something like it, remained a major fear in eighteenth-century Britain. Anxieties about epidemics and the drive for self-protection influenced eighteenth-century culture in ways that deserve much more attention. Britons, especially urban ones, understood their communities according to zones of safety and danger, locales that overlapped with areas of wealth and poverty. Contact zones like courtrooms or parish vestries that drew rich and poor together were particularly troubling. Preliminary evidence in the form of popular practices like vinegar sniffing suggests that this fear influenced daily life and thus needs to be written more deeply into our histories of eighteenth-century social interaction. Anxieties were episodic, intensifying at key moments like the great London plague, the Marseilles epidemic, or the 1750 Old Bailey outbreak.

This last event was particularly animating, ushering in a period of roughly four decades when jails represented the most threatening domestic biohazard. Filthy and crammed with bodies thought to be both impoverished and immoral, prisons became the site of a disease that was both real and imaginary and which by the 1770s had captured national attention. Yet even from the time of the Oglethorpe commission of the late 1720s we saw that prison reform was already powerfully driven by the fear that disease would cross class lines. For so long the plight of the debtor, the once-propertied prisoner reduced to poverty and forced to live among vagrants, dominated calls for action. Historians of prison reform regard the period before the 1770s as one of little action. But Parliament acted again and again, and its doing so reveals just how the political nation perceived and addressed the challenge. The problem was not that prisons were filthy or that felons died in them. The problem was that *other* people took ill, like debtors and their families, and that fever might spread more widely among their circles. So in the era before Howard, national action on prisons amounted to one

Insolvency Act after another, freeing debtors but leaving prison structures largely alone.

The 1750 outbreak began to demonstrate the need for more action, but again primarily because of who died and where. Elite men died in their homes from a fever allegedly caught in a courtroom. Jail fever was not a problem in jails; it was a problem outside of jails. After all, Newgate deaths happened frequently and caused little stir. The Old Bailey outbreak was much more terrifying. Newspapers and medical treatises demonstrate heightened awareness after 1750 about the disease now nicknamed jail fever. Yet the rebuilding of Newgate languished, and it took a second Old Bailey outbreak in 1772 to spark a national conversation about prisons, bodies, and disease, and to set John Howard on his mission. The situation would worsen before it improved, due largely to the interruption of transportation occasioned by the American Revolution, precipitating a full-blown crisis in English prisons. The scale of the Jail Fever Panic might be best measured by the scope of hero worship for Howard. His celebration is often couched in the language of sentimentality, with Howard demonstrating a superior capacity to care for the vulnerable. But Howard's masculine bravery was every bit as important as his big heart. Howard's heroics consisted of doing precisely what terrified so many propertied Britons: willingly exposing his body to filthy plebeian ones for the sake of the nation. In this Howard embodied a unique combination, the sensitive man of feeling and the courageous man of action. Through Howard, moreover, we can see just how close to the surface plague remained. For it was to lazarettos that he turned, the logic embedded in theories of jail fever pointing him directly to continental plague ports in his search for strategies to protect public health.

Just as Howard looked beyond jails, so too did his compatriots, who never forgot that the principles believed to produce fever in prisons necessarily generated it in slums as well. As they refocused their attention to the sites of pathogenesis identified in plague treatises so long ago, polite Britons brought the logic of the lazaretto to bear on the lives of the working class. Surveillance, quarantine, disinfection: the strategies of the 1790s were at once throwbacks to a bygone age and portents of public health things to come. Moreover, because the underclass was apprehended as a health hazard, with fever presented as endemic—a standard feature of the plebeian world—claims about putridity and danger were extended quite widely. So often discussions of the poor compartmentalized them: the working poor or the idle, the deserving or undeserving poor, the able- or non-able-bodied, the worthy or the wicked. However, we have seen that doctors discussing plague and fever rarely made such distinctions. Instead they tossed out unreflective generalizations that exploded widely and allowed their readers to define "the poor" however they liked. Did the fever-prone poor include artisans? Or were they strictly abject paupers on relief? Doctors never said. For them "the poor" was a flexible category that expanded and contracted with each reader's imagination. Although such claims were intellectually lazy, they were invested with all the importance of Enlightenment-era scientific facts, the social rank of bodies offered as a key medical variable in theories of pathology for two centuries. Class was thus simultaneously ubiquitous but uninvestigated. Doctors clearly felt little need to specify who they did and didn't mean. Instead, there was a silent agreement between writer and reader that such clarifications were unnecessary. They knew who they meant. Thus doctors' laziness to define their categories in ways that might satisfy traditional social historians provides an important clue for the cultural historian of the body. Though they usually spoke of it in terms of a simplistic binary, class was a distinction that clearly mattered to them. I contend that generalizations about social rank in theories of plague and fever are sufficiently sweeping to support the conclusion that class was understood as having a physiological component during the seventeenth and eighteenth centuries. Plague and fever texts treated the poor as an undifferentiated mass with distinct physiological characteristics that rendered them dangerous. It is for this reason that I wish to spend the rest of this Conclusion not summarizing *Rotten Bodies'* findings but rather contemplating, tentatively, experimentally even, their implications for the larger project of the history of the body. How does the kind of evidence explored in this book relate to the early science underpinning modern identity categories, and thus how might we incorporate class into the history of eighteenth-century ideas about human variety?

Pathology and Difference

For these findings to be important it is necessary to demonstrate that they were not aberrations: interesting examples, but too rare to support larger assertions. Thankfully, this is easy to do. Plague and jail fever were not the only diseases linked to class during the long eighteenth century. For example, one could apply the same analysis to the skin disease known as the itch, and in fact, I have done so. In the same category of "putrid diseases" as plague and pestilential fever, the itch was rooted in corrupt blood. The poor were predisposed to it for the same reasons that they were to plague and fever: living in filth, consuming a poor diet, and failing to sweat out their impurities because of idleness. Moreover, diseases were also linked to wealth. Porter and Rousseau have expertly charted how eighteenth-century theories of gout presented that disease as endemic to the rich, proclaiming it "the Patrician Disease." Here, doctors invoked a similar bevy of factors like diet and behavior to warn against the physiological implications of luxury. If the diets of the poor were rotten, those of the wealthy were too rich. If paupers were idle because they shirked work, the spoiled rich could be just as sedentary. Moreover, we know that theories on nervous diseases similarly linked pathology to class in suggestions that the delicate nerves of elites rendered them prone to mental disorders. George Cheyne perhaps most famously asserted that as many as one third of the English upper class suffered from nervous disease. Porter, moreover, has further shown that consumption was similarly believed to prey on the rich thanks to a related etiology.[1]

Enlightenment doctors thus clearly used predisposition to particular diseases as a tool to distinguish socioeconomic groups. Moreover, we know that they used this same tool to differentiate bodies in other ways, for example by gender. While anatomists have rightly received most of the attention from scholars exploring the period's increasingly rigid models of gender difference, pathologists—doctors discussing disease—contributed significantly to this project. Anatomical texts increasingly stressed that men's and women's bodies were composed of different structures, but treatises on disease performed some of the cultural heavy lifting by pathologizing (and thereby politicizing) those structures. Hysteria is the obvious example, though greensickness, nymphomania, and other nervous disorders are among the range of diseases used to distinguish the sexes in the eighteenth century.[2] Predisposition for particular diseases was thus a key physiological feature used to distinguish bodies in the Enlightenment.

It is also significant that many of the diseases linked to class were said to be transmissible from parent to child. The hereditary passage of traits is a central element in the science of identity characteristics believed to be fixed and essential rather than arbitrarily acquired. We have already seen that one of the many factors thought to predispose poor bodies to fevers was a so-called "taint" in the blood, the remnants of disease imperfectly cured that lingered to reignite or spark new diseases years later and which could be inherited from one's parents or even grandparents. The putrid diseases of the poor like fever, pox, or scurvy were strongly linked to such taints, with the "scorbutick taint" offering one of the more common iterations of this idea. Such ideas presage discussions of the scorbutic and other "diatheses" that typified constitutional thinking in the Victorian period with links to early eugenics. Charles Rosenberg showed how nineteenth-century thought about heredity continued to draw heavily on the flexible early modern model that we have explored: "Heredity was a dynamic process . . . [which] assumed that the inheritance of character, disease, and temperament was a protean affair of tendency and predisposition, not of discrete and unitary qualities." Indeed, he shows that the fluid quality of early thinking on heredity allowed it to be harnessed to moral agendas quite readily. While scholars of heredity have presented the turn of the nineteenth century as a key moment when ideas about heredity hardened, they have faced the nagging problem that early modern discussions of hereditary *diseases* were robust much earlier, as our exploration of Willis demonstrated in Chapter 1. It is also telling that independently exploring the topic of hereditary disease in the Enlighten-ment brings one straight back to class. Because in addition to the putrid diseases of the poor, the predominant hereditary diseases of the period were ones strongly associated with wealth: gout and madness. This is not a coinci-dence. When eighteenth-century doctors tried to explain how predisposition for a disease passed from parents to children, they inevitably fell into discus-sions of families, of which one of the most identifiable characteristics was economic status. The apparently gouty and nervous aristocracy was espe-cially useful in this regard. John Waller, for example, has helpfully argued that hereditary diseases in the period were often those deemed incurable, as both madness and gout were. When doctors' best efforts failed, they often attributed it to a disease being incurably rooted in the constitution since birth, and diseases that ran in families seemed to confirm this model. Thus when doctors sought to understand how and why diseases seemed to prevail in particular subgroups, the rich and the poor—as ever, vaguely defined—stood out as sufficiently identifiable to trace epidemiological patterns. Indeed, one of the leading thinkers on the topic was Charles Darwin's grandfather, Erasmus Darwin, who punctuated his discussion of hereditary disease with a warning that demonstrates not only how such thinking addressed class but how it could drift toward quasi-racialized presentations that became associated with eugenic degeneration fears a century later: "A scrophulous race is frequently produced among the poor from a deficient stimulus of bad diet, or of hunger; and among the rich, by a deficient irritability from their having been long accustomed to too great stimulus, as of vinous spirit." More work is needed here, but it certainly seems that eighteenth-century thought on hereditary disease linked it strongly to class.[3]

Pathology, therefore, demonstrates two key factors that make it relevant to the larger history of the science of human variety: 1) it was used to categorize human difference, and 2) it contained the potential to present physiological features as heritable. Here the role of disease susceptibility in emerging discussions of race can be especially enlightening. Indeed, I contend that a good way to understand the biological constructions of class in the period is to compare them to contemporary understandings of race. For not only did race and class function in quite similar fashion in this regard, but, we will see, they intersected in telling ways that cry out for further study.

Pathology and Race

Eighteenth-century thinkers contemplating human variety had so many properties they could compare: size, skin color, hair, bones, the structure and qualities of particular organs, reproductive capacities, and, thanks to the nerves' role connecting mind to body, even mental and moral faculties. The list was long, but predisposition to particular diseases was assuredly on it. Historians like Roxann Wheeler have demonstrated that the category of race remained quite flexible in the eighteenth century. Theories about climate dominated explanations of why bodies appeared so different globally. Traits could be passed hereditarily, but a "soft hereditarianism" pervaded, in which numerous factors had influence. Eighteenth-century bodies were, as I have termed them elsewhere, pliable, adapting to environmental forces. Monogenism, the belief that all humans descended from Adam and Eve, ruled the day and worked to inhibit the kinds of hard, fixed theories of racial difference that would become so influential in the nineteenth century. Pathology influenced such thinking as doctors sought to explain diseases incident to different locales. Medical historians like Mark Harrison argue for a "weak transmutationism," by which eighteenth-century colonial medicine cast bodies not as essentially formed, but malleable, succumbing to or fending off diseases based on how well or poorly they acclimated to new conditions.

However, like soft hereditarianism, weak transmutationism held that climatically influenced traits could become fixed over generations, an idea that Harrison suggests became more pronounced in the late eighteenth century. (Moreover, it is noteworthy that Harrison stresses the centrality of the putrefactive theory of disease to the early tropical medicine he explores.)[4]

Indeed, there was churning debate on the question of race in the Enlightenment, with early polygenistic positions emerging and considerable scientific activity aimed at identifying fixed features of racial difference, whether measuring skulls or examining black skin under the microscope. Pathology played a role in these efforts. Hans Sloane, the well-known English physician who spent time in Jamaica, argued against the prevailing climatic theory of corporeal difference. Speaking to the Royal Society in 1690, he addressed the topic of "the Colours of Animalls, and particularly of the Negroes, whether it was the product of this climate or that they were a Distinct race of Men." Intriguingly, he used disease to argue for essential racial difference: "Dr. Sloan said he had observed the Cuticular Diseases, and Ulcers of Negrows are much harder to cure than those of Europeans, and these argued a specific Difference as to the Skin." This, from a physician whom Wendy Churchill shows was influenced more by class than by race in his colonial medical practice. Sloane's seventeenth-century contemporary Thomas Trapham offered one of the earliest medical treatises on Jamaica, which attributed numerous diseases to Africans and Native Americans, whom he called "animal people" worthy of slavery and conquest because of their pathogenic degeneration. The clearest discussion centers on yaws, a near cousin to syphilis that he argued was endemic to blacks and "indians," they having acquired a permanent "taint" in their blood through bestiality. Trapham references heritability due to "the taint of their spermatick original," and suggested that said taint also explained their predisposition to the disease of "guinny worm" and their heightened power to pass syphilis to Europeans. Of course, the similar attribution of syphilis to Amerindians has been long known.[5]

Eighteenth-century thinkers continued this exploration. Norris Saakwa-Mante has explored the theory of naval surgeon and polygenist John Atkins on Africans' predisposition to "Sleepy Distemper," which eschewed environmental factors and emphasized innate characteristics. Indeed, he did so in part by applying the theory of depauperated blood.[6] A more important thinker in the history of race, polygenist Edward Long, provides numerous similar examples. The British colonial administrator is infamous for his three-volume *History of Jamaica* (1774), in which he explicitly declared that blacks and whites constituted different races, and implied a wide gulf between them: "I think there are extremely potent reasons for believing, that the White and the Negroe are distinct species." Scholars like Wheeler and Suman Seth have demonstrated Long's role as an early crafter of what Seth calls eighteenth-century "race science." What matters here is that the issue so crucial to the physiology of class—predisposition to disease—contributed to Long's polygenism. In his chapter on health, Long espoused typical climatic views. Indeed, he repeatedly suggested that Africans and Europeans were influenced by climate or diseases similarly, and that differences in pathology were explained by diet or behavior. However, he was inconsistent, and elsewhere highlighted susceptibility to disease as a key racial distinction. In his chapter "On Negroes," for example, he used health to compare different ethnic groups and included predisposition to particular diseases among their essential identifying features. Africans in general, claimed Long, were more prone to dropsy than Europeans, and their women predisposed to menstrual obstructions. Moreover, following Trapham (whom he cited), he wrote that their blood was tainted by yaws, a disease he expressly compared to putrid fevers. "These Negroes are few of them exempt from the venereal taint; and very many have, at the time of their arrival, that dreadful disorder, the *yaws*, lurking in their blood." Sean Quinlan has shown that similar arguments were advanced by influential French physicians such as Jean Barthélemy Dazille, who asserted: "There must be . . . in Negroes, a particular, predisposing cause, one that is not found in Whites, or that is not found in the same proportion, since if pians [yaws] is not an illness from which Whites are excluded, it is always very rare among them, while it is very common with the former. It is necessary, by consequence, that a humor exists which has an analogy more particular with the nature of this virus." By stating that Africans' humours were predisposed because analogous to the disease, Dazille here advances a claim clearly reminiscent of the early modern assertion that paupers' predisposition to plague rested on the "similitude" between their blood and plague itself.[7]

Susceptibility also worked in the reverse, for Long elsewhere suggested that African constitutions were less susceptible to certain ailments. Africans' pores were said to be wider than Europeans', providing "a free transpiration to bad humours"; that is, they enjoyed the virtues of healthy perspiration, the deficiency of which we saw contributed to putrid fevers. Moreover, he cited

Benjamin Franklin's discussion of these same alleged racial differences in perspiration to suggest that although their pores benefited them in hot climates (and thus suited them to labor in Jamaica), they rendered them prone to the disease of frostbite farther north. Indeed, the theories about putrid fever at the heart of this book influenced him: "The fluids in the human body will become putrescent, if due exercise is too long neglected: hence we may conclude, that habitual indolence and inactivity are likewise to be reckoned among the predisposing causes of bad fevers." Thus, in repeatedly describing Africans as naturally "indolent," he suggested that the health benefits offered to Africans by their unique skin may have been offset because of other inherent failings.[8]

Writers of lesser renown agreed, for example James Grainger, a Scottish physician who settled on the island of St. Kitts. In his 1764 treatise on West Indian diseases he aimed to explain the ailments of plantation slaves and sustained a comparison of white and black bodies throughout. "Negros" were more prone than Europeans to more than a dozen diseases. Focused primarily on the practical issues of diagnosis and treatment, Grainger admitted that he was often "waving theory" and rarely explained why black constitutions differed. But he gave hints, as when explaining that Creoles were predisposed to a wasting disease because of their "watery poverty of the blood." Moreover, a later edition called leprosy and elephantiasis "hereditary," warning white readers that their children could be infected if they used black wet nurses who "have this taint in their constitution." Predisposition to fever also differed: "White people in the West Indies are liable to remitting fevers. The fever of Negroes is inflammatory"—though Grainger also noted that because of Africans' natural indolence their fevers (rather like those of idle workers) often "became putrid, malignant or nervous." Racial distinction was equally demonstrated by the diseases to which Africans were inherently *less* prone: aphthae (oral ulcers), bladder stones, heartburn, constipation, and the Flour Albus.[9]

The belief in Africans' reduced susceptibility to certain ailments leads us to an important disease with close links to pestilential fever, namely yellow fever, a disease that terrorized numerous American cities in the 1790s and to which Africans were believed immune.[10] Colin Chisholm's 1795 treatise on the epidemic is particularly useful for beginning to bring together different threads of our (admittedly wide-ranging) discussion. A Scottish surgeon who settled in Grenada, Chisholm mimicked Grainger in listing ten diseases that were "fortunately confined to the Negro race," including leprosy, elephantiasis, yaws, and putrid sore throat. Chisholm identified yellow fever as a "malignant pestilential fever" that developed on a ship anchored for too long off the African coast, communicated to the Americas when it arrived in the West Indies. Chisholm begins to demonstrate how race and class could sit side by side in such discussions. For example, he affirmed mainstream ideas about class when he offered the status of the ships' passengers as a scientific fact proving that the ship could not have begun its journey with seeds of the disease: "As the [settlers] were in general of the middling class of people . . . no suspicion whatever can be entertained of the existence of latent infection among them." (And Chisolm's reference to the middling class here means that his vision went slightly beyond the typical binary to conceive of at least three classes, upper, middle, and lower.) Like so many jail fever theorists, he identified the disease as "partaking of the nature of the true plague" and thus presumed the poor most susceptible: "It will not appear extraordinary that the lower classes of men, and those more especially of loose and debauched manners, should be the most subject to this disease." However, he made a bold claim about race. "Some were more obnoxious to it than others; and the colour had evidently much influence in determining its violence." According to Chisholm's figures, black inhabitants, whether free or enslaved, had much lower infection and mortality rates than various categories of whites. To explain the phenomenon Chisholm wandered—like so many doctors discussing the poor—between behavioral factors and essential constitutional predisposition. "Although the contagion seemed to vary much in different descriptions of people, it is highly probable that the virus of the contagion was uniformly the same, only variously modified by peculiar constitutions, habits or modes of living. Thus among sailors, perhaps a scorbutic taint, joined to extreme irregularity and imprudence, rendered the disease infinitely more fatal than among any other class of men. On the other hand, among field-negroes, who certainly possess an idiosyncrasy peculiar to themselves, and whose mode of living is generally temperate and regular in a remarkable degree, the virus was so blunted, as to act in the mildest form." White sailors and black slaves experienced the same *contagia* differently, partially because of their modes of living, but partially because of distinct physiologies. Thus an exploration of fever allowed here for the physiological qualities of working-class bodies (with their "scorbutic taint") and black bodies (with their "peculiar idiosyncrasy") to be discussed in tandem.

Chisholm never identifies that "idiosyncrasy," but he did reiterate the point later, noting that it "is probable that the negro race possess something constitutional which resists the action of contagion in a very great degree."[11]

As is well known, the American physician Benjamin Rush ascribed to a version of this theory. That is, he did until the epidemic in Philadelphia proved it glaringly false. As scholars have noted, Rush was influenced by doctors like John Lining, who had also argued for black immunity to yellow fever decades earlier. The disease struck whites of both sexes, "Indians," and even mulattoes. However, "There is something very singular in the constitution of the Negroes which renders them not liable to this fever." Prevailing theory held that yellow fever was associated with hyperproduction of bile. And bile, we now know, was responsible for the very essence of blackness in considerable eighteenth-century thought. Quinlan and Andrew Curran have shown that French physicians like Alexis Littré and Pierre Barrère advanced an influential theory that excess bile accounted for black skin, as well as black blood and even black brains, a point that we will see has salience for our discussion. Rush had excerpts from Lining's work, including the passage above, printed in newspapers to call upon black Philadelphians to take up the dangerous work of tending the sick, since their unique bilious constitutions would protect them. When little distinguished black and white mortality rates, Rush was forced to admit his terrible mistake, although, against all evidence, he and others continued to hold that "the disease was lighter in them, than in white people." As Rush moved away from a bilious explanation of skin color, he advanced an idea that even more firmly demonstrates the importance of pathology to theories of race. Although an abolitionist who tends to be presented as progressive on the question of slavery, Rush asserted that blackness was rooted in systemic leprosy—rendering race literally into an ailment, what Winthrop Jordan called "the Disease of Color." Focusing on colonial medicine, Mark Harrison has offered the fullest study of the role played by the science of pathology to the early formation of race, including, for example, James Johnson's belief that blackness was attributed to "permanent hereditary jaundice." Climate still played a role in explaining race, but as racial ideas hardened theories of pathology—including those regarding predisposition, fever, and putrid decay—were significant.[12]

We have had to skirt over very large issues here, but the salient point is that levels of susceptibility to diseases, including forms of fever closely associated with jail fever, clearly provided important markers of racial difference in the eighteenth century—mirroring the role that similar ideas played for the construction of class at the same point in history.

The Mingling of Class and Race

Rush advanced his leprosy theory as part of an ongoing debate on race, specifically as a response to the ideas of leading American monogenist Samuel Stanhope Smith. Smith's *Essay on the Causes of Variety of Complexion and Figure in the Human Species* (1787) still held that overabundance of bile accounted for dark skin and attributed said bile production to variable factors like climate. Smith's bodies were thus versions of the pliable, adaptable bodies that typified so much early modern thought on human variety. However, he is worth our attention because he consistently brought race and class into direct conversation with each other. But unlike the thinkers above he did not emphasize the inherent differences between white paupers and people of color but rather suggested fundamental similarities.

Such interaction between race and class in eighteenth-century texts is historiographically noteworthy because scholarship on gender and race has demonstrated how significantly these identity markers influenced one another during the Enlightenment. We now know that race and gender were not formulated in isolation but rather, as scholars like Londa Schiebinger, Felicity Nussbaum, and Kathleen Wilson have shown, they cross-fertilized throughout the eighteenth century. Anne McClintock has shown for the nineteenth century that class can be integrated into this kind of analysis, and here I wish to make the case that the sort of evidence explored in this book may allow seventeenth- and eighteenth-century scholars to begin working toward a deeper integration of class within the history of ideas about human variation. Dror Wahrman's history of the self is notable for its attempt to incorporate class directly into the discussion of the Enlightenment processes that produced modern race and gender, demonstrating that class, like these other categories, came to be understood as more fixed during the last third of the century. When he addresses class, however, Wahrman moves away from the kind of scientific, natural history texts that underpin so much of the work on race and gender and instead analyzes class as strictly political. But now that we have evidence that Enlightenment doctors *did* speak of class in physiological terms—again, at least to the extent of a dualistic rich/poor binary—it becomes possible to move toward an even more integrated history in which class can join race and gender in a dynamic conversation based on the same kinds of scientifically grounded texts. An analysis of Stanhope Smith can offer a brief demonstration of what this might look like, but we must first contextualize important roots of his thought that connected class and race profoundly.[13]

Smith was responding directly to influential polygenist Henry Home, Lord Kames, and was thus entering the discussion of what has come to be known as stadial or "four stages" theory. A product of the Scottish Enlightenment, this body of thought suggested that the world's peoples existed on a continuum characterized by stages of historical development, stages that were linked closely to different economic systems. It has been extensively studied by historians studying race, but it is crucial to note that ideas about social rank were central to the theory. Put simply, the earliest or "savage" states of man were understood as impoverished. Stadial thinkers virtually all attributed the progression of the races to their having developed more sophisticated economies and thereby acquiring greater wealth. Thinkers like Kames, Adam Ferguson, or John Millar presented poverty, usually in the forms of hunger, nakedness, or homelessness, as essential to the savage state. One of the most basic qualities of savages was that they were poor, and it was through efforts to overcome that poverty that new forms of economic activity emerged and racial progress was achieved. Thus the hunting of the savage gave way to herding, farming, and finally commerce, and stadial theorists presented the differences between races—whether manners, intelligence, morals, or physical traits—as direct results of these different economic states and corresponding levels of wealth. While we know that Enlightenment philosophers explored the state of nature as a kind of looking glass into Europeans' own mythic past, making it a profoundly historical mode of thought, it was equally economic, as Wheeler has noted.[14] Ronald Meek, for example, has shown that stadial theorists such as William Robertson gave economics primacy in their evaluations of the world's peoples: said Robertson, "In every enquiry concerning the operations of men when united together in society, the first object of attention should be their modes of subsistence."[15] Stadial theory was thus classist in the sense that eighteenth-century Britons understood themselves as not just historically or technologically advanced beyond savages, but *wealthier* than them. Poverty was essential to savagery, and wealth was critical to civilization. Assumptions of racial difference were thus hopelessly bound up in assumptions of economic difference. The possession of property, that deus ex machina for so much Enlightenment thought, and the different economic activities—forms of labor—needed to acquire it, lay at the very heart of the most influential eighteenth-century theory about the causes of human variety. Moreover, while many of the claims about what I have called class in this book tended to draw upon and reproduce a fairly simplistic binary that Corfield aptly termed rich-poor dualism, the stadial thinkers offered a more developed hierarchy, typically with at least four distinct stages, each set off from one another by different forms of labor and clear gradations of wealth.

Consider Ferguson, for example, who presented the development out of savagery as a kind of social mobility, with savage peoples moving from a state of poverty to "a station more affluent." Racial distinctions flowed directly from there: "The peculiar genius of nations . . . arise from the state of their fortunes." The role of class is particularly clear in Ferguson, who presented the *awareness* of class distinction not just as a marker of different stages of civilization but as itself a driving force for material difference. What it meant to be civilized, for Ferguson, was to have a class structure. Savages have "little attention to property" and consequently "scarcely any beginnings of subordination or government." He went on, "Others having possessed themselves of herbs, and depending for their provision on pasture, know what it is to be poor and rich. They know the relations of patron and client, of servant and master, and by the measures of fortune determine their station. This distinction must create a material difference of character, and may furnish two separate heads, under which to consider the history of mankind in their rudest state; that of the savage, who is not yet acquainted with property; and that of the barbarian, to whom it is, although not ascertained by laws, a principal object of care and desire." Class distinctions—not only levels of wealth, but power relations relative to production (those between "servant and master")—created "a material difference of character." New methods of acquiring property coupled with the social relations that new economic systems produced moved "rude" peoples away from their inherent "disposition" (note the term) to sloth and toward industry, a claim that would have been just as applicable to the English poor as it was to imaginary savages. Indeed, Kames elsewhere applied his same argument about hunger driving savages toward industry (and thus civilization) directly to the English poor within his lengthy discussion of domestic politics. For Ferguson, Native Americans remained savages because, although they labored, they did so communally and hence lacked conceptions of private property. As a result, "they admit of no distinctions of rank or condition." They knew no class: "Among the Iroquois, and other nations of the temperate zone, the titles of *magistrate* and *subject*, of *noble* and *mean*, are as little known as those of *rich* and *poor*." Fellow stadial theorist John Millar shows the centrality of class to this body of thought in his decision to title his book *Observations Concerning the Distinction of Ranks*. For Millar, race, nation, and class collapse in on one another. The acquisition of property drives progress as savage nations transform from a state in which they "feel the want of almost every thing" toward more complex societies characterized by "affluence" and "opulence." This thinking was rife. Wheeler notes the importance of poverty in David Hume's influential essay "Of National Characters" (1742), functioning both as a defining feature of the savage state and as a motivation for economic, and therefore racial, development. Adam Smith described savages as "the poorest of all nations." When comparing Native Americans with the allegedly more advanced Chinese, he called the latter "much richer, better cultivated, and more advanced in the arts and manufactures." All of this would seem to suggest that David Cannidine's insight—that class powerfully framed how nineteenth-century Britons saw their empire—offers considerable food for thought for eighteenth-century scholars. Indeed, even earlier theorists about the so-called state of nature formulated a vision of a deep historical past characterized by poverty. It is often overlooked that Hobbes's state of nature was not merely "nasty, brutish and short," as we so often hear, but rather, lacking "industry" or "commodities," it was "*poore*, nasty, brutish and short." The associations between conceptions of race and class in stadial thought deserve far more probing analysis than can be attempted in the space available here. However, it should be clear that this body of thought forged profound links between savagery and pauperism, and this was the literature Stanhope Smith engaged in his treatise on human variety.[16]

Although a Presbyterian minister, Stanhope Smith grounded his ideas about human variation firmly in medical thinking. He attributed racial difference—physical, moral, and intellectual—to two factors: climate and, with fellow stadial thinkers, "the state of society." Climate worked in its usual medical ways, but a people's level of civilization either protected against or augmented climate's impact. Lacking material possessions, savages were exposed to climate's brutal effects, so their bodies transformed more radically. Their poverty, in other words, left them helpless against climate and thus contributed significantly to mold their constitutions. Consider this explanation of dark skin, which frames savages as impoverished (naked and homeless) and draws both on theories about bile that we met earlier and on medical doctrines of putridity. "A naked savage, seldom enjoying the protection of a miserable hut, and compelled to lodge on the bare ground and under the open skies, imbibes the influence of the sun and atmosphere at every pore. He inhabits an uncultivated region filled with stagnant waters, and covered with putrid vegetables, that fall down and corrupt on the spot where they have grown. . . . The vapour of rivers, the exhalations of marshes, and the noxious effluvia of decaying vegetables, fill the whole atmosphere in an unimproved country, and tend to give a dark and bilous hue to the complexion." This passage leaves little doubt that Smith had absorbed the sorts of medical discourse explored in this book. "Putrid exhalations" transformed the bile and darkened it. Indeed, his later explanation of dark skin invoked several causes that we have seen were also said to render paupers' blood putrid: "The vapours of stagnant waters with which uncultivated regions abound; all great fatigues and hardships; poverty and nastiness, tend, as well as heat, to augment the bile," which in turn darkened the skin. Thus the same factors that made the blood putrid made the skin dark. According to Smith there were two prevailing theories about bile; either it darkened because it was itself putrid or else the body released excess bile as "a corrector of putridity."[17] He wasn't sure which was right, but either way the black body was black because it was putrid.

Although as a monogenist he disagreed with Kames that the races represented different species, he did see racial difference as quite stark. Savages were "liable to be considered as an inferior grade in the descent from the human to the brute creation," and their features, while not permanent, were extremely sturdy. He estimated that it took a thousand years for Europeans to become "polished" from their savage roots, and he presented features like skin color as practically eternal: "The negroe colour, for example, may by the exposure of a poor and servile state, be rendered almost perpetual." Of course, that claim nicely highlights Smith's belief that Africans' poverty contributed to their racial degeneration. Their hot climate made them dark, but their poverty fixed that characteristic in a much more lasting way. Smith believed that American slaves offered a fruitful example to demonstrate the impact of class on race, one that he believed deserved much more attention. "If white inhabitants of America afford us less conspicuous instances, than some other nations, of the power of society, and of the difference of ranks, in varying the human form, the blacks, in the southern republics, afford one that is highly worthy the attention of philosophers." Rank varied the human form: few claims made the point as succinctly. Smith held up field slaves and house slaves as parallels for the classes among whites. Like the lives of the rich and poor, those of field laborers and house servants were distinguished by the quality of their housing, food, clothing, activities, and exposure to "manners." Field slaves, as a result of their poor conditions, were "slow in changing the aspect and figure of Africa," and thus remained practically as savages. By comparison their better-fed, -clothed, and -educated—we must thus say richer—counterparts in domestic service, who, notably, performed what would have been considered more refined forms of labor, "have advanced far before them in acquiring the agreeable and regular features, and the expressive countenance of civilized society." These changes were not just behavioral but physiological as well. "The former are frequently ill shaped. They preserve, in a great degree, the African lips, and nose, and hair. Their genius is dull, and their countenance sleepy and stupid—the latter are straight and well-proportioned; their hair extended to three, four, and sometimes even to six or eight inches; the size and shape of their mouth handsome, their features regular, their capacity good, and their look animated." His accompanying footnote stressed that the power of rank could even *exceed* climate in inscribing racialized features on the body. Many of the improvements among house slaves "depend[] more on the state of society than on the climate." This offered what Smith believed to be tantalizing proof that if Africans lived in prosperity rather than poverty, their racial transformation would be much accelerated. "The great difference between the domestic and field slaves, gives reason to believe that, if they were perfectly free, enjoyed property, and were admitted to a liberal participation of the society, rank and privileges of their masters, they would change their African peculiarities much faster." Levels of wealth—by way of the living conditions and forms of labor associated with them—drove racial development, just as stadial theory had suggested.[18]

Notwithstanding claims as pronounced as these, Smith went much further to connect race and class. For not only were savages poor, but the poor were a whole lot like savages. Logic demanded that it work both ways. For instance, and as Joanna Brooks has noted, Smith asserted that the white poor were quickest to degenerate back toward a savage state. In his explanation of how putridity discolored the bile and skin, he noted that the disorders that "leave the blood impoverished, and shed a yellow appearance over the skin" disproportionately affected the poor. Furthermore, the same bevy of factors that darkened the skin of Native Americans wrought a "sallowness" on white Americans—but one that was unevenly distributed: "It is more observable . . . in the lower and laboring classes of people, than in families of easy fortune who possess the means and the inclination to protect their complexion." Precisely like savages, then, "the Poor and laboring classes . . . are always first and most deeply affected by the influence of climate." As a result, the poor of Georgia and Carolina had "degenerate[d] to a complexion that is but a few shades lighter than that of the Iroquois. Not only is their complexion but their whole constitution seems to be changed. So thin and meagre is the habit of the poor, and of the overseers of their slaves that, frequently, their limbs appear to have a disproportioned length to the body, and the shape of the skeleton is evidently discernable through the skin."[19]

Smith attached a revealing footnote to this point. It was meant to refute Kames and the polygenists. However, it broadcast just how profound he believed the constitutional effects of poverty to be. "If these men had been found in a distant region where no memory of their origin remained the philosophers who espouse the hypothesis of different species of men would have produced them in proof." In other words, the white poor were distinct enough from their richer neighbors that he understood why some might consider them a different species. He repeated this bold claim several times. Discussing beauty, he later contrasted "the soft and elegant tints of complexion in genteel life, and the course ruddiness of the vulgar." So profound were these distinctions that "some writers would pronounce them different races." In a more elaborate example he discussed the poor in Scotland but began with broader general claims:

> The poor and laboring part of the community are usually more swarthy and squalid in their complexion, more hard in their features, and more coarse and ill-formed in their limbs, than persons of better fortune, and more liberal means of subsistence. . . . Such distinctions become more considerable by time, after families have held for ages the same stations in society. They are most conspicuous in those countries in which the laws have made the most complete and permanent

division of ranks. What an immense difference exists, in Scotland, between the chiefs and the commonality of the highland clans? If they had been separately found in different countries, the philosophy of some writers would have ranged them in different species.

Smith's monogenism would not allow him to go quite that far, but he could see why others might arrange the classes taxonomically.[20]

Indeed, the racial proximity between people of color and the white poor was so close as to allow them to stand in for each other in comparative examples. On at least six occasions Smith slipped from the one to the other, supporting claims about blacks or natives with examples of the white poor. The last quotation, for example, followed an open assertion of the evidentiary value the European poor could provide for scientific claims about Native Americans. To support the assertion that the poverty of Native Americans "naturally" produced their "most distinguishing features," he proclaimed: "I shall derive my first illustration from the several classes of men in polished nations," and proceeded to make the claim we have seen about Scottish Highlanders. He did it for smaller points as well. To support the contention that Africans' practice of bringing their children into the fields demonstrated poor parental instincts, he invoked "a similar negligence among the poor, who suffer their children to lie in ashes, or on the naked ground." This practice damaged, of all things, poor children's hair, which he quickly compared to Africans' hair. It was likewise "short, and thin, and frittered," a point that seemed to offer physiological evidence of their shared moral failings. Of course, such claims relied on readers accepting that paupers and savages could serve as analogues for each other. Smith obviously trusted that they would, for the examples continued to flow. The dark complexion of savages was said to be augmented by their exposure to smoky fires in their huts, a point supported with the evidence that smoke similarly "discolours the skin of . . . labourers and mechanics." Drawing on physiognomy, he lengthily compared the state of savages' and paupers' facial features: "The rustic state, by its solitude and want of thought and emotion, bears some analogy to the savage. And we see it accompanied by similar effects on the visage. The countenance vacant, the lips thick, the face broad and spread, and all its muscles lax and swelling." He called the structure of the savage face "rude and uncouth," adding immediately that "a similar negligence among the vulgar adds exceedingly to that disgusting coarseness which so many other causes contribute to create." For proof of Native Americans' licentiousness he offered the example of impoverished frontiersmen who "approach[] the roughness and simplicity of savage manners." At times, as here, the comparisons flowed breezily from savage to pauper and back again.

> The hardships of their condition, that weaken and exhaust the principle of life—their scanty and meagre fare, which wants the succulence and nourishment which gives freshness and vigor to the constitution—the uncertainty of their provision, which sometimes leaves them to languish in want, and sometimes enables them to overstrain themselves by a surfeit—and their entire inattention to personal and domestic cleanliness, all have a prodigious effect to darken the complexion, to relax and emaciate the constitution, and to render their features coarse and deformed. Of the influence of these causes we have an example in persons reduced to extreme poverty, who are usually as much distinguished by their thin habit, their uncouth features, and their swarthy and squalid aspects, as by the meanness of their garb. Nakedness, exposure, negligence of appearance, want of cleanliness, bad lodging, and meagre diet, so discolour and injure their form, as to enable us to frame some judgement of the degree in which such causes will contribute to augment the influence of climate in savage life. Independently on climate, these causes will render it impossible that a savage should ever be fair. And the co-operation of both, will usually render men in that state of society extremely dark in their complexion.

Though he here discussed physical appearances rather than predisposition to disease, his claims about the constitutional impacts of various forms of poverty—insufficient nutrition, filth, meager clothing, and decrepit housing—would have fit any plague or fever treatise.[21]

The racialized construction of the poor intensified even further when Smith commented on the heritable nature of working-class features. This time, instead of vacillating between workers and savages he shifted into a discussion of animals. "Every remarkable change of feature that has grown into a habit of body, is transmitted with other personal properties, to offspring. The coarse features of laboring people, created by hardships, and by long exposure to the weather are communicated.—The broad feet of the rustic, that have been spread by often treading the naked ground; and the large hand and arm, formed by constant labour, are discernable in children. . . . We continually see the effect of this principle on the inferior animals." Note again that here it is not merely poverty but the impact of manual labor itself that transforms physiology in ways that become heritable. Smith then discusses horse breeding and the process of selecting traits to produce desirable breeds. However, when he segues back to humans, he makes a claim that clearly adumbrates eugenics—claiming not merely that desirable traits could be selected but that the process could be usefully managed by the state: "If men in the affair of marriage were as much under management as some other animals, an absolute ruler might accomplish in his dominions almost any idea of the human form." Given the British eugenics movement's later fascination with poverty and degeneration, it is more than a little interesting that Smith's examples to support this point emphasized class rather than race. Was it not obvious, he asked, that the European nobility have, by their ability to select the most desirable mates, improved their features and constitutions immensely? "The superior ranks will always be first, and, in general, most improved . . . because they have it, more than others, in their power to form matrimonial connexions favourable to this end." Through selective breeding, he claimed, the Persian nobility had nearly eradicated all traces of their ancestor Tartars, "the most deformed and stupid nations upon earth." So, too, had the Greek nobility molded itself, as well as, via Captain Cook's enormously influential travelogue, elite Pacific Islanders. Smith quoted Cook directly: "The same superiority which is observable in the *Erees* [nobles] through all the other islands, is also found here. Those who, we saw were, without exception, perfectly well formed; whereas the lower sort, besides their general inferiority, are subject to all the variety of make and figure that is seen in the populace of other countries." At the end of this claim we see that even Cook slipped quickly from the particular to the universal, extending the point to stake a claim for physiological class distinctions the world over. Smith thus offered evidence from around the globe and across time to hint at the eugenic potential of class-based selective breeding.[22]

⁂

We have come a long way from the British poor and their diseases. Or have we? A string of episodes that we encountered along the way now read a little differently: Mead's ability to move seamlessly back and forth between Africans and poor Britons in his explanation of plague; Ferriar's use of stadial language to explain that paupers suffered fever because they still lived as in "earlier states of society"; Clerke's framing of public health interventions in slums as a civilizing mission. We can revisit with fresh eyes Figure 3, the 1803 engraving of the Oglethorpe Gaol Committee. The destitute prisoner, depicted in rags, on bended knee—and with a strikingly dark complexion—supplicates before the committee's beaming white faces. When set against a text like Stanhope Smith's, its eerie similarities to contemporary depictions of New World peoples or even Josiah Wedgewood's famous abolitionist image *Am I not a Man and Brother?* take on potentially new significance.

Certainly, such racialized constructions of the working class will be familiar to scholars of the nineteenth century. Louis Chevalier long ago explored the tendency of the middle classes to look upon the poor as savages. *Barbare, sauvages,* and *nomades,* these were the terms used to characterize the underclass in nineteenth-century Paris, while for Britain, Gareth Stedman Jones called attention to the racist language underpinning what he called Urban Degeneration Theory. Gertrude Himmelfarb has argued that such presentations of the working class were embodied through a Victorian "moral physiognomy" that emphasized physiological difference. Explorers of the urban underworld such as Henry Mayhew or William Booth saw their tours of slums as a kind of civilizing mission, with an aim to improving people they described repeatedly as a "race" or "tribe." Even such sympathetic Victorians as Engels, who just a generation later toured the very fever-ridden neighborhoods of Manchester that we explored in Chapter 7, called the poor "a race apart," a claim anticipated by Tocqueville, who described these same slums as sites where "civilized man is turned back almost into a savage." Henrika Kuklick has shown that nineteenth-century evolutionary anthropologists referred to the urban underclass as a "new city race," and "a primitive people in our midst," while Alastair Bonnett has suggested that the British working class became white only in the twentieth century. Himmelfarb and others have linked this racialization of the working class directly to medical discussions of disease and public health, while Walkowitz has shown that popular accounts voiced fears of Lamarckian degeneration that characterized urban poverty as itself a disease. Indeed, Pickstone alerts us to the importance of medical discourses about poverty and fever to these constructions, noting that in the 1830s fever experts like James Kay-Shuttlesworth approached the poor as an "alien mass" and a "community of savages," one that—tellingly for our purposes—he presented as the "rotting tissue of the social body." Moreover, medical historians like Pauline Mazumdar have demonstrated just how obsessed the British eugenics movement became with pauperism. It is thus not difficult to see where eighteenth-century discourses were heading.[23]

Make no mistake; class would never attain the sense of fixed immutability of either race or gender. Instead it is well characterized by the soft hereditarianism that usefully describes the still-flexible quality of race before the nineteenth century. However, in that sense, class was probably just as developed as race was at that point in history—perhaps even more developed, since we have not even touched on the convention of presenting class as hereditarily rooted in the blood: the tradition of claims about "royal blood" or "noble blood" stretched back centuries. It thus made considerable eighteenth-century sense that social rank might express itself physiologically. The project to identify the essential qualities of nations, races, and genders constituted one of the Enlightenment's greatest thought-experiments. It probably should not surprise us that some thinkers would try out these ideas on a category like the poor or that there would be dynamic interplay between them and other groups. Moreover, in plague and fever Britain faced a major social problem—one rooted in bodies—that drew considerable attention to the question and at times raised medical debates to levels of national importance. It is certainly likely that as scientific racism hardened in the nineteenth century, its own logic worked to *limit* the extent to which class could ever be seen as firmly fixed in biology. Yet Daniel Bender's work on the biological and racial constructions of the working class in the early twentieth century, and Samuel Kelton Robert Jr.'s analysis of the intersection of physiological constructions of race and class in Jim Crow America—both of which focus on anxieties about epidemic disease[24]—offer telling examples suggesting that this story was far from over in 1800, that class remained deeply woven into theoretical formulations about human variation, and that the developments charted in *Rotten Bodies* echoed long into the modern age.

All of this was one more element of plague's massive bequeathal to modernity. Plebeian putridity was always just one of many factors that doctors linked to the frightening specter of disease. But it was a consistent factor. For two centuries a line of thought pervaded in medicine, reinforced generation after generation. The bodies of the poor had unique qualities that were cause for considerable concern. Susceptibility to fever has offered us one way to explore the early scientific construction of class. Perhaps now we can pursue others.

Notes

Introduction

1. On the topic of epidemic disease the eighteenth century can boast nothing like the deep bodies of work on the centuries that surround it. For plague see Paul Slack, *The Impact of Plague in Tudor and Stuart England* (Oxford: Oxford University Press, 1985); A. Lloyd Moote and Dorothy Moote, *The Great Plague: The Story of London's Most Deadly Year* (Baltimore: Johns Hopkins University Press, 2004); Samuel Cohn, *Cultures of Plague: Medical Thinking at the End of the Renaissance* (Oxford: Oxford University Press, 2009); Ernest B. Gilman, *Plague Writing in Early Modern England* (Chicago: University of Chicago Press, 2009); and Margaret Healy, *Fictions of Disease in Early Modern England* (New York: Palgrave, 2001), 101–122. On epidemic disease and the poor in the nineteenth century see Christopher Hamlin, *Public Health and Social Justice in the Age of Chadwick* (Cambridge: Cambridge University Press, 1998); Margaret Pelling, *Cholera, Fever, and English Medicine, 1825–1865* (Oxford: Oxford University Press, 1978); Anne Hardy, *The Epidemic Streets: Infectious Diseases and the Rise of Preventative Medicine, 1856–1900* (Oxford: Clarendon, 1993); and Graham Mooney, *Intrusive Interventions: Public Health, Domestic Space, and Infectious Disease Surveillance in England, 1840–1914* (Rochester, NY: University of Rochester Press, 2015).
2. Christopher Hamlin suggests a similar relationship between plague and eighteenth-century fever. *More than Hot: A Short History of Fever* (Baltimore: Johns Hopkins University Press, 2014), 90. That said, we see change over time differently, and I will contend that there was greater continuity across the seventeenth and eighteenth centuries than he allows.
3. Roy Porter, *English Society in the Eighteenth Century* (New York: Penguin, 1982), 80–81.
4. On poor relief and welfare see Steven King, *Poverty and Welfare in England, 1700–1850: A Regional Perspective* (Manchester: Manchester University Press,

2000); David Green, *Pauper Capital: London and the Poor Law, 1790–1870* (Burlington, VT: Ashgate, 2010); Paul Slack, *From Reformation to Improvement: Public Welfare in Early Modern England* (Oxford: Clarendon, 1998); Steven King and Allanah Tomkins, eds., *The Poor in England, 1750–1840: An Economy of Makeshifts* (Manchester: Manchester University Press, 2003); Alysa Levene, *The Childhood of the Poor: Welfare in Eighteenth-Century London* (London: Palgrave Macmillan, 2012); and Lynn Hollen Lees, *The Solidarities of Strangers: The English Poor Laws and the People, 1700–1948* (Cambridge: Cambridge University Press, 2006). On voluntary charity see Donna Andrew, *Philanthropy and Police: London Charity in the Eighteenth Century* (Princeton: Princeton University Press, 1989), and Sarah Lloyd, *Charity and Poverty in England, c. 1680–1820: Wild and Visionary Schemes* (Manchester: Manchester University Press, 2009). On crime and disorder see Robert Shoemaker, *The London Mob: Violence and Disorder in Eighteenth-Century England* (London: Hambledon, 2004); Peter Linebaugh, *The London Hanged: Crime and Civil Society in the Eighteenth Century* (1991; New York: Verso, 2003); Peter King, *Crime and Law in England, 1750–1850: Remaking Justice at the Margins* (Cambridge: Cambridge University Press, 2006); and John Beattie, *Policing and Punishment in London, 1660–1750* (Oxford: Oxford University Press, 2001). On hospitals and institutions see Mary Fissell, *Patients, Power, and the Poor in Eighteenth-Century Bristol* (Cambridge: Cambridge University Press, 1991); Guenter Risse, *Hospital Life in Enlightenment Scotland* (Cambridge: Cambridge University Press, 1986); Susan Lawrence, *Charitable Knowledge: Hospital Pupils and Practitioners in Eighteenth-Century London* (Cambridge: Cambridge University Press, 2002); Kevin Siena, *Venereal Disease, Hospitals, and the Urban Poor: London's Foul Wards, 1600–1800* (Rochester, NY: University of Rochester Press, 2004); Jonathan Reinarz and Leonard Schwarz, eds., *Medicine in the Workhouse* (Rochester, NY: University of Rochester Press, 2013); Jeremy Boulton and John Black, "Paupers and Their Experience of a London Workhouse: St Martins-in-the-Fields, Westminster, 1725–1824," in *Residential Institutions in Britain, 1725–1950: Inmates and Environments*, ed. J. Hamlett, L. Hoskins, and R. Preston, 79–92 (London: Pickering and Chatto, 2013); Jeremy Boulton and Leonard Schwarz, "The Medicalisation of a Parish Workhouse in Georgian Westminster: St Martin in the Fields, 1725–1824," *Family and Community History* 17 (2014): 122–140; Alysa Levene, *Childcare, Health, and Mortality at the London Foundling Hospital* (Manchester: Manchester University Press, 2007); and Mary Fissell, "Charity Universal, Institutions, and

Moral Reform in Eighteenth-Century Bristol," in *Stilling the Grumbling Hive: The Response to Social and Economic Problems in England, 1689–1750*, ed. Lee Davidson, Tim Hitchcock, Tim Keirn, and Robert Shoemaker, 121–144 (New York: St. Martin's Press, 1992). On intellectual trends see Gertrude Himmelfarb, *The Idea of Poverty: England in the Early Industrial Age* (New York: Knopf, 1984); Slack, *From Reformation to Improvement;* and Paul Fideler, *Social Welfare in Pre-Industrial England* (London: Palgrave Macmillan, 2006). On social science see Andrea Rusnock, *Vital Accounts: Quantifying Health and Population in Eighteenth-Century England and France* (Cambridge: Cambridge University Press, 2002).

5. Thomas Laqueur, *Making Sex: Body and Gender from the Greeks to Freud* (Cambridge: Harvard University Press, 1992); Londa Schiebinger, *The Mind Has No Sex? Women in the Origins of Modern Science* (Cambridge: Harvard University Press, 1989); Roxann Wheeler, *Categories of Difference in Eighteenth-Century British Culture* (Philadelphia: University of Pennsylvania Press, 2000); David Bindman, *Ape to Apollo: Aesthetics and the Idea of Race in the Eighteenth Century* (Ithaca, NY: Cornell University Press, 2002); Kathleen Wilson, *The Island Race: Englishness, Empire, and Gender in the Eighteenth Century* (London: Routledge, 2002); Felicity Nussbaum, *The Limits of the Human: Fictions of Anomaly, Race, and Gender in the Long Eighteenth Century* (Cambridge: Cambridge University Press, 2003); Dror Wahrman, *The Making of the Modern Self: Identity and Culture in Eighteenth-Century England* (New Haven: Yale University Press, 2005); and Londa Schiebinger, *Nature's Body: Gender in the Making of Modern Science* (New Brunswick, NJ: Rutgers University Press, 1995).

6. The field of epigenetics studies modifications in how genes are expressed rather than alterations of the genetic code itself. It does so through analysis of methyl groups, which are chemical tags on the exterior of genes that alter DNA structure and regulate how genes are expressed—a process often described in lay terms as determining whether a gene is turned "off" or "on." In this case, numerous researchers have tested for the impact of stressors associated with poverty, such as malnourishment. Nada Borghol, Matthew Suderman, Wendy McArdle, Ariane Racine, Michael Hallett, Marcus Pembrey, Clyde Hertzman, Chris Power, and Moshe Szyf, "Associations with Early-Life Socio-Economic Position in Adult DNA Methylation," *International Journal of Epidemiology* 41, no. 1 (2012): 62–74; J. R. Swartz, A. R. Hariri, and D. E. Williamson, "An Epigenetic Mechanism Links Socioeconomic Status to Changes in Depression-Related Brain Function

in High-Risk Adolescents," *Molecular Psychiatry*, May 24, 2016, http://dx.doi.org/10.1038/mp.2016.82; and L. L. Lam, E. Emberly, H. B. Fraser, S. M. Neumann, E. Chen, G. E. Miller, and M. S. Kobor, "Factors Underlying Variable DNA Methylation in a Human Community Cohort," *Proceedings of the National Academy of Sciences* 109, supplement 2 (2012): 17253–17260. For overviews of this research in the popular press see Sara Reardon, "Poverty Linked to Epigenetic Changes and Mental Illness," *Nature*, May 24, 2016, https://www.nature.com/news/poverty-linked-to-epigenetic-changes-and-mental-illness-1.19972; Andy Coghlan, "Childhood Poverty Leaves Its Mark on Adult Genetics," *New Scientist*, October 26, 2011, https://www.newscientist.com/article/dn20255-childhood-poverty-leaves-its-mark-on-adult-genetics/; and Alison Gopnik, "Poverty's Vicious Cycle Can Affect Our Genes," *Wall Street Journal*, September 24, 2014.

7. The literature is vast. Classic studies include Asa Briggs, "The Language of 'Class' in Early Nineteenth Century England," in *Essays in Labour History*, ed. Asa Briggs and John Savile, 43–73 (London: Macmillan, 1960); Harold Perkin, *The Origins of Modern English Society* (Toronto: University of Toronto Press, 1969); John Foster, *Class Struggle and the Industrial Revolution: Early Industrial Capitalism in Three English Towns* (London: Weidenfeld and Nicolson, 1974); and, from a somewhat different perspective, Peter Laslett, *The World We Have Lost* (London: Scribner, 1965). Debates about whether to use the language of class versus that of "orders" and "ranks" for the period are well covered in Keith Wrightson, "Estates, Degrees, and Sorts: Changing Perceptions of Society in Tudor and Stuart England," in *Language, History, and Class*, ed. Penelope J. Corfield, 30–52 (Oxford: Basil Blackwell, 1991), and Peter Burke, "The Language of Orders in Early Modern Europe," in *Social Orders and Social Classes in Europe since 1500: Studies in Social Stratification*, ed. M. L. Bush, 1–12 (London: Routledge, 1992). On language, see Gareth Stedman Jones, *Languages of Class: Studies in English Working Class History, 1832–1982* (Cambridge: Cambridge University Press, 1983); Patrick Joyce, "The End of Social History?" *Social History* 20, no. 1 (1995): 73–91; and Patrick Joyce, *Visions of the People: Industrial England and the Question of Class, 1840–1914* (Cambridge: Cambridge University Press, 1991). For counterpoints see Bryan Palmer, *Descent into Discourse: The Reification of Language and the Writing of Social History* (Philadelphia: Temple University Press, 1990), and Geoff Ely and Keith Nield, *The Future of Class in History: What's Left of the Social?* (Ann Arbor: University of Michigan Press, 2007).

8. This is hardly surprising considering, as Andy Wood reminds us, that in the 1980s such leading early modern English historians as Anthony Fletcher, John Stevenson, John Morrill, David Underdown, Perez Zagorin, and J. C. D. Clark rejected the applicability of the concept, in some cases out of hand. *The Politics of Social Conflict: The Peak Country, 1520–1770* (Cambridge: Cambridge University Press, 2004), 16, and the works he cites in note 19.

9. Penelope Corfield, "Class by Name and Number in Eighteenth-Century Britain," in Corfield, *Language, Class, and History*, 101–130, 114; Porter, *English Society*, 63; Wrightson, "Estates, Degrees, and Sorts," 52; Keith Wrightson, "The Social Order of Early Modern England: Three Approaches," in *The World We Have Gained*, ed. Lloyd Bonfield, Richard M. Smith, and Keith Wrightson, 177–202 (Oxford: Basil Blackwell, 1986); and Keith Wrightson, " 'Sorts of People' in Tudor and Stuart England," in *The Middling Sort of People: Culture, Society, and Politics in England, 1500–1800*, ed. Jonathan Barry and Christopher Brooks, 28–51 (New York: St. Martin's Press, 1994).

10. Dror Wahrman, *Imagining the Middle Class: The Political Representation of Class in Britain, c. 1780–1840* (Cambridge: Cambridge University Press, 1995). See also Jerrold Seigel, *Modernity and Bourgeois Life: Society, Politics, and Culture in England, France, and Germany since 1750* (Cambridge: Cambridge University Press, 2012), 156–159. Important here as well is foundational scholarship from a feminist perspective such as Leonore Davidoff and Catherine Hall, *Family Fortunes: Men and Women of the English Middle Class, 1780–1850* (Chicago: University of Chicago Press, 1987), and Anna Clark, *Struggle for the Breeches: Gender and the Making of the British Working Class* (Berkeley: University of California Press, 1997). Here it is worth noting that traditional accounts of the timing and scope of economic change have been challenged with significant implications for the history of sixteenth- and seventeenth-century social relations. See Jan Luiten van Zanden, "The 'Revolt of the Early Modernists' and the 'First Modern Economy': An Assessment," *Economic History Review* 55 (2002): 619–641.

11. E. P. Thompson, "Patrician Society, Plebeian Culture," *Journal of Social History* 7 (1974): 382–405; E. P. Thompson, "Eighteenth-Century English Society: Class Struggle without Class?" *Social History* 3 (1978): 133–165; and Thompson's response to critics in *Customs in Common* (New York: New Press, 1991), 87–96. On the middling sort see Barry and Brooks, *The Middling Sort of People;* Peter Earle, *The Making of the English Middle Class: Business, Society, and Family Life in London, 1660–1730* (Berkeley:

University of California Press, 1989); Margaret Hunt, *The Middling Sort: Commerce, Gender, and the Family in England, 1680–1780* (Berkeley: University of California Press, 1996); H. R. French, *The Middle Sort of People in Provincial England, 1600–1750* (Oxford: Oxford University Press, 2007); and H. R. French, "The Search for the 'Middle Sort of People' in England, 1600–1800," *Historical Journal* 43, no. 1 (2000): 277–293. Like these scholars, Corfield also demonstrates that these polar formulations coexisted with tripartite visions of lower, middle, and upper, which were also common throughout the century. Corfield, "Class by Name and Number," 117–119. We will see that doctors discussing contagion overwhelmingly opted for the former. Wrightson, "Social Order," 183; Wood, *Politics of Social Conflict*, 9, 22–24; and Craig Muldrew, "Class and Credit: Social Identity, Wealth, and the Life Course in Early Modern England," in *Identity and Agency in England, 1500–1800*, ed. Henry French and Jonathan Barry, 147–177, 149 (London: Palgrave Macmillan, 2004). Summarizing the literature Alexandra Shepard similarly acknowledges that work on the middling orders likewise showcases a tendency to frame identity in moral terms, especially through negative distinction: "Middling-sort identities were more negatively founded on their distinction from morally reprehensible 'others' (that is, the poorer, meaner, vulgar, baser sorts) than positively articulated through assertions of belonging to a clearly bounded social group." *Accounting for Oneself: Worth, Status, and the Social Order in Early Modern England* (Oxford: Oxford University Press, 2015), 7.

12. Lees, *Solidarities of Strangers*, 23; Steve Hindle, "Civility, Honesty, and the Identification of the Deserving Poor in Seventeenth-Century England," in French and Barry, *Identity and Agency in England*, 38–59; Jeremy Boulton, "The 'Meaner Sort': Labouring People and the Poor," in *A Social History of England, 1550–1750*, ed. Keith Wrightson, 310–329 (Cambridge: Cambridge University Press, 2017); and A. L. Beier, *Masterless Men: The Vagrancy Problem in England, 1560–1640* (London: Methuen, 1985). For the most recent exploration of the subtle gradients by which the poor described themselves, see Shepard, *Accounting for Oneself*, 114–146.

13. Wahrman, *Imagining the Middle Class*, 16; John L. Austin, *How to Do Things with Words* (Cambridge: Harvard University Press, 1962), lecture VIII, 94–108; Timothy McInerney, "The Better Sort: Nobility and Human Variety in Eighteenth-Century Great Britain," *Journal for Eighteenth-Century Studies* 38, no. 1 (2015): 47–63; Timothy McInerney, "Race and Nobility in the Works of Johann Reinhold and Georg Forster," *Études anglaises* 66, no. 2

(2013): 250–266; and Roy Porter and G. S. Rousseau, *Gout: The Patrician Malady* (New Haven: Yale University Press, 2000), 98.

14. As Laura Gowing asserts for the period, "The term 'gender' is a modern and contested one. It depends on a distinction between biological sex and cultural gender which was crucial to feminism, but which was not made by historians of a hundred years ago, and which does not necessarily describe the way sexual difference was understood before about 1750." *Gender Relations in Early Modern England* (London: Routledge, 2012), 4. I discuss the literature on race in the Conclusion.

15. Wood, *Politics of Social Conflict*, 9. On the sixteenth century see Andy Wood, *The 1549 Rebellions and the Making of Early Modern England* (Cambridge: Cambridge University Press, 2007).

16. It is telling of the need for a study such as this one that an excellent survey of the Enlightenment like Dorinda Outram's devotes an entire chapter to the question of gender and two to the issue of race, yet nowhere explores the eighteenth-century ideological constructions of class. *The Enlightenment* (Cambridge: Cambridge University Press, 2013), see chapters 5–7, 43–83.

17. Here Alexandra Shepard's and Andy Wood's explorations of how early modern men and women described themselves in court documents represent major steps forward. Shepard, *Accounting for Oneself*, and Wood, *The Memory of the People: Custom and Popular Senses of the Past in Early Modern England* (Cambridge: Cambridge University Press, 2013). See also John Smail, *The Origins of Middle Class Culture: Halifax, Yorkshire, 1660–1780* (Ithaca, NY: Cornell University Press, 1994.)

18. For statements on the approach see Tim Hitchcock, "A New History from Below," *History Workshop Journal* 57 (2004): 294–298, and Tim Hitchcock, *Down and Out in Eighteenth-Century London* (London: Hambledon, 2004), especially "The History of the Poor," 233–240. A sample of this research includes Peter King and Pamela Sharpe, eds., *Chronicling Poverty: The Voices and Strategies of the English Poor, 1640–1840* (Basingstoke: Macmillan, 1997); Jeremy Boulton, " 'It Is Extreme Necessity That Makes Me Do This': Some Survival Strategies of Pauper Households in London's West End during the Eighteenth Century," *International Review of Social History* 45 (2000): 47–69; King and Tomkins, *The Poor in England;* Steven King, Thomas Nutt, and Alannah Tomkins, eds., *Narratives of the Poor in Eighteenth-Century England,* vol. 1, *Voices of the Poor* (London: Pickering and Chatto, 2006); Shoemaker, *The London Mob;* Alannah Tomkins, *The Experience of Urban Poverty, 1723–82: Parish, Charity, and Credit* (Manchester: Manchester University Press,

2006); Lynn MacKay, *Respectability and the London Poor, 1780–1870: The Value of Virtue* (London: Pickering and Chatto, 2013); and Steven King and Peter Jones, eds., *Obligation, Entitlement, and Dispute under the Poor Laws* (Newcastle upon Tyne: Cambridge Scholars Press, 2015). The potential of the approach has been most recently demonstrated by Tim Hitchcock and Robert Shoemaker's magisterial *London Lives: Poverty, Crime, and the Making of a Modern City, 1690–1800* (Cambridge: Cambridge University Press, 2015).

19. The best surveys are Keith Wrightson's: *English Society, 1580–1680* (London: Hutchison, 1982) and *Earthly Necessities: Economic Lives in Early Modern Britain* (New Haven: Yale University Press, 2002). See also Robert Jütte, *Poverty and Deviance in Early Modern Europe* (Cambridge: Cambridge University Press, 1994); Beier, *Masterless Men;* David Hitchcock, *Vagrancy in English Culture and Society, 1650–1750* (London: Bloomsbury, 2016); and Audrey Eccles, *Vagrancy in Law and Practice under the Old Poor Law* (New York: Routledge, 2016).

20. For studies of numerous expressions of concern by such organizations as the Society for the Reformation of Manners, see the contributions to Davidson et al., *Stilling the Grumbling Hive,* as well as Faramerz Dabhoiwala, "Sex and Societies for Moral Reform, 1688–1800," *Journal of British Studies* 46, no. 2 (2007): 290–319; Joanna Innes, "Politics and Morals: The Reformation of Manners Movement in Later Eighteenth-Century England," in *The Transformation of Political Culture: England and Germany in the Late Eighteenth Century,* ed. Eckhart Hellmuth, 57–118 (Oxford: Oxford University Press, 1990); and Jessica Warner, *Craze: Gin and Debauchery in an Age of Reason* (London: Profile, 2003).

21. Lees, *Solidarities of Strangers,* 41, 94–100; Himmelfarb, *Idea of Poverty,* passim. Alysa Levene usefully summarizes these trends in her introduction to *Narratives of the Poor in Eighteenth-Century Britain,* vol. 1 (London: Pickering and Chatto, 2006), vii–xvi. Hitchcock, *Vagrancy in English Culture and Society,* 20, 27, 149–152.

22. Hans Zinsser, *Rats, Lice, and History* (Boston: Little Brown, 1935), and Charles Creighton, *A History of Epidemics in Britain,* 2 vols. (Cambridge: Cambridge University Press, 1891). For an introduction to retrospective diagnosis see Jon Arrizabalaga, "Problematizing Retrospective Diagnosis in the History of Disease," *Asclepio* 54 (2002): 51–70.

23. T. R. McKeown and R. G. Brown, "Medical Evidence Relating to English Population Changes in the Eighteenth Century," *Population Studies* 9 (1955): 115–141; and T. R. McKeown, *The Modern Rise of Population* (London:

Edward Arnold, 1976). McKeown's nutrition thesis was challenged by R. Schofield, "Population Growth in the Century after 1750: The Role of Mortality Decline," and A. Perrenoud, "Mortality Decline in Its Secular Setting," both in *Pre-Industrial Population Change: The Mortality Decline and Short-Term Population Movements*, ed. Tommy Bengtsson et al., 17–39 and 41–69, respectively (Stockholm: Almsquist and Wiksell International, 1984); Stephen J. Kunitz, "Speculations on the European Mortality Decline," *Economic History Review* 36 (1983): 349–364; and Simon Szreter, "The Importance of Social Intervention in Britain's Mortality Decline, c. 1850–1914: A Re-Interpretation of the Role of Public Health," *Social History of Medicine* 1 (1988): 1–38.

24. John Landers, *Death and the Metropolis: Studies in the Demographic History of London, 1670–1830* (Cambridge: Cambridge University Press, 1993), 240; E. A. Wrigley and Roger Schofield, *The Population of England, 1541–1871: A Reconstitution* (London: Edward Arnold, 1981), 244; and Alexander Mercer, *Infections, Chronic Disease, and the Epidemiological Transition: A New Perspective* (Rochester, NY: University of Rochester Press, 2014), 43–47, 56, 61, 77–81.

25. Stephen J. Kunitz, "Making a Long Story Short: A Note on Men's Heights and Mortality in England from the First through the Nineteenth Centuries," *Medical History* 31 (1987): 269–280, and Roderick Floud, Annabel Gregory, and Kenneth Wachter, *Height, Health, and History: Nutritional Status in the United Kingdom, 1750–1980* (Cambridge: Cambridge University Press, 1991). Peter Razzell has challenged the consensus opinion that height is a useful indicator of health for various social groups in the late eighteenth and nineteenth centuries. *Population and Disease: Transforming English Society, 1550–1850* (London: Caliban, 2007), 273.

26. Landers, *Death and the Metropolis*, 258, 265–266, 284–350. As Landers notes, the nutritional impact on resistance to typhus appears to have been modest, as evidenced by the frequency of weak relations between fever deaths and prices. However, extreme price rises could have a stronger effect, often by way of a "lagged response," leading to his conclusion that the effects of high prices probably "reflected underlying changes in the determinants of exposure" rather than weakened immunity from malnourishment (266). See also A. B. Appleby, "Nutrition and Disease: The Case of London, 1550–1750," *Journal of Interdisciplinary History* 6 (1975): 1–22; Razzell, *Population and Disease*, 111–119.

27. Landers, *Death and the Metropolis*, 356–357; J. D. Chambers, *Population, Economy, and Society in Pre-Industrial England* (Oxford: Oxford University

Press, 1972), 102–106; Razzell, *Population and Disease*, 19–22, 140–142, 168–176; James Riley, *The Eighteenth-Century Campaign to Avoid Disease* (London: Macmillan, 1987), 113–138.

28. On theories of fever in the period see relevant chapters in W. F. Bynum and Vivian Nutton, *Theories of Fever from Antiquity to the Enlightenment* (London: Wellcome Institute for the History of Medicine, 1981), and Riley, *Eighteenth-Century Campaign to Avoid Disease*. On fever in tropical and military medicine see Mark Harrison, *Climates and Constitutions: Health, Race, Environment, and British Imperialism in India, 1600–1850* (Oxford: Oxford University Press, 1999), and Mark Harrison, *Medicine in an Age of Commerce and Empire: Britain and Its Tropical Colonies, 1660–1830* (Oxford: Oxford University Press, 2010). On childbed fever see Margaret DeLacy, "Puerperal Fever in Eighteenth-Century Britain," *Bulletin of the History of Medicine* 63 (1989): 521–556; Christine Hallett, "The Attempt to Understand Puerperal Fever in the Eighteenth and Early Nineteenth Centuries: The Influence of Inflammation Theory," *Medical History* 49, no. 1 (2005): 1–28; and Irvine Loudon, *The Tragedy of Childbed Fever* (Oxford: Oxford University Press, 2000). On yellow fever see J. Worth Estes and Billy G. Smith, eds., *A Melancholy Scene of Devastation: The Public Response to the 1793 Philadelphia Yellow Fever Epidemic* (Canton, MA: Science History Publications, 1997); J. H. Powell, *Bring Out Your Dead: The Great Plague of Yellow Fever in Philadelphia in 1793* (Philadelphia: University of Pennsylvania Press, 1993); and Margaret Humphreys, *Yellow Fever and the South* (Baltimore: Johns Hopkins University Press, 1992).

29. Hamlin, *More than Hot*, 163; Candace Ward, *Desire and Disorder: Fevers, Fictions, and Feeling in English Georgian Culture* (Lewisburg, PA: Bucknell University Press, 2007), 100–148; Pelling, *Cholera, Fever, and English Medicine;* and Christopher Hamlin, *Public Health and Social Justice in the Age of Chadwick* (Cambridge: Cambridge University Press, 1998).

30. Erwin H. Ackerknecht, "Anticontagionism between 1821 and 1867," *Bulletin of the History of Medicine* 22 (1948): 562–593. Ackerknecht's thesis that nations' political systems influenced their prevailing disease theories has been tested and reassessed in Peter Baldwin, *Contagion and the State in Europe, 1830–1930* (Cambridge: Cambridge University Press, 1999); Margaret DeLacy, "Nosology, Mortality, and Disease Theory in the Eighteenth Century," *Journal of the History of Medicine and Allied Sciences* 54, no. 2 (1999): 261–284. Hamlin, *More than Hot*, 69–86, 110–112; and Arnold Zuckerman, "Plague and Contagionism in Eighteenth-Century England:

The Role of Richard Mead," *Bulletin of the History of Medicine* 78, no. 2 (2004): 273–308.

31. Pelling, *Cholera, Fever, and English Medicine*, 18; Hamlin, *Public Health and Social Justice*, 60–61.

32. Margaret DeLacy, *The Germ of an Idea: Contagionism, Religion, and Society in Britain, 1660–1730* (New York: Palgrave Macmillan, 2016), and Margaret DeLacy, *Contagionism Catches On: Medical Ideology in Britain, 1730–1800* (New York: Palgrave Macmillan, 2016).

33. Charles MacLean, *The Plague not Contagious; or, A Dissertation on the Source of Epidemic and Pestilential Diseases* (London: The Author, 1800), 39–40.

34. John V. Pickstone, "From Ferriar's Fever to Kay's Cholera: Disease and Social Structure in Cottonopolis," *History of Science* 22 (1984): 401–419; John V. Pickstone, "Dearth, Dirt, and Fever Epidemics: Rewriting the History of British 'Public Health,' 1780–1850," in *Epidemics and Ideas: Essays on the Historical Perception of Pestilence*, ed. Terrance Ranger and Paul Slack, 125–148 (Cambridge: Cambridge University Press, 1992); and John V. Pickstone, *Medicine and Industrial Society: A History of Hospital Development in Manchester and Its Region, 1752–1946* (Manchester: Manchester University Press, 1985), 23–41.

35. DeLacy, *Contagionism Catches On*, chapters 7 and 8.

36. Roy Porter, "Cleaning up the Great Wen: Public Health in Eighteenth-Century London," *Medical History* 11 (1991): 61–75.

1. *Plague, Putrefaction, and the Poor*

1. By pursuing the story to the 1720s Paul Slack's seminal *The Impact of Plague in Tudor and Stuart England* (Oxford: Oxford University Press, 1985) shows its importance yet again. See 311–337. Studies of Richard Mead or Daniel Defoe explore select eighteenth-century topics, though primarily for the 1720s. Arnold Zuckerman, "Plague and Contagionism in Eighteenth-Century England: The Role of Richard Mead," *Bulletin of the History of Medicine* 78, no. 2 (2004): 273–308. On Defoe's plague writing see Wayne Wild, " 'Due Preparations': Defoe and Dr. Mead and the Threat of Plague," in *Liberating Medicine, 1720–1835*, ed. Tristanne Connolly and Steve Clark, 55–68 (London: Pickering and Chatto, 2009); Robert Mayer, "The Reception of *A Journal of the Plague Year* and the Nexus of Fiction and History in the Novel," *English Literary History* 57, no. 3 (1990): 529–555; Ernest B. Gilman, *Plague Writing in Early Modern England* (Chicago: University of Chicago Press, 2009), 229–243; and John Bender, *Imagining the Penitentiary: Fiction*

and the Architecture of the Mind in the Eighteenth Century (Chicago: University of Chicago Press, 1987), 63–86.

2. Margaret Healy, *Fictions of Disease in Early Modern England* (New York: Palgrave, 2001), 101–122. On the poor as both bearers and victims of plague see Brian Pullan, "Plague and Perceptions of the Poor in Early Modern Italy," in *Epidemics and Ideas: Essays on the Historical Perception of Pestilence,* ed. Terrance Ranger and Paul Slack, 101–124, esp. 107 (Cambridge: Cambridge University Press, 1992); Robert Jütte, *Poverty and Deviance in Early Modern Europe* (Cambridge: Cambridge University Press, 1994); Samuel Cohn, *Cultures of Plague: Medical Thinking at the End of the Renaissance* (Oxford: Oxford University Press, 2009), 210–215. John Henderson, "Charity and Welfare in Early Modern Tuscany," in *Health Care and Poor Relief in Counter Reformation Europe,* ed. Ole Peter Grell, Andrew Cunningham, and Jon Arrizabalaga, 56–86, 78 (London: Routledge, 1999); Slack, *Impact of Plague,* 239. This is not to argue that medieval commentators never made the link. Carol Rawcliffe notes charges of plague as *"morbus pauperum"* in the late Middle Ages. *Medicine for the Soul: The Life, Death, and Resurrection of an English Hospital: St. Giles Norwich, c. 1249–1550* (Stroud, UK: Sutton, 1999), 215.

3. Slack, *Impact of Plague,* 111–143, 199–226, 252–253, 284–310, 336–337; F. P. Wilson, *The Plague in Shakespeare's London* (Oxford: Oxford University Press, 1963), 18, 22–26, 51, 89, 115, 120, 133, 162, 165–166; Ann Carmichael, *Plague and the Poor in Renaissance Florence* (Cambridge: Cambridge University Press, 1986), 108–126; Cohn, *Cultures of Plague,* 223–227; and Pullan, "Plague and Perceptions." Jane Stevens Crawshaw sees the connection coming slightly later in Venice, not until the seventeenth century. *Plague Hospitals: Public Health for the City in Early Modern Venice* (London: Routledge, 2012), 79–108. Michael J. Braddick, *State Formation in Early Modern England, c. 1550–1700* (Cambridge: Cambridge University Press, 2001), 103–135. Also Michel Foucault, *Discipline and Punish: The Birth of the Prison,* trans. Alan Sheridan (New York: Pantheon, 1977), 195–200, and Michel Foucault, *Abnormal: Lectures at the College de France, 1974–1975,* trans. G. Burchell (London: Verso, 2003), 43–48. J. A. I. Champion, "Epidemics and the Built Environment in 1665," in *Epidemic Disease in London,* ed. J. A. I. Champion, 35–52 (London: Centre for Metropolitan History Working Papers Series, no. 1, 1993); J. A. I. Champion, *London's Dreaded Visitation: The Social Geography of the Great Plague of London, 1665* (London: Centre For Metropolitan History, 1995), passim; A. Lloyd Moote

and Dorothy Moote, *The Great Plague: The Story of London's Most Deadly Year* (Baltimore: Johns Hopkins University Press, 2004), 46–50, 60–61. Vanessa Harding, "The Changing Shape of Seventeenth-Century London," in *Imagining Early Modern London: Perceptions and Portrayals of the City from Stow to Stype, 1593–1720*, ed. J. F. Merritt, 133–135 (Cambridge: Cambridge University Press, 2001). For an overview of mortality statistics in the birth of political economy see Andrea Rusnock, *Vital Accounts: Quantifying Health and Population in Eighteenth-Century England and France* (Cambridge: Cambridge University Press, 2002), 15–41. Raymond A. Anselment, *The Realms of Apollo: Literature and Healing in Seventeenth-Century England* (Newark: University of Delaware Press, 1994), 95; Healy, *Fictions of Disease*, 109; Paula Pugliatti, *Beggary and Theatre in Early Modern England* (Aldershot, UK: Ashgate, 2003), 107–122.

4. On contagion and miasma theories in England see Slack, *Impact of Plague*, 26–28, 36–47; Andrew Wear, *Knowledge and Practice in English Medicine, 1550–1680* (Cambridge: Cambridge University Press, 2000), 298–303; Ann Carmichael, "Contagion Theory and Contagion Practice in Fifteenth-Century Milan," *Renaissance Quarterly* 44 (1991): 197–256; Carlo M. Cipolla, *Public Health and the Medical Profession in the Renaissance* (Cambridge: Cambridge University Press, 1976); Carlo M. Cipolla, *Miasmas and Disease: Public Health and the Environment in the Pre-Industrial Age*, trans. Elizabeth Potter (New Haven: Yale University Press, 1992); and Vivian Nutton, "The Reception of Fracastoro's Theory of Contagion: The Seed That Fell among Thorns?" *Osiris* 6 (1990): 126–234. On the difficulty of cleanly dividing these camps see Margaret DeLacy, "Nosology, Mortality, and Disease Theory in the Eighteenth Century," *Journal of the History of Medicine and Allied Sciences* 54, no. 2 (1999): 261–284; Dorothy Porter, *Health, Civilization, and the State: A History of Public Health from Ancient to Modern Times* (London: Routledge, 1999), 54–56; and Annemarie Kinzelbach, "Infection, Contagion, and Public Health in Late Medieval and Early Modern German Imperial Towns," *Journal of the History of Medicine and Allied Sciences* 61, no. 3 (2006): 369–389. On plague and disorder see Slack, *Impact of Plague*, 295–307; Carmichael, *Plague and the Poor*, 116–126; Healy, *Fictions of Disease*, 89–97, and Margaret Healy, "Discourses of the Plague in Early Modern London," in Champion, *Epidemic Disease in London*, 19–34; Jütte, *Poverty and Deviance*, 22–23, 109.

5. Wear, *Knowledge and Practice*, 275–276, 282.

6. Ibid., 136–141, 414–415; Patricia Crawford, "Attitudes to Menstruation in Seventeenth-Century England," *Past and Present* 91 (1981): 47–73; Audrey

Eccles, *Obstetrics and Gynaecology in Tudor and Stuart England* (Kent, OH: Kent State University Press, 1982), 49–50; Hilda Smith, "Gynecology and Ideology in Seventeenth-Century England," in *Liberating Women's History: Theoretical and Critical Essays,* ed. Berenice A. Carroll, 97–114 (Urbana: University of Illinois Press, 1976); Alexandra Lord, " 'The Great Arcana of the Deity': Menstruation and Menstrual Disorders in Eighteenth-Century British Medical Thought," *Bulletin of the History of Medicine* 73 (1999): 38–63; Kaara L. Peterson, "Re-Anatomizing Melancholy: Burton and the Logic of Humouralism," in *Textual Healing: Essays on Medieval and Early Modern Medicine,* ed. Elizabeth Lane Furdell, 149–167 (Leiden: Brill, 2005); Gail Kern Paster, "The Unbearable Coldness of Female Being: Women's Imperfection and the Humoral Economy," *English Literary Renaissance* 28, no. 3 (1998): 416–440; and Carlo Ginzburg, *The Cheese and the Worms: The Cosmos of a Sixteenth-Century Miller,* trans. John Tedeschi and Anne Tedeschi (Baltimore: Johns Hopkins University Press, 1980), xi.

7. Christopher Hamlin, *More than Hot: A Short History of Fever* (Baltimore: Johns Hopkins University Press, 2014), 45–48, 119; Cohn, *Cultures of Plague,* 213, 216, 222. Also excellent is chapter 3, "Plague, Poison, and Putrefaction" in Frederick Gibbs, "Medical Understandings of Poison circa 1250–1600," Ph.D. diss., University of Wisconsin, 2009, 116–156; Mark Jenner, "Early Modern English Conceptions of 'Cleanliness' and 'Dirt,' as Reflected in the Environmental Regulation of London, c. 1530–c. 1700," D.Phil. thesis, Oxford University, 1991; Mark Jenner, " 'Nauceious and Abominable'? Pollution, Plague, and Poetics in John Gay's *Trivia,*" in *Walking the Streets of Eighteenth-Century London: John Gay's "Trivia,"* ed. Clare Brant and Susan Whyman, 90–104 (Oxford: Oxford University Press, 2007); Mark Jenner, "Death, Decomposition, and Dechristianization? Public Health and Church Burial in Eighteenth-Century England," *English Historical Review* 120, no. 487 (2005): 615–632; Vanessa Harding, "Burial of the Plague Dead in Early Modern London," in Champion, *Epidemic Disease in London,* 53–64; and Vanessa Harding, *The Dead and the Living in Paris and London, 1500–1670* (Cambridge: Cambridge University Press, 2002), 82–83, 112–113. On the slippage between physical and nonphysical forms of corruption see Gilman, *Plague Writing,* 42–48, 129–162, 210; Healy, "Discourses of the Plague"; Anselment, *Realms of Apollo,* 96–98; and Slack, *Impact of Plague,* 29–50.

8. Mary Douglas, *Purity and Danger: An Analysis of Concepts of Pollution and Taboo* (London: Routledge and Kegan Paul, 1966); and Alain Corbin, *The Foul and the Fragrant: Odor and the French Social Imagination* (Cambridge:

Harvard University Press, 1986). For an extensive review of this approach
see Mark Jenner, "Follow Your Nose: Smell, Smelling, and Their Histories,"
American Historical Review 16, no. 2 (2011): 335–351. Leona J. Skelton, *Sanita-
tion in Urban Britain, 1560–1700* (New York: Routledge, 2016), 36–40; Cohn,
Cultures of Plague, 215–218; Gibbs, "Medical Understandings of Poison";
Wear, *Knowledge and Practice,* 303–313; Margaret DeLacy, *The Germ of an
Idea: Contagionism, Religion, and Society in Britain, 1660–1730* (New York:
Palgrave Macmillan, 2016), 10–12, 26–27, 40–41, 154–165; Kevin Siena,
"Pollution, Promiscuity, and the Pox: English Venereology and the Early
Modern Medical Discourse on Social and Sexual Danger," *Journal of the
History of Sexuality* 8, no. 4 (1998): 553–574, esp. 562–570. Richard Mead
provided the authoritative account of poisons for the eighteenth century, *A
Mechanical Account of Poisons* (London: R. J. for Richard Smith, 1702). On
Mead see Zuckerman, "Plague and Contagionism"; Hamlin, *More than Hot,*
83–84; William Austin, *Epiloimia epe; or, The anatomy of the pestilence, a poem
in three parts* (London: Nath. Brooke, 1666), 6. Fracastoro similarly
compared the infected heart to a rotten apple. Nutton, "Reception of Fracastoro's Theory," 212.

9. Paul Barbette, *Thesaurus Chirurgiae . . . together with a treatise of the Plague*
(London: Henry Rhodes, 1687), 121; Thomas Brasbridge, *The Poore Mans
Jewel, that is to say, A Treatise of the Pestilence* (London: George Byshop,
1578), Caps. 3, 8, 10; Hamlin, *More than Hot,* 48.

10. Barbette, *Thesaurus Chirurgiae,* chapter 4; Vivian Nutton, "The Seeds of
Disease: An Explanation of Contagion and Infection from the Greeks to the
Renaissance," *Medical History* 27, no. 1 (1983): 1–34; Nutton, "Reception of
Fracastoro's Theory," 201, 205, 208, 210–213, 222–223; Gibbs, "Medical
Understandings of Poison," 190.

11. Carmichael, *Plague and the Poor,* 127–131; Nutton, "Seeds of Disease," 4, 6,
15–16, 26; also Nutton, "Reception of Fracastoro's Theory," 212, 226;
Girolamo Fracastoro, *De Contagione et Contagiosis Morbis et Eorum Cura-
tione, Libri III,* trans. Wilmer Cave Wright (New York: Putnam, 1930),
83–87.

12. Wear, *Knowledge and Practice,* 154–209; Peter H. Niebyl, "The Non-
Naturals," *Bulletin of the History of Medicine* 45 (1971): 486–492; Louise
Curth, "Lessons from the Past: Preventative Medicine in Early Modern
England," *Medical Humanities* 29 (2003): 16–21; Roy Porter, "The Patient in
England, c. 1660–1800," and Guenter Risse, "Medicine in the Age of
Enlightenment," both in *Medicine in Society: Historical Essays,* ed. Andrew

Wear, 91–118 and 149–196, respectively, esp. 99, 108, 150–152 (Cambridge: Cambridge University Press, 1992).

13. See "De Pestilentibus Febribus," in Fracastoro, *De Contagione*, 83–87.

14. Nutton, "Seeds of Disease," 27–28, 31; Hamlin, *More than Hot*, 61; Nathaniel Hodges, *Loimologia: or, an Historical Account of the Plague in London in 1665* (London, 1721), 86, originally published as *Loimologia, sive, Pestis nuperæ apud populum Londinensem grassantis narratio historica* (London: Gul. Godbid, 1671). Gideon Harvey defined plague thus: "The Plague is a most Malignant and Contagious Feaver." *A Discourse of the Plague containing the Nature, Causes, Signs, and Presages of the Pestilence in general, together with the state of the present contagion* (London, 1665), 2; Thomas Willis, *A Plain and Easie Method for Preserving (by God's blessing) those that are well from the infection of the Plague, or any contagious distemper in city, camp, fleet, &c* (London: W. Crook, 1691), 25.

15. Thomas Sydenham, *Collections of Acute Diseases, the second and third part* (London: J. R., 1688), 3, 21–22, 66. See also Harvey, *Discourse of the Plague*, 2–3. On the influence of these ideas in the eighteenth century see William Grant, *An Essay on the Pestilential Fever of Sydenham, commonly called the Gaol, Hospital, Ship and Camp-Fever* (London: T. Cadell, 1775); Mark Harrison, *Medicine in an Age of Commerce and Empire: Britain and Its Tropical Colonies, 1660–1830* (Oxford: Oxford University Press, 2010), 31–32. On the early modern diseases' ability to morph into other ailments see Claudia Stein, *Negotiating the French Pox in Early Modern Germany* (Burlington, VT: Ashgate, 2009), 55–56, 142–143, 171, 177.

16. Cohn, *Cultures of Plague*, 209; William Bullein, *A Dialogue bothe Pleasaunte and Pietifull wherein is a Goodly Regimente against the Feuer Pestilence with a Consolacion and Comfort against Death* (London: Ihon, Kingston, 1564), fol. 4, and Brasbridge, *Poore Mans Jewel*, Cap. 9.

17. Steven Bradwell, *A Watch-Man for the Pest. Teaching the True Rules of Preservation from the Pestilent Contagion, at this time fearefully over-flowing this famous Citie of London* (London: Iohn Dawson and George Vincent, 1625), 4, 18, 36, 43.

18. Ibid., 45–46; and Cohn, *Cultures of Plague*, 221.

19. Bradwell, *Watch-Man for the Pest*, 45; Hodges, *Loimologia*, 56.

20. Bradwell, *Watch-Man for the Pest*, 8–11, 13, 18, 23–31, 37, 44, 48; A. L. Beier, *Masterless Men: The Vagrancy Problem in England, 1560–1640* (London: Methuen, 1985), 4–7, 38, 86, 151, 165; Pugliatti, *Beggary and Theatre*, 55–63; Abigail Rachel Scherer, "Idleness in Early Modern English Literature,"

Ph.D. diss., University of Alabama, 2004; David Hitchcock, *Vagrancy in English Culture and Society, 1650–1750* (London: Bloomsbury, 2016), 21–54; Sarah Jordan, *The Anxieties of Idleness: Idleness in Eighteenth-Century British Literature and Culture* (Lewisburg, PA: Bucknell University Press, 2003).

21. Tommasi quoted in Cohn, *Cultures of Plague*, 213; Michelle DiMeo, "Openness and Secrecy in the Hartib Circle: Revisiting 'Democratic Baconianism' in Interregnum England," in *Secrets and Knowledge in Medicine and Science, 1500–1800*, ed. Elaine Leong and Alisha Rankin, 105–124, 113 (London: Routledge, 2011); and Michael MacDonald, *Witchcraft and Hysteria in Elizabethan London: Edward Jorden and the Mary Glover Case* (London: Routledge, 1991), xv–xvi. Lauren Kassell identifies him as Banister's son-in-law, although Jonathan Sanderson suggests he was Banister's grandson. Kassell, "Casebooks in Early Modern England: Medicine, Astrology, and Written Records," *Bulletin of the History of Medicine* 88, no. 4 (2014): 595–625, 617, and Jonathan Sanderson, "Nicholas Culpeper and the Book Trade: Print and the Promotion of Vernacular Medical Knowledge, 1649–65," Ph.D. diss., Leeds University, 1999, 22–23. Sanderson further notes that Bradwell got into trouble with the college in 1609 and 1610, a point supported by Margaret Pelling, *Medical Conflicts in Early Modern London: Patronage, Physicians, and Irregular Practitioners, 1550–1640* (Oxford: Clarendon, 2003), 70n50, 291; Jonathan Gil Harris, *Sick Economies: Drama, Mercantilism, and Disease in Shakespeare's England* (Philadelphia: University of Pennsylvania Press, 2004), 112–114; Stephen [*sic*] Bradwell, *Helps for suddain accidents endangering life. By which those that live farre from physitions or chirurgions may happily preserve the life of a poore friend or neighbour, till such a man may be had to perfect the cure* (London: Thomas Purfoot, 1633), as well as Stephan [*sic*] Bradwell, "Mary Glovers Late Woeful Case, Together with her Joyfull Deliverance," printed in MacDonald, *Witchcraft and Hysteria*, 3. See also Laura Gowing, *Common Bodies: Women, Touch, and Power in Seventeenth-Century England* (New Haven: Yale University Press, 2003), 79–80.

22. Harvey, *Discourse of the Plague*, 8–9; Hodges, *Loimologia*, 20, 58–59; and Nathaniel Hodges, *Vindiciae Medicinae & Medicorum* (London: John Field, 1665), 232.

23. Slack, *Impact of Plague*, 305. On anxieties about alehouses see Beier, *Masterless Men*, 11, 38, 85, and Peter Clark, "The Alehouse and the Alternative Society," in *Puritans and Revolutionaries: Essays in Seventeenth-Century History Presented to Christopher Hill*, ed. Donald Pennington and Keith Thomas, 47–72 (Oxford: Oxford University Press, 1978). On tensions

NOTES

surrounding the deserving vs. undeserving poor see Jütte, *Poverty and Deviance;* Paul Slack, *From Reformation to Improvement: Public Welfare in Early Modern England* (Oxford: Clarendon, 1998); Paul Fideler, *Social Welfare in Pre-Industrial England* (New York: Palgrave, 2006), 8–67; Patricia Fumerton, *Unsettled: The Culture and Mobility of the Working Poor in Early Modern England* (Chicago: University of Chicago Press, 2006); Clare Schen, "Constructing the Poor in Seventeenth-Century London," *Albion* 32, no. 3 (2000): 450–463; Steve Hindle, "Dependency, Shame, and Belonging: Badging the Deserving Poor," *Cultural and Social History* 1, no. 1 (2004): 6–35.

24. Harvey, *Discourse of the Plague,* 5.

25. Ibid., 16–18, 21–22.

26. The OED gives the etymology: "Greek κακόχῡμος with unhealthy humours, < κακο-bad + χῡμός juice, humour."

27. Thomas Cock, *Advice for the Poor by way of cure & caution* (London, 1665), 1–3; Harvey, *Discourse of the Plague,* 15–16.

28. Thomas Lodge, *A Treatise of the Plague* (London, 1603), sig. A2, fol. F1v; Wear, *Knowledge and Practice,* 282; Penelope Corfield, "Class by Name and Number in Eighteenth-Century Britain," in *Language, Class, and History,* ed. Penelope J. Corfield, 101–130, 117–119 (Oxford: Basil Blackwell, 1991).

29. Corporation of London, *By the mayor the right honourable the lord mayor . . . considering how the infection of the plague is dispersed,* 1.

30. Carmichael, *Plague and the Poor,* 131.

31. Hodges, *Vindiciae Medicinae,* 161–162; Thomas Elyot, *The Dictionary of Sir Thomas Elyot Knyght* (London: Thomae Bertheleti, 1538), [n. p.]; Thomas Blount *Glossographia, or, A Dictionary* (London: T. B., 1661), [n.p.]; Early English Books Online, https://eebo.chadwyck.com/home, searched July 15, 2011.

32. On the debates generated by the rise of the new science see Harold Cook, "Physicians and the New Philosophy: Henry Stubbe and the Virtuosi-Physicians," in *The Medical Revolution of the Seventeenth Century,* ed. Andrew Cunningham and Roger French, 246–271 (Cambridge: Cambridge University Press, 1989); Harold Cook, "The Society of Chemical Physicians, the New Philosophy, and the Restoration Court," *Bulletin of the History of Medicine* 61 (1987): 61–77; and Harold Cook, *The Decline of the Old Medical Regime in Stuart London* (Ithaca, NY: Cornell University Press, 1986), esp. 150–155; Wear, *Knowledge and Practice,* 353–398. On Thomson see Charles Webster, "The Helmontonian George Thomson and William

Harvey: The Revival and Application of Slpenectomy to Physiological Research," *Medical History* 15 (1971): 154–167; Cook, "Society of Chemical Physicians," 71. Webster elsewhere called Thomson "the most active Helmontonian pamphleteer." *The Great Instauration: Science, Medicine, and Reform, 1626–1660* (London: Duckworth, 1975), 282.

33. Hodges, *Vindiciae Medicinae*, 161–162; George Thomson, *Galeno-pale; or, a chymical trial of the Galenists* (London: R. Wood, 1665), 67, and George Thomson, *Loimotomia, or, The pest anatomized* (London: Nath. Crouch, 1666), 157. For a literary analysis of *Loimotomia*, see Gilman, *Plague Writing*, 117–125.

34. John Smith, *Gerochomia vasilike: King Solomons portraiture of old age* (London: J. Hayes, 1666), 108–109, 184–185. My emphasis.

35. Harris, *Sick Economies*, passim. On hepatitis see 142–145, 160–162.

36. Thomas Willis, *Diatribae duae medico-philosophicae quarum prior agit de fermentatione* (London: Tho. Roycroft, 1659), 23, 33, 44, 47, 51. In *De Febribus*'s independent pagination, 11, 59, 76, 85, 86, 87, 209, 212.

37. Robert Martensen, "Habit of Reason: Anatomy and Anglicanism in Restoration England," *Bulletin of the History of Medicine* 66, no. 4 (1992): 511–533, esp. 518–524. Also germane is Martensen's conclusion about Willis's tendency to infuse his neuroanatomy with metaphors stemming from the sociopolitical hierarchy.

38. For this discussion I have used the 1684 English translation of Willis's works. Thomas Willis, *Dr. Willis's Practice of Physick being the whole works of that renowned and famous physician* (London: T. Dring, 1684), 11. See also 19–20, 23, 70, 77–79. My emphasis. Here the term *consume* may bring to mind flammable combustion. However, given the predominance of mercantilist rhetoric, the economic connotations of consumption are just as pertinent. On consumption as another example of "semantic cross-pollination" between seventeenth-century medicine and economics, see Harris, *Sick Economies*, 163–185.

39. On Willis see John Trevor Hughes, *Thomas Willis, 1621–1675* (London: Royal Society of Medicine, 1991); Robert Gregg Frank, *Harvey and the Oxford Physiologists: Scientific Ideas and Social Interaction* (Berkeley: University of California Press, 1980); Robert Gregg Frank, "Thomas Willis and His Circle: Brain and Mind in Seventeenth-Century Medicine," in *The Languages of Psyche: Mind and Body in Enlightenment Thought*, ed. G. S. Rousseau, 107–146 (Berkeley: University of California Press, 1990); and Donald G. Bates, "Thomas Willis and the Epidemic Fever of 1661: A Commentary," *Bulletin of the History of Medicine* 39, no. 5 (1965): 393–414.

40. Willis, *A Plaine and Easie Method*, 27, and *Practice of Physick*, 20, 78.

41. Willis, *Practice of Physick*, 51, 52, 64, 78, 82, 149–151; William Harvey, "Second Anatomical Essay to Jean Riolan," quoted in Gail Kern Paster, *The Body Embarrassed: Drama and the Disciplines of Shame in Early Modern England* (Ithaca, NY: Cornell University Press, 1993), 72–73.

42. Smith, *Gerochomia vasilike*, 184–185.

43. George Acton, *Physical Reflections upon a Letter written by J. Denis . . . concerning a new way of curing sundry diseases by transfusion of blood* (London: T. R. for J. Martyn, 1668), 6–7, 9; Thomas Coxe, *A Discourse wherein the Interest of the Patient in Reference to Physick and Physicians is Soberly Debated* (London: C.R., 1669), 95–98.

44. Bernard Capp, *When Gossips Meet: Women, Family, and Neighbourhood in Early Modern England* (Oxford: Oxford University Press, 2003), 189, also 88, 252. Jonathan Lamb's cultural history of the disease confirms its connection to the diseases explored in *Rotten Bodies*, especially its connections to putrescence. *Scurvy: The Disease of Discovery* (Princeton: Princeton University Press, 2017), 49–51; Willis, *Practice of Physick*, 175–179.

45. Cock, *Advice for the Poor*, 1–3; Willis, *Practice of Physick*, 175–176. Faulty perspiration as a cause of fever was a mainstay of classical thought. Hamlin, *More than Hot*, 18, 25, 37, 46; Lamb, *Scurvy*, 12; and Slack, *From Reformation to Improvement*, 9.

46. Willis, *Practice of Physick*, 156.

47. Ibid., 156, 203–204. It is worth noting that Willis also here implicated a "taint of the blood [that] is either hereditary or acquired." P.L., *Letter from an Apothecary* (London: M. Cooper, 1752), 34.

48. Willis, *Practice of Physick*, 170; Bradwell, *Watch-Man for the Pest*, 45–46; Theophilus Garencières, *A Mite cast into the Treasury of the Famous City of London: being a brief and methodical discourse of the nature, causes, symptomes, remedies and preservation from the plague, in this calamitous year, 1665* (London: Thomas Ratcliffe, 1665), 3, 12, 15; Anon., *A Treatise Concerning the Plague and the Pox* (London: Gartrude Dawson, 1652), 14. This doctor further warned of the "hereditable" nature of predisposition to putrid diseases and attributed it to the menstrual blood, arguing in his section on measles and smallpox, "The conjunct cause is the menstruall bloud, which from the beginning in our mothers womb wee received, the which mixing it self with the rest of our bloud, doth cause an Ebullition of the whole" (51–52).

49. Thomas Laqueur, *Making Sex: Body and Gender from the Greeks to Freud* (Cambridge: Harvard University Press, 1992); Londa Schiebinger, *The Mind*

Has No Sex? Women in the Origins of Modern Science (Cambridge: Harvard University Press, 1989), 160–213; Robert Martensen, "The Transformation of Eve: Women's Bodies, Medicine, and Culture in Early Modern England," in *Sexual Knowledge, Sexual Science: The History of Attitudes to Sexuality*, ed. Roy Porter and Mikulas Teich, 107–133 (Cambridge: Cambridge University Press, 1994). See also Mary Fissell, "Gender and Generation: Representing Reproduction in Early Modern England," *Gender and History* 7, no. 3 (1995): 433–456; Michael Stolberg, "A Woman Down to Her Bones: The Anatomy of Sexual Difference in the Sixteenth and Early Seventeenth Century," along with Laqueur and Schiebinger's responses "Sex in the Flesh" and "Skelettestreit," all in *Isis* 94, no. 2 (2003): 274–299, 300–306, and 307–313, respectively; Winfried Schleiner, "Early Modern Controversies about the One Sex Model," *Renaissance Quarterly* 53, no. 1 (2000): 180–191; Wendy Churchill, "The Medical Practice of the Sexed Body: Women, Men, and Disease in Britain, *circa* 1600–1740," *Social History of Medicine* 18, no. 1 (2005): 3–22; Mary Fissell, *Vernacular Bodies: The Politics of Reproduction in Early Modern England* (Oxford: Oxford University Press, 2004), 53–89; Lord, " 'The Great Arcana of the Deity,' "; and Siena, "Pollution, Promiscuity, and the Pox," 563.

50. Willis, *Practice of Physick*, 126–127. Here early modern discussions of menstruating men are also pertinent. Men were thought not to need menstruation because their labor caused them to sweat out impurities that women had to purge. Inadequate perspiration thus appears to have offered medical writers a multipurpose tool for constructing both class and gender ideals. See Michael Stolberg, "Menstruation and Sexual Difference in Early Modern Medicine," in *Menstruation: A Cultural History*, ed. Andrew Shail and Gillian Howie, 90–101 (New York Palgrave, 2005), and Lisa Wynne Smith, "The Body Embarrassed? Rethinking the Leaky Male Body in Eighteenth-Century England and France," *Gender and History* 23, no. 1 (2010), 27.

51. I address race extensively in the Conclusion, where the relevant works are cited.

52. Gail Kern Paster, "Laudable Blood" in *The Body Embarrassed*, 64–112, esp. 68, 78–80, also 127.

53. Schiebinger, *The Mind Has No Sex?* 189–213; Michel Foucault, *The History of Sexuality*, vol. 1, *An Introduction*, trans. Robert Hurley (New York: Vintage, 1980), 104, 116–117, 121; Sander Gilman, Helen King, Roy Porter, G. S. Rousseau, and Elaine Showalter, eds., *Hysteria beyond Freud* (Berkeley: University of California Press, 1993); Guenter Risse, "Hysteria at the Edin-

burgh Infirmary: The Construction and Treatment of a Disease, 1770–1800," *Medical History* 32, no. 1 (1988): 1–22.

54. For discussion of one such example, see Chapter 4, note 10.

55. Jütte, *Poverty and Deviance*. For work on this issue specific to medicine see the companion volumes Ole Peter Grell and Andrew Cunningham, eds., *Health Care and Poor Relief in Protestant Europe 1500–1700* (London: Routledge, 1997), and Grell, Cunningham, and Arrizabalaga, *Health Care and Poor Relief in Counter Reformation Europe*. For influence on the gendered body see Fissell, *Vernacular Bodies*, 35–52, 86–89.

56. Slack, *Impact of Plague*, 29–44; Gilman, *Plague Writing*, 247; Kevin Siena, "Pliable Bodies: The Moral Biology of Health and Disease," in *A Cultural History of the Human Body in the Enlightenment*, ed. Carole Reeves, 33–52 (Oxford: Berg, 2010).

57. Hodges, *Loimologia*, 56.

58. Theodore Brown long ago demonstrated that Willis's theory of fevers was instrumental to the acceptance of the new science by mainstream physicians largely because its language had become fashionable. "The College of Physicians and the Acceptance of Iatromechanism in England, 1665–1695," *Bulletin of the History of Medicine* 44 (1970): 12–30.

2. Reframing Plague after 1666

1. Paul Slack, *The Impact of Plague in Tudor and Stuart England* (Oxford: Oxford University Press, 1985), 311–337.

2. All newspapers cited in the following discussion were consulted through the British Library's 17th and 18th Century Burney Collection Database, accessed during July 2011. Examples from the period include John Seller, *The History of England: giving a true and impartial account of the most considerable transactions in Church and State* (London, 1702), 18, 311, 332–335, 361, 389, 480, 518, 547, 619, 637; and Anon., *The History of England. Faithfully Extracted from Authentick Records, Approved Manuscripts, and the most Celebrated Histories of this Kingdom* (London, 1702), 20–21, 113–116, 129, 174–175, 187, 221, 390.

3. For a thorough account of strategies to protect against importing plague by sea see John Booker, *Maritime Quarantine: The British Experience, c. 1650–1900* (Aldershot, UK: Ashgate, 2007); *Post Boy*, June 23–25, December 12–15, 1696, August 24–26, November 16–18, December 2–4, December 9–11, 1697, January 1–4, April 14–16, June 4–7, July 16–19, August 20–23, 1698, July 4–6, 1699, January 18–20, April 9–11, 1700, and March 4–6, April

24–26, 1701; *Post Man and the Historical Account,* September 2–4, 1697, and
April 9–11, 1700; *Post Man and the Historical Account,* April 30-May 1, July
28–30, 1696, November 13–16, 1697, and August 27–30, 1698; *Flying Post or
The Post Master,* July 16–19, 1698, and September 21–24, 1700; and *English
Post with News Foreign and Domestick,* January 10, 1701.

4. *Post Man and the Historical Account,* September 26–28, September 28–30, and
September 30–October 3, 1699.

5. *Post Man and the Historical Account,* August 27–30, 1698, and September
28–30, 1699; *Flying Post or The Post Master,* May 19–21, 1698, and July 3–5,
1701; *London Post with Intelligence Foreign and Domestick,* April 2–4 and July
4–7, 1701; *English Post with News Foreign and Domestick,* July 18–21, 1701;
New State of Europe Both As to Publick Transactions and Learning, July 19–22,
1701; and *Post Boy,* March 29–31, 1698.

6. Slack, *Impact of Plague,* 327–335; C. F. Mullet, "The English Plague Scare of
1720–23," *Osiris* 2 (1936): 484–516; Mark Harrison, *Contagion: How
Commerce Has Spread Disease* (New Haven: Yale University Press, 2012),
24–49; Booker, *Maritime Quarantine,* 85–122; Arnold Zuckerman, "Plague
and Contagionism in Eighteenth-Century England: The Role of Richard
Mead," *Bulletin of the History of Medicine* 78, no. 2 (2004): 273–308; Wayne
Wild, " 'Due Preparations': Defoe and Dr. Mead and the Threat of Plague,"
in *Liberating Medicine, 1720–1835,* ed. Tristanne Connolly and Steve Clark,
55–68 (London: Pickering and Chatto, 2009).

7. *Applebee's Original Weekly Journal,* September 3, 1720; *Post Boy,* November
5–8, 1720; *Evening Post,* November 24–26, 1720; Nathaniel Hodges, *Loimologia: or, an Historical Account of the Plague in London in 1665* (London, 1721),
86; Thomas Willis, *A Preservative from the infection of the Plague . . . Written
in the year 1666* (London: A. Bettesworth, 1721), 23.

8. Richard Blackmore, *A Discourse upon the Plague, with a preparatory account of
Malignant Fevers* (London: John Clark, 1721); Anon., *The Great Bill of
Mortality: or, the late dreadful plague at Marseilles* (Bristol: Sam. Farley, 1721),
4; Phil-anthropos, *A Brief Essay on the Small-Pox and Measles, Plague,
Malignant and Pestilential fevers* (London: n.p., 1721).

9. On Mead see Arnold Zuckerman, "Dr. Richard Mead (1673–1754): A
Biographical Study," Ph.D. diss., University of Illinois, 1965.

10. In this discussion I will draw from, and distinguish between, Mead's first
edition (1720) and his revised eighth edition (1722). Richard Mead, *A Short
Discourse concerning Pestilential Contagion, and the Methods to be used to
Prevent it* (London: Sam. Buckley, 1720), 3–11, 18, 21–30, 45, 58; Richard

Mead, *A Short Discourse concerning the Pestilential Contagion, and the Methods to be used to Prevent it*, 8th ed. (London: Sam. Buckley, 1722), 8, 43.

11. Mead, *Short Discourse* (1720), 4, 6, 9, 12, 18, 20, 45, 48. On medical theories about heat and climate see Alan Bewell, *Romanticism and Colonial Disease* (Baltimore: Johns Hopkins, 1999), 35–46; Mark Harrison, *Medicine in an Age of Commerce and Empire: Britain and Its Tropical Colonies, 1660–1830* (Oxford: Oxford University Press, 2010), 1–88; James Riley, *The Eighteenth-Century Campaign to Avoid Disease* (London: Macmillan, 1987), 31–51. The most influential eighteenth-century text was assuredly James Lind, *An Essay on Diseases Incidental to Europeans in Hot Climates* (London: T. Becket, 1768). On the example of syphilis in this regard see Kevin Siena, "Pollution, Promiscuity, and the Pox: English Venereology and the Early Modern Medical Discourse on Social and Sexual Danger," *Journal of the History of Sexuality* 8, no. 4 (1998): 553–574, esp. 569–571.

12. Mead, *Short Discourse* (1720), 2, 6–17; and Mead, *Short Discourse* (1722), 20.

13. Mead, *Short Discourse* (1722), 29, 32–34.

14. Mead, *Short Discourse* (1720), 38, 40–41, 43.

15. Ibid., 44, and Mead, *Short Discourse* (1722), xxi–xxii.

16. Pichatty de Croissainte, *A Brief Journal of what passed in the City of Marseilles, While it was Afflicted with the Plague, in the Year 1720* (London: J. Roberts, 1721), 6–10.

17. Blackmore, *Discourse upon the Plague*, 24.

18. Ibid., 25–26; The Explainer, *Distinct Notions of the Plague, with the Rise and Fall of Pestilential Contagion* (London: J. Peele, 1722), 119–121; J.S., *An Historical Account of the Plague at Marseilles* (London: J. Billingsley, 1722), 11.

19. Slack, *Impact of Plague*, 329–333; Zuckerman, "Plague and Contagionism," 273–308; Margaret DeLacy, "Nosology, Mortality, and Disease Theory in the Eighteenth Century," *Journal of the History of Medicine and Allied Sciences* 54, no. 2 (1999): 261–284. On this debate during the Marseilles epidemic see Margaret DeLacy, *The Germ of an Idea: Contagionism, Religion, and Society in Britain, 1660–1730* (New York: Palgrave Macmillan, 2016), 147–162.

20. George Pye, *A Discourse of the Plague; Wherein Dr. Mead's Notions are Consider'd and Refuted* (London: J. Darby, 1721), 4, 7–10, 12–13, 22–26, 28. My emphasis. As will be evident, *goal* was a common misspelling of *gaol*.

21. John Pringle, *A Rational Enquiry into the Nature of Plague* (London: J. Peele, 1722), 15–23.

22. On this body of thought see DeLacy, *Germ of an Idea*, 37–40, 69–76; M. J. Ratcliff, *The Quest for the Invisible: Microscopy in the Enlightenment*

(Burlington, VT: Ashgate, 2009), 25; R. Mead, "An Abstract of Part of a Letter from Dr Bonomo to Sigmor Redi," *Philosophical Transactions* 23, no. 283 (1702): 1296–1299.

23. K. Codell Carter, *The Rise of Causal Concepts of Disease: Case Studies* (Aldershot, UK: Ashgate, 2003), and DeLacy, *Germ of an Idea*.

24. Anon., *A New Discovery of the Nature of the Plague* (London: T. Bickerton, 1721), Dedication [n. p.], 4–6, 9–12, 22–23, 27, 29.

25. Ibid., 16–17, 19–20, 27, 29–30, 35.

26. Ibid., 39–40.

27. The literature is vast. Starting points include Robert Mayer, "The Reception of *A Journal of the Plague Year* and the Nexus of Fiction and History in the Novel," *English Literary History* 57, no. 3 (1990): 529–555; Maximillian Novak, "Defoe and the Disordered City," *PMLA* 92, no. 2 (1977): 241–252; Frank Ellis, "Defoe's Journal of the Plague Year," *Review of English Studies* 45, no. 177 (1994): 76–82.

28. Daniel Defoe, *Due Preparations for the Plague, as well for Soul as Body* (London: E. Matthews, 1722), 5–10.

29. Ibid., 25–36, 41, 47, 55.

30. Ibid., 22.

31. Ibid., 19–24.

32. Andrew Wear, Introduction to *Due Preparations for the Plague* and *Mere Nature Delineated*, vol. 5 of *The Works of Daniel Defoe*, ed. W. R. Owens and P. N. Furbank (London: Pickering and Chatto, 2002), 8.

3. Prisons, Debtors, and Disease in the Early Eighteenth Century

1. For commentary on the alleged lack of health reform that argues for seeing prison reform as a public health initiative, see Roy Porter, "Cleaning up the Great Wen: Public Health in Eighteenth-Century London," *Medical History* 11 (1991): 61–75, 69, 73. Note that although there were distinctions between different categories of institution, as will be discussed, I use the terms *prison* and *jail* interchangeably.

2. Sidney Webb and Beatrice Webb, *English Prisons under Local Government* (1922; rpt. Hamden, CT: Archon, 1963); R. S. E. Hinde, *The British Penal System, 1773–1950* (London: Gerald Duckworth, 1951), 12–13; Sean McConville, *A History of English Prison Administration*, vol. 1 (London: Routledge, 1981), 49–54. Christopher Harding et al., *Imprisonment in England and Wales: A Concise History* (Beckenham, UK: Croom Helm, 1985), 93–96.

3. Michel Foucault, *Discipline and Punish: The Birth of the Prison,* trans. Alan Sheridan (New York: Pantheon, 1977); Michael Ignatieff, *A Just Measure of Pain: The Penitentiary in the Industrial Revolution, 1750–1850* (New York: Penguin, 1978), esp. chapter 3, 44–79.

4. Margaret DeLacy, *Prison Reform in Lancashire, 1700–1850: A Study in Local Administration* (Stanford: Stanford University Press, 1986), 81, 93–94; Roy Porter, "Howard's Beginning: Prisons, Disease, Hygiene," in *The Health of Prisoners: Historical Essays,* ed. Richard Creese, W. F. Bynum, and J. Bearn (Amsterdam: Rodopi, 1995), 16; Robin Evans, *The Fabrication of Virtue: English Prison Architecture, 1750–1840* (Cambridge: Cambridge University Press, 1982), 94–117; and Harding et al., *Imprisonment in England and Wales,* 95.

5. DeLacy, *Prison Reform in Lancashire,* 80–94; Joe Sim, *Medical Power in Prisons: The Prison Medical Service in England, 1774–1989* (Milton Keynes: Open University Press, 1990); Peter McRorie Higgins, *Medical Care in English Prisons, 1770–1850* (Bloomington, IN: Trafford, 2007). On earlier prison reform efforts see Webb and Webb, *English Prisons,* 18–31; Harding et al., *Imprisonment in England and Wales,* 87–88, 90, 96–102; McConville, *History of English Prison Administration,* 19, 54–56, 65–66. For a discussion specific to health see Wayne Joseph Sheehan, "The London Prison System, 1666–1795," Ph.D. diss., University of Maryland, 1975, 311–347.

6. Anon., *A New Discovery of the Nature of the Plague* (London: T. Bickerton, 1721), 47–49. It is indicative of the frequent lack of clear theoretical distinctions in this period that this animalculist still afforded causative significance to quasi-miasmatic "steams" and "mists."

7. For London the best survey remains Sheehan, "London Prison System"; Daniel Defoe, *A Tour Through the Whole Island of Great Britain,* ed. P. N. Furbank and W. R. Owens, (1724; New Haven: Yale University Press, 1991), 157; J. M. Beattie, *Crime and the Courts in England, 1660–1800* (Princeton: Princeton University Press, 1986), 497–500, 546–548, 560–564; John Beattie, *Policing and Punishment in London, 1660–1750* (Oxford University Press, 2001), 362–365; Robert Shoemaker, *Prosecutions and Punishment: Petty Crime and the Law in London and Rural Middlesex, c. 1660–1725* (Cambridge: Cambridge University Press, 1991), 166–197. The data on incarceration rates come from the associated dataset "Old Bailey Punishment Sentences, 1690–1800," available through the e-book version of Tim Hitchcock and Robert Shoemaker, *London Lives: Poverty, Crime, and the Making of a Modern City, 1690–1800* (Cambridge: Cambridge University Press, 2015), 79.

8. Randall McGowan, "The Well-Ordered Prison: England, 1780–1865," in *The Oxford History of the Prison*, ed. Norval Morris and David J. Rothman, 71–99 (Oxford: Oxford University Press, 1998), 73; Joanna Innes, "Prisons for the Poor: English Bridewells, 1555–1800," in *Labour, Law, and Crime: An Historical Perspective*, ed. Francis Snyder and Douglas Hay, 42–122 (London: Tavistock, 1987). The best survey of workhouses remains Timothy V. Hitchcock, "The English Workhouse: A Study in Institutional Poor Relief in Selected Counties, 1696–1750," D.Phil. thesis, Oxford University, 1985; Anon., *New Discovery*, 48; and Richard Mead, *A Short Discourse concerning Pestilential Contagion, and the Methods to be used to Prevent it* (London: Sam. Buckley, 1720), 41–42.

9. Margot Finn, *Character of Credit: Personal Debt in English Culture c. 1740–1914* (Cambridge: Cambridge University Press, 2003), 109–112; Joanna Innes, *Inferior Politics: Social Problems and Social Policies in Eighteenth-Century Britain* (Oxford: Oxford University Press, 2009); Craig Muldrew, *The Economy of Obligation: The Culture of Credit and Social Relations in Early Modern England* (London: Macmillan, 1998), 183 and 288–290; Paul Hess Haagen, "Imprisonment for Debt in England and Wales," Ph.D. diss., Princeton University, 1986, 77–78. Peter Earle estimates that in the early eighteenth century 10–15 percent of London's wealthiest tradesmen had to declare bankruptcy at some point in their careers. *The Making of the English Middle Class: Business, Society, and Family Life in London, 1660–1730* (Berkeley: University of California, 1989), 129–130.

10. Innes, *Inferior Politics*, 232–234; McGowan, "The Well-Ordered Prison," 74, 116–117; Finn, *Character of Credit*, 57, 109–151; Muldrew, *Economy of Obligation*, 287; Defoe, *Tour*, 157; Ian Duffy, *Bankruptcy and Insolvency in London during the Industrial Revolution* (New York: Garland, 1985), 56; Philip Woodfine, "Debtors, Prisons, and Petitions in Eighteenth-Century England," *Eighteenth-Century Life* 30, no. 2 (2006): 1–31, 4.

11. Innes, *Inferior Politics*, 227–278. There were no fewer than sixty-two failed attempts to amend laws pertaining to debtors in the eighteenth century. Julian Hoppit, ed., *Failed Legislation, 1660–1800* (London: Hambledon, 1997); McConville, *History of English Prison Administration*, 56.

12. Sheehan, "London Prison System," 17; DeLacy, *Prison Reform in Lancashire*, 15–55.

13. Moses Pitt, *The Cry of the Oppressed. Being a True and Tragical Account of the Unparrallel'd Sufferings of Multitudes of poor Imprisoned Debtors* (London: Moses Pitt, 1691), "Epistle Dedicatory," Preface [n.p.], fol. A3 and A4.

14. Ibid., 89, 92.
15. Ibid., 10, 16–17, 21–22, 24–25, 30–35, 38–40, 45–46.
16. Ibid., 11–12, 18–19, 21–22, 32, 38–48. On filth and human waste in the period see Emily Cockayne, *Hubbub: Filth, Noise, and Stench in England* (New Haven: Yale University Press, 2007), 181–205; Mark Jenner, "Early Modern English Conceptions of 'Cleanliness' and 'Dirt,' as Reflected in the Environmental Regulation of London, c. 1530–c. 1700," D.Phil. thesis, University of Oxford, 1991. The work on filth has been informed by important theoretical works such as Mary Douglas, *Purity and Danger: An Analysis of Concepts of Pollution and Taboo* (London: Routledge and Kegan Paul, 1966); Alain Corbin, *The Foul and the Fragrant: Odor and the French Social Imagination* (Cambridge: Harvard University Press, 1986); and Dominique Laporte, *History of Shit*, trans. Rodolphe el-Khoury (1978; Cambridge: MIT Press, 2000).
17. McGowan, "Well-Ordered Prison," 73–75; Harding et al., *Imprisonment in England and Wales*, 91–92; Evans, *Fabrication of Virtue*, 23–268; DeLacy, *Prison Reform in Lancashire*, 28–34; Sheehan, "London Prison System," 313; and Wayne Joseph Sheehan, "Finding Solace in Eighteenth-Century Newgate," in *Crime in England, 1550–1800*, ed. J. S. Cockburn (London: Methuen, 1977), 236. Sander Gilman reflects on the history of the melancholy pose in early modern depictions of disease in *Disease and Representation: Images of Illness from Madness to AIDS* (Ithaca, NY: Cornell University Press, 1988), 252–254. On the skin as a text, especially for revealing stigmatized diseases associated with poverty, see the eighteenth-century contributions to Jonathan Reinarz and Kevin Siena, eds., *A Medical History of Skin: Scratching the Surface* (London: Pickering and Chatto, 2013).
18. Pitt, *Cry of the Oppressed*, 21–22, 45–46, 57–59.
19. These are loose petitions collected but unnumbered and usually not dated. Archivists date them to the period c. 1675–1700. LMA, CLA/032/01/021, "Petitions of prisoners, offices of Newgate and the Compters, and other persons relating to prisons life, repairs of prisons, collections, ill-health, abuse by offices, for discharge, &c."
20. Innes, *Inferior Politics;* Finn, *Character of Credit*, 109–151; Margaret Dorey, "Reckliss Endangerment: Feeding the Poor Prisoners of London in the Early Eighteenth Century," in *Experiencing Poverty in Medieval and Early Modern England*, ed. Anne M. Scott (Aldershot, UK: Ashgate, 2012), 183–198; Woodfine, "Debtors, Prisons, and Petitions"; and Jerry White, "Pain and Degradation in Georgian London: Life in the Marshalsea Prison," *History Workshop Journal* 68, no. 1 (2009): 69–98.

21. All references LMA, CLA/032/01/021. Dorey notes similar complaints that poor water supply at the Wood Street Compter "may breed infection." "Reckliss Endangerment," 188.

22. 22 and 23 Charles II c. 20, quoted in Harding et al., *Imprisonment in England and Wales*, 95–96 (my emphasis); DeLacy, *Prison Reform in Lancashire*, 23; Haagen, "Imprisonment for Debt," 138–139.

23. Leslie F. Church, *Oglethorpe: A Study of Philanthropy in England and Georgia* (London: Epworth, 1932), 11–12; John Bender, *Imagining the Penitentiary: Fiction and the Architecture of the Mind in the Eighteenth Century* (Chicago: University of Chicago Press, 1987), 108–115; White, "Pain and Degradation," 76; Hugh Barty-King, *The Worst Poverty: A History of Debt and Debtors* (Stroud, UK: Alan Sutton, 1991), 62–65; Rodney M. Baine, "The Prison Death of Robert Castell and Its Effect on the Founding of Georgia," in *James Edward Oglethorpe: New Perspectives on his Life and Legacy*, ed. John C. Inscoe (Savannah: Georgia Historical Society, 1997), 35–46. On the makeup of the committee see White, "Pain and Degradation," 77.

24. John Mackay, *A True State of the Proceedings of the Prisoners in the Fleet-Prison* (London: A. Campbell, 1729); Anon., *The Miseries of Goals, and the Cruelty of Goalers: being a narrative of several persons now under confinement* (London: Tho. Payne, 1729); Sheehan, "London Prison System," 206 and 386–387; Baine, "Prison Death of Robert Castell," 35–46.

25. House of Commons, *A Report from the Committee appointed to enquire into the state of the goals of this kingdom: relating to the Fleet Prison* (London: Robert Knaplock et al., 1729), 8, 13; House of Commons, *A Report from the Committee appointed to enquire into the state of the goals of this kingdom: relating to the Marshalsea Prison* (London: Robert Knaplock et al., 1729), 4.

26. House of Commons, *Report from the Committee . . . relating to the Marshalsea Prison*, 4, 8, 17–18; House of Commons, *Report from the Committee . . . relating to the Fleet Prison*, 10.

27. Anon., *The Tryal of William Acton, Deputy-Keeper and Lessee of the Marshalsea Prison in Southwark* (London: J. Smith, 1729); White, "Pain and Degradation," 90–93; House of Commons, *A Report from the Committee . . . relating to the Marshalsea Prison*, 3–4; House of Commons, *Report from the Committee . . . relating to the Fleet Prison*, 9.

28. Samuel Wesley, *The prisons open'd. A poem occasion'd by the late glorious proceedings of the committee appointed to enquire into the state of the goals of this Kingdom* (London: J. Roberts, 1729), 8, 16; James Thomson, "Winter" in *The Seasons. A Hymn* (London: J. Millan, 1730), 23; Bender, *Imagining the*

Penitentiary, 18. The engraver Thomas Cook is mistaken in portraying the image as Bambridge's trial at the Old Bailey. The original oil on canvas painting survives at the National Portrait Gallery. However, it is extremely dark and reproduces poorly.

29. Anon., *Tryal of William Acton,* 18–19; *Proceedings of the Old Bailey,* Thomas Bambridge, Killing, murder, May 21, 1729, ref # t17290521–50; Alex Pitofsky, "The Warden's Court Martial: James Oglethorpe and the Politics of Eighteenth-Century Prison Reform," *Eighteenth-Century Life* 24, no. 1 (2000): 88–102, 95–99; McConville, *History of English Prison Administration,* 56.

30. 2 Geo. II, c. 20, 2 Geo. II, c. 22, and 3 Geo. II, c. 27; 5 Geo. II, c. 27; 8 Geo. II, c. 24; 14 Geo. II, c. 34; 10 Geo. II, c. 26; 11 Geo. II, c. 9; 16 Geo. II, c. 17; 21 Geo. II, c. 31; 21 Geo. II, c. 33; 11 Geo II, c. 20; House of Commons, *Report from the Committee Appointed to Enquire into the State of the Goals of this Kingdom. Relating to the Kings-Bench Prison* (London: Robert Knaplock et al., 1730), 10; Haagen, "Imprisonment for Debt," 35; McConville, *History of English Prison Administration,* 56; Sheehan, "London Prison System," 130–137; Duffy, *Bankruptcy and Insolvency,* 65, 75–78; Barty-King, *The Worst Poverty,* 67–68; and Innes, *Inferior Politics,* 235–238.

31. Harding et al., *Imprisonment in England and Wales,* 96.

32. 9 Geo. III, c. 12.

33. Finn, *Character of Credit,* 25–105; Muldrew, *Economy of Obligation,* 183.

34. The classic studies are Douglas Hay, "Property, Authority, and the Criminal Law," in *Albion's Fatal Tree: Crime and Society in Eighteenth-Century England,* ed. Douglas Hay et al., 17–63 (London: Penguin, 1975), and E. P. Thompson, *Whigs and Hunters: Origins of the Black Act* (New York: Pantheon, 1975). For a response to Hay see John H. Langbein, "Albion's Fatal Flaws," *Past and Present* 98 (1983): 96–120.

35. On contemporary commentary regarding the tensions between debt laws and Insolvency Acts, see Duffy, *Bankruptcy and Insolvency,* 78–79.

4. Jail Fever Comes of Age

1. On the case see the Tim Hitchcock and Robert Shoemaker, *Tales from the Hanging Court* (London: Hodder Arnold, 2006), 54–60; Robert Shoemaker, "The Taming of the Duel: Masculinity, Honour, and Ritual Violence in London, 1660–1800," *Historical Journal* 45, no. 3 (2002): 525–545, 533; Nicholas Rogers, "London's Marginal Histories," *Labour/Le Travail* 60 (2007): 232–233; Anon., *The Trial of Captain Edward Clark . . . for the Murder of Captain Thomas Innes . . . in a Duel in Hyde Park March 12, 1749: at*

Justice-Hall in the Old Bailey (London: M. Copper, 1750); Trial of Edward Clark, *Proceedings of the Old Bailey*, April, 25, 1750 (t17500425–19). *Whitehall Evening Post or London Intelligencer*, May 17–19, 22–24, 26–29, 1750; *General Advertiser*, May 2, 1750; *Old England*, May 5, 1750.

2. *London Evening Post*, May 12–15, 15–17, 19–22, 22–24, 1750; *Whitehall Evening Post or London Intelligencer*, May 14–17, 17–19, 19–22, 22–24, 1750; *General Advertiser*, May 17, 19, 21, 1750; *Old England*, May 19, 1750; *Read's Weekly Journal or British Gazetteer*, May 19, 1750. On fever rates see *London Evening Post*, April 24–26, May 15–17, 29–31, June 5–7, 1750.

3. *Whitehall Evening Post or London Intelligencer*, May 17–19, 19–22, 22–24, 26–29, 1750; *Remembrancer*, May 26, 1750; *General Advertiser*, May 26, 1750; *Read's Weekly Journal or British Gazetteer*, May 26, 1750.

4. James Riley, *Eighteenth-Century Campaign to Avoid Disease* (London: Macmillan, 1987).

5. *London Evening Post*, May 24–26, 1750; *Whitehall Evening Post or London Intelligencer*, May 24–26, 1750; *General Advertiser*, May 26, 1750.

6. Priscilla Wald, *Contagious: Cultures, Carriers, and the Outbreak Narrative* (Durham: Duke University Press, 2008), 1–28.

7. Ibid., 68–113, 213–263; Richard A. McKay, " 'Patient Zero': The Absence of a Patient's View of the Early North American AIDS Epidemic," *Bulletin of the History of Medicine* 88, no. 1 (2014): 161–194; Laura McGough, "Quarantining Beauty: The French Disease in Early Modern Venice," in *Sins of the Flesh: Responding to Sexual Disease in Early Modern Europe*, ed. Kevin Siena (Toronto: Centre for Reformation and Renaissance Studies, 2005), 211–237.

8. Robert Parsons, *An Epistle of the Persecution of Catholickes in Englande* (Rouen: Parsons, 1582), 149–150. Also, Thomas Cogan, *The Haven of Health Chiefly gathered for the Comfort of Students . . . Hereunto is added a preservation from the pestilence, with a short censure of the late sicknes at Oxford* (London: Anne Griffin, 1636), 317–319; Anthony Wood, *The history and antiquities of the University of Oxford*, vol. 2 (London, Printed for the editor, 1792), 188–192, first published as *Historia et antiquitates universitatis Oxoniensis duobus voluminibus compreheniae* (Oxford: E. Theatro Sheldoniano, 1674); Jeremiah Whitaker Newman, *The lounger's common-place book; or, miscellaneous anecdotes*, vol. 4 (London: Kerby, 1799), 42–45. On plague spreaders see William Naphy, *Plagues, Poisons, and Potions: Plague-Spreading Conspiracies in the Western Alps, c. 1530–1640* (Manchester: Manchester University Press, 2002).

9. Richard Baker, *A Chronicle of the Kings of England* (London: Daniel Frere, 1643), "The Raigne of Queen Elizabeth," 44. See also John Stow, *The*

Abridgement of the English Chronicle (London: Company of Stationers, 1618), 324.

10. Physicians like Charles White who emphasized putridity made these kinds of connections. White noted that Thomas Willis had intriguingly presented poor women as less susceptible than rich ones, because their labor promoted healthy sweating while the lazy rich retained impurities. But White, a Manchester Infirmary physician who boasted of experience with "all ranks of women," argued a century later that Willis's argument no longer held: "It is well known that they [the poor] are very liable to this fever both in the hospitals, and in their own houses, especially if they are situated in the middle of large manufacturing towns and cities. . . . [Willis wrote] at a time when there was no hospital for lying-in-women in the British dominions, our manufactures were in their infancy, and the diet and mode of living amongst the poor people, were totally different from what they are at this time." Explaining the "great inclination to putridity," he compared women's crowded birthing chambers to slums and jails. "When the woman is in labour, she is often attended by a number of her friends in a small room with a large fire, which, together with her own pains. Throw her into profuse sweats; by the heat of the chamber, and the breath of so many people, the whole air is rendered foul, and unfit for respiration; this is the case in all confined places, hospitals, jails and small houses inhabited by many families, where putrid fevers are apt to be generated, and proportionally the more so where there is the greatest want of free air. Putrid fevers thus generated are infectious, *witness the black assize, as it is usually called.*" Charles White, *A Treatise on the Management of Pregnant and Lying-in Women* (London: W. Johnston, 1772), xvi, 2–5, also 155. My emphasis. Christine Hallett has shown that the dominant debate on puerperal fever pitted proponents of theories of putrescence against others emphasizing inflammation. "The Attempt to Understand Puerperal Fever in the Eighteenth and Early Nineteenth Centuries: The Influence of Inflammation Theory," *Medical History* 49, no. 1 (2005): 1–28. Puerperal fever may thus offer a rich venue to explore the ways in which gender and class may have mingled in medical theories of fever.

11. Francis Bacon, *Sylva Sylvarum: or A Naturall Historie In Ten Centuries* (London: W. Lee, 1627), 243, 246, 248; and Wood, *History and antiquities,* 190–191. Bacon's contemporary Thomas Cogan called the Oxford sickness a "neere cosin to the plague," Cogan, *Haven of Health,* 315. Raphael Holinshed, *The Third Volume of Chronicles, Beginning at Duke William the Norman, Commonlie called the Conqueror; and Descending by Degrees of Yeeres to all the*

Kings and Queenes of England in their Orderlie Successions (London: H. Denham, 1586), 1547–1548. Notably, Holinshed identified poverty as its main cause. The disease was spawned, he said, in the bodies of "certaine poor Portingals," that is, Portuguese, imprisoned in the Exeter jail. He emphasized their poverty, filth and "hungar starved" condition when they were thrust into a "stinking dungeon," where they sickened before spreading infection to other prisoners, then judges and jurors in court, and through them to the whole shire. Richard Izacke confirms this picture, describing the poverty of the Portuguese sailors as being "by diseases (chiefly occasioned through want of Victals and Necessaries) were all wornt out." *Antiquities of the City of Exeter* (London: Tyler and Holt, 1677), 138.

12. Richard Mead, *A Short Discourse concerning Pestilential Contagion, and the Methods to be used to Prevent it* (London: Sam. Buckley, 1720), 42.

13. Using variant spellings, none of the terms created by combining the word *goal, gaol, goale, gaole, jail,* or *jayl* with *fever, feaver, distemper, disease, sickness,* or *sicknesse* (thus "goal fever," "jail fever," "gaol distemper," "jayl sickness," and so on) yielded any texts using the terms. Nor did a search for all those pairs employing proximity searching, a function that locates texts in which the terms occur near one another. Of course, not all texts in the *EEBO* database are available for such searching. Still, it is telling that the terms do not appear in the more than sixty thousand sixteenth- and seventeenth-century books that are full-text searchable. Searched June 27, 2016.

14. John Allen, *A Full and True account of the Behaviors, Confessions, and Last Dying Speeches of the Condemn'd Criminals that were executed at Tyburn, on Friday the 24th of May, 1700* (London: E. Mallet, 1700), 1. None of the aforementioned accounts on the Oxford Assizes assigns a name to the disease beside the "stench" of the prisoners. A search of *Early English Books Online* brings up not a single text using the term "jail/gaol fever" or "distemper."

15. Richard Mead, *A Short Discourse concerning the Pestilential Contagion, and the Methods to be used to Prevent it,* 8th ed. (London: Sam. Buckley, 1722), 149, and *Short Discourse* (1720), 38 and 41–44.

16. Peter Kennedy, *A Second Discourse, by way of Supplement to Dr. Kennedy's First, on Pestilence and Contagion, &c.* (London: T. Bickerton, 1721), 11–12, and Peter Kennedy, *A Discourse on Pestilence and Contagion in General; containing the cause, prevention, and cure* (London: J. Hooke, 1721), 5, 19. Kennedy additionally emphasized predisposition, idleness as a predisposing factor, the need to cleanse poor neighborhoods, and the incitement by plague

of a kind of class warfare in the blood, recommending medicines that "defend the nobler Parts." *Discourse on Pestilence*, 9, 26–27, 29, 36, 37.

17. *Parker's London News or the Impartial Intelligencer*, May 6, 1724; Anon., *The Tryal of William Acton, Deputy-Keeper and Lessee of the Marshalsea Prison in Southwark* (London: J. Smith, 1729), 16–18; John Everett, *A genuine narrative of the memorable life and actions of John Everett* (London: John Applebee, 1730), 24; *Dublin Evening Post*, January 3, 1736, vol. 4, issue 51; *Old Common Sense: or The Englishman's Journal*, June 10, 1738; and *The Ordinary of Newgate, his account of the behaviour, confession, and dying words of the male-factors who were executed at Tyburn, on Friday the 21st of October, 1743* (London: John Applebee, 1743), 5.

18. Charles Creighton, *A History of Epidemics in Britain*, 2 vols. (Cambridge: Cambridge University Press, 1891), 2: 92–93; Candace Ward, *Desire and Disorder: Fevers, Fictions, and Feeling in English Georgian Culture* (Lewisburg, PA: Bucknell University Press, 2007), 101; *London Evening Post*, April 7–9, 11–14, 14–16, 16–18, 1730; *Daily Post*, April 9, 1730; *Daily Journal*, April 15, 1730; *Weekly Journal or British Gazetteer*, April 11, 1730; *Daily Courant*, April 15, 1730; *Monthly Chronicle*, April 1730; and *Grub Street Journal*, April 16, 23, 1730.

19. On the same page that announced Pengelly's death, the *London Evening Post* reported the worrying story that a colonel, a captain, and a justice of the peace had all been infected when they visited a prisoner in Newgate. *London Evening Post*, April 28–30, 1730. Death notices in the *Monthly Chronicle*, April 1730, identify the dead as Colonel Edward Riley and Colonel John Ellis and specify the presence of "Goal Fever." Creighton, *History of Epidemics; London Evening Post*, April 18–21, 1730; *Monthly Chronicle*, April 1730.

20. British Library, *17th and 18th Century Burney Collection Newspapers*, and *Eighteenth Century Collections Online*, searched June 28, 2016.

21. *London Evening Post*, May 29–31, June 2–5, 1750; John Pringle, *Observations on the Nature and Cure of Hospital and Jayl-Fevers. In a Letter to Doctor Mead, Physician to his Majesty, &c.* (London: A. Millar and D. Wilson in the Strand, 1750). For a similar testimonial that was also accompanied with a separate advertisement on the same page see *General Advertiser*, June 16, 1750. For the classic study of empirics see Roy Porter, *Health for Sale: Quackery in England, 1660–1850* (Manchester: Manchester University Press, 1989).

22. On Pringle see Erich Weidenhammer, "Patronage and Enlightened Medicine in the Eighteenth-Century British Military: The Rise and Fall of Dr. John Pringle, 1707–1782," *Social History of Medicine* 29, no. 1 (2016): 21–43, and

Erich Weidenhammer, "Air, Disease, and Improvement in Eighteenth-Century Britain: Sir John Pringle (1707–1782)," Ph.D. diss., University of Toronto, 2014; Stephen C. Craig, "Sir John Pringle MD, Early Scottish Enlightenment Thought, and the Origins of Modern Military Medicine," *Journal for Eighteenth-Century Studies* 38, no. 1 (2015): 99–114; Sydney Selwyn, "Sir John Pringle: Hospital Reformer, Moral Philosopher, and Pioneer of Antiseptics," *Medical History* 10, no. 3 (1966): 266–274; Margaret DeLacy, *Contagionism Catches On: Medical Ideology in Britain, 1730–1800* (New York: Palgrave Macmillan, 2016), 55–66.

23. Pringle, *Hospital and Jayl-Fevers*, 1–3.

24. Riley provides an excellent survey of the ideas in *Eighteenth-Century Campaign to Avoid Disease*, 89–112. See more recently Christopher Hamlin, *More than Hot: A Short History of Fever* (Baltimore: Johns Hopkins University Press, 2014), 114–124. The fullest study of the impact of jail fever on penal institutions is Robin Evans, *The Fabrication of Virtue: English Prison Architecture, 1750–1840* (Cambridge: Cambridge University Press, 1982), 94–117.

25. Hamlin usefully reminds us that despite the rise of iatromechanistic models in the early part of the century or increased attention to the nerves, putridity would "reign over fever discourse" well into the nineteenth century. *More than Hot*, 67–70, 120; Pringle, *Hospital and Jayl-Fevers*, 4–5, 8–10, 15, 50. My emphasis.

26. Pringle, *Hospital and Jayl-Fevers*, 11–12, 16, 18, 20–25, 32, 36, also 43–44. On smell, to take just one of the most important examples, William Cullen presented it as a matter of fact in his influential textbook. He listed four tell-tale symptoms of "the putrescent state of the fluids": the appetite, qualities of the mass of blood, the state of excretions, and finally "the cadaverous smell of the whole body." William Cullen, *First lines of the practice of physic, for the use of students in the University of Edinburgh*, vol. 1 (Edinburgh: J. Murray, 1777), 84. See also Anon., *A collection of very valuable and scarce pieces relating to the last plague in the year 1665* (London: J. Roberts, 1721), 18–19; John Ball, *A Treatise of Fevers* (London: H. Cock, 1758), 114; William Grant, *An Essay on the Pestilential Fever of Sydenham, commonly called the Gaol, Hospital, Ship and Camp-Fever* (London: T. Cadell, 1775), 142; John Clark, *Observations on Fevers* (London: T. Cadell, 1780), 20; John Barker, *Epidemicks* (Birmingham: E. Piercy, 1795), 63.

27. Pringle, *Hospital and Jayl-Fevers*, 2, 9–10, 51–52.

28. John Pringle, *Observations on the Diseases of the Army* (London: A. Millar, 1752), 270. Similar claims about class litter the text. See, for example, 82, 343,

352, 407. Indeed, Pringle's discussion of the Old Bailey outbreak in his chapter on malignant fever (in which he quoted Bacon and invoked 1577) immediately followed an explanation of why dysentery was frequent among the poor; he drew class to his readers' minds by attributing the 1750 epidemic to the pent-up perspiration "of all sorts of people" in the courtroom that day (345–349).

29. Hamlin, *More than Hot*, 48. Elsewhere he tries to suggest that ideas about putridity did not so much fade as change, becoming "observational rather than theoretical," a point that is neither supported nor explored (120–121). Margaret DeLacy, *The Germ of an Idea: Contagionism, Religion, and Society in Britain, 1660–1730* (New York: Palgrave Macmillan, 2016), x.

30. Dale Ingram, *An Historical Account of the Several Plagues that have appeared in the World since the year 1346* (London: R. Baldwin, 1755), 26, also 68–69, 172; John Gregory, *Elements of the Practice of Physick*, 3rd ed. (Edinburgh: Strahan and Cadell, 1788), 130–131.

31. Daniel Peter Layard, *Directions to Prevent the contagion of Jail Distemper, commonly called the Jail-Fever* (London: James Robson, 1772), 1–7; James Lind, *A Treatise of the Scurvy, in Three Parts* (Edinburgh: Sands, Murray and Cochrane, 1753), and James Lind, *An Essay on the Most Effectual Means of Preserving the Health of Seamen . . . Together with Observations on the Jail Distemper, and the proper Methods of preventing and stopping its Infection* (London: Wilson and Nicol, 1774), 3. Mark Harrison, *Medicine in an Age of Commerce and Empire: Britain and Its Tropical Colonies, 1660–1830* (Oxford: Oxford University Press, 2010), 72. On Lind's importance as a theorist of fevers see also Hamlin, *More than Hot*, 119–125, and DeLacy, *Contagionism Catches On*, 66–74; Anon., *A Treatise on Fevers; wherein their Causes are exhibited in a new Point of View* (London: Scratcherd and Whitaker, 1788). This author presented a unique take on the old saw about paupers being immune vectors—highly infectious, yet themselves healthy—by arguing that their bodily filth made them unappealing fare for the tiny bugs: "The animalcules avoid preying upon such nauseous bodies" (65–67). On animalculist views of fever in this period, including their heavy reliance on theories of putridity, see DeLacy, *Contagionism Catches On*, 100–103, 108–109.

32. On the nervous body see G. S. Rousseau, *Nervous Acts: Essays on Literature, Culture, and Sensibility* (New York: Palgrave, 2004); Christopher Lawrence, "The Nervous System and Society in the Scottish Enlightenment," in *Natural Order: Historical Studies of Scientific Culture*, ed. Barry Barnes and Steven Shapin (London: Sage, 1979), 19–40. Understandings of the nervous body should now be read in tandem with what Hisao Ishizuka has recently termed

the "Fibre Body": "Enlightening the Fibre-Woven Body: William Blake and Eighteenth-Century Fibre Medicine," *Literature and Medicine* 25, no. 1 (2006): 72–92; and " 'Fibre Body': The Concept of Fibre in Eighteenth-Century Medicine, c. 1700–1740," *Medical History* 56, no. 4 (2012): 562–584. Hamlin, *More than Hot*, 127–133. On Cullen's thought as it applied to fever see W. F. Bynum, "Cullen and the Study of Fevers in Britain, 1760–1820," and Dale C. Smith, "Medical Science, Medical Practice, and the Emerging Concept of Typhus in Mid-Eighteenth-Century Britain," both in *Theories of Fever from Antiquity to the Enlightenment*, ed. W. F. Bynum and Vivian Nutton, 121–134 and 134–148, respectively (London: Wellcome Institute for the History of Medicine, 1981); W. F. Bynum, "Cullen and the Nervous System," in *William Cullen and the Eighteenth-Century Medical World*, ed. A. Doig et al. (Edinburgh: Edinburgh University Press, 1993), 152–162; Guenter Risse, *Mending Bodies, Saving Souls: A History of Hospitals* (Oxford: Oxford University Press, 1999), 243–251.

33. Hamlin, *More than Hot*, 120; DeLacy, *Contagionism Catches On*, 137, 146; Smith explores the influences of mid-eighteenth-century doctors like Huxham on Cullen's conception of typhus. "Medical Science," esp. 131–134; William Cullen was explicit that "it can hardly be doubted that human and marsh effluvia are of the same quality." *First Lines of the Practice of Physic*, 3rd ed., vol. 1 (Edinburgh: William Creech, 1781), 74–75. It is also worth pointing out that Cullen toed the traditional line on the generation of the disease called jail fever, attributing it to "the effluvia constantly arising from the living body, if long retained." And while he noted that climate or seasons could affect the characteristics of fevers, so, too, did "the peculiar constitutions of the several persons affected." Cullen's students were thus still encouraged to take into account the quality of different bodies when evaluating fevers. *First Lines of the Practice of Physic*, 69–72. Also quoted in John Alderson, *An Essay on the Nature and Origin of the Contagions of Fevers* (Hull: G. Prince, 1788), 6. My emphasis.

34. Physician Lewis Mansey specified ten names for the same disease. In his chapter on "The Putrid or Malignant Fever" he noted, "This fever is also called the Pestilential Fever," adding a footnote to declare that it was "Otherwise called the Violent, Putrid, Malignant, Gaol, Camp, Hospital or Spotted fever." *The Practical Physician; or, medical instructor* (London: W. Stratford, 1800), 75.

35. Erica Charters, *Disease, War, and the Imperial State: The Welfare of the British Armed Forces during the Seven Years War* (Chicago: University of Chicago Press, 2014). As late as 1801 influential Quaker physician John Coakley

Lettsom still linked plague and fever: "Many circumstances, and among others, that of malignant fever preceding and following, plague, seem to prove that the plague is merely an aggravated malignant fever." *Hints Designed to Promote Beneficence, Temperance, & Medical Science,* vol. 1 (London: J. Mawman, 1801), 326; John Beattie, *Crime and the Courts in England, 1660–1800* (Oxford: Oxford University Press, 1986), 213–235. Also Nicholas Rogers, "Confronting the Crime Wave: The Debate over Social Reform and Regulation, 1749–1753," in *Stilling the Grumbling Hive: The Response to Social and Economic Problems in England, 1689–1750,* ed. Lee Davison et al. (New York: St. Martin's, 1989), 77–98.

36. Nicholas Rogers, *Mayhem: Post-War Crime and Violence in Britain, 1748–53* (New Haven: Yale University Press, 2013), 36; Rogers, "Confronting the Crime Wave," 81–85; Tim Hitchcock and Robert Shoemaker, *London Lives: Poverty, Crime, and the Making of a Modern City, 1690–1800* (Cambridge: Cambridge University Press, 2015), 198; Peter Clark, "The Mother Gin Controversy in the Early Eighteenth Century," *Transactions of the Royal Historical Society* 38 (1988): 63–84; Lee Davison, "Experiments in the Social Regulation of Industry: Gin Legislation, 1729–1751," in Davison et al., *Stilling the Grumbling Hive,* 25–48; and Jessica Warner, *Craze: Gin and Debauchery in an Age of Reason* (London: Profile, 2003).

37. Beattie, *Crime and the Courts,* 220. Beattie's figures came from Surrey, which accounted for perhaps one sixth of greater London at the time.

38. John Huxham, *Observationes de aëre et morbis epidemicis* (London: S. Austen, 1739); John Huxham, *An Essay on Fevers, and their Various Kinds, as depending on the Different Constitutions of the Blood* (London: S. Austen, 1750), 56, 61, 79–80, 131–132. The book was advertised in the *London Evening Post,* August 9–11, 1750. It would go through ten editions by 1785. DeLacy, *Contagionism Catches On,* 32. Grant, *Essay on the Pestilential Fever of Sydenham,* 9, also 68, 115, 165–166.

39. William Black, to take just one example, attributed sterility both to "too frequent coition" and to "excessive chastity." *An arithmetical and medical analysis of the diseases and mortality of the human species* (London: John Crowders, 1789), 155–156; Anon., *The Practical Scheme. Explaining the Symptoms and Nature of the Venereal or Secret Disease, a Broken Constitution & a Gleet* (London: H. Parker, 1725). For references to a "venereal taint" in fever treatises see Jean Astruc, *Academical lectures on fevers* (London: J. Nourse, 1747), 131; Simon Mason, *The nature of an intermitting fever and ague consider'd* (London: J. Hodges, 1745), 245–256; and James Sims,

Observations on epidemic disorders, with remarks on nervous and malignant fevers (London: J. Johnson, 1773), 123. Lind, *Treatise of the Scurvy*, 176, and Lind, *Health of Seamen*, 141.

40. Layard, *Directions to Prevent the contagion of Jail Distemper*, 5–8, 19–20. My emphasis.

41. John Mason Good, *Dissertation on the Diseases of Prisons and Poor Houses* (London: C. Dilly, 1795), 25–26, 29–30, 33.

42. Ibid., 26–27.

43. Ibid., 73.

44. Ibid., 31–32, 68, 73. By 1795 typhus was becoming an increasingly common name for the disease. Mason Good made the point to clarify that he meant the same disease described by Huxham almost fifty years earlier (91–92).

45. Ibid., 74–76.

5. Jail Fever and Prison Reform

1. *Remembrancer*, May 26, 1750; *Whitehall Evening Post or London Intelligencer*, May 26–29, 1750; *Public Advertiser*, February 20, 1755.

2. Stephen Theodore Janssen, *A Letter to the Right Honourable the Lord-Mayor, The Worshipful the Aldermen, The Recorder, and the Gentlemen of the Committee, Appointed for the Rebuilding of Newgate* (London: n.p., 1767). 20–22, 34, 38–39 and 56. The exporting of Newgate's waste would be remembered for years. *Public Advertiser*, February 20, 1755, and *Gazetteer and New Daily Advertiser*, December 6, 1771. On waste management see Emily Cockayne, *Hubbub: Filth, Noise, and Stench in England* (New Haven: Yale University Press, 2007), 181–205, and Leona J. Skelton, *Sanitation in Urban Britain, 1560–1700* (New York: Routledge, 2016).

3. *Public Advertiser*, February 20, 1755; Janssen, *Letter*, 57–58.

4. *Whitehall Evening Post or London Intelligencer*, May 19–22, 22–24, 1750; *Read's Weekly Journal or British Gazetteer*, May 26, 1750; *London Evening Post*, June 7–9, 1750; *Old England*, June 2, 1750.

5. Anthony Babington, *The English Bastille: A History of Newgate Gaol and Prison Conditions in Britain, 1188–1902* (New York: St. Martin's, 1971); John Murray, *The Gaol: The Story of Newgate—London's Most Notorious Prison* (London: John Murray, 2008); Gary Kelly, General Introduction to *Newgate Narratives*, vol. 1, ed. Gary Kelly, ix–xciii (London: Pickering and Chatto 2008).

6. Janssen, *Letter*, 4–5, 8, 14–19. Janssen dates O'Connor's report as March 24, but given the course of events it is likely that he meant May 24; *Read's Weekly Journal or British Gazetteer*, June 9, 1750.

7. Stephen Hales, *Statical Essays: containing Hæmastatics*, vol. 2 (London: W. Innys, 1740), 100, 104–107, 115, 126–127 and 213–214; D. G. Allan and Robert E. Schofield, *Stephen Hales: Scientist and Philanthropist* (London: Scolar Press, 1980), 30–47, 65–99; A. E. Clark-Kennedy, *Stephen Hales, D.D., F.R.S.: An Eighteenth-Century Biography* (Cambridge: Cambridge University Press, 1929), 90–110, 151–207; James Riley, *The Eighteenth-Century Campaign to Avoid Disease* (London: Macmillan, 1987), 20–21, 97–108; Robin Evans, *The Fabrication of Virtue: English Prison Architecture, 1750–1840* (Cambridge: Cambridge University Press, 1982), 96–103.

8. Stephen Hales, *A Description of Ventilators, Whereby Great Quantities of Fresh Air May with Ease be conveyed into Mines, Goals, Hospitals, Work-Houses and Ships, in Exchange for their Noxious Air* (London: W. Innys, 1743), 39, quoted in Evans, *Fabrication of Virtue*, 100–102; Clark-Kennedy, *Stephen Hales*, 151–169 and 189–191.

9. *Whitehall Evening Post or London Intelligencer*, August 11–14, 1750; *Old England*, August 18, 1750; *Read's Weekly Journal or British Gazetteer*, August 18, 1750; *Daily Advertiser*, March 20, 1752; *Read's Weekly Journal or British Gazetteer*, April 4, 1752; *London Daily Advertiser*, April 14, 1752, May 5, 1752. Janssen, *Letter*, 21, 22, 25, 29; Clark-Kennedy, *Stephen Hales*, 199–201; Evans, *Fabrication of Virtue*, 102; John Pringle, "An Account of several Persons seized with Goal-Fever, working in Newgate; and of the Manner, in which the Infection was communicated to one intire Family," *Philosophical Transactions* 48 (1753): 42–55.

10. Stephen Hales, "A Description of Dr. Halel's [*sic*] Ventilators fixed in Newgate," *Gentleman's Magazine, and Historical Chronicle, Volume XXII for the Year MDCCLII* (London, 1752), 179–182. Hales used similar language in a report to Janssen that same year. Janssen, *Letter*, 36; Riley, *Eighteenth-Century Campaign to Avoid Disease*.

11. *Whitehall Evening Post or London Intelligencer*, August 7–9, 1750; *Read's Weekly Journal or British Gazetteer*, July 6, 1754; *Public Advertiser*, February 6, 1753, March 18, 1754; Stephen Hales, "A Further account of the Success of Ventilators, &c.," *Gentleman's Magazine or Monthly Chronologer* 23 (1754): 123; and Stephen Hales, "An Account of the Great Benefit of Ventilators in many Instances, in preserving the Health and Lives of People, in Slave and other Transport Ships," *Philosophical Transactions* 49 (1755): 312–332.

12. *Daily Advertiser* (not to be confused with the *London Daily Advertiser*), March 17, 1752; *London Daily Advertiser*, May 25, June 14, 1753; *London Evening Post*, June 12–14, 1753, February 1–4, 1755; *Read's Weekly Journal or British*

Gazetteer, June 16, 30, 1753; *Public Advertiser,* February 5, 20, 28, 1755; Janssen, *Letter,* 45.

13. *Whitehall Evening Post or London Intelligencer,* June 12–14, 1755. LMA, Corporation of London, Court of Common Council: Newgate Gaol Committee, Minutes, COL/CC/NGC/01/01/001, 1–2.

14. LMA, Newgate Gaol Committee, Minutes, COL/CC/NGC/01/01/001, 2–3, 8–9; LMA, Newgate Gaol Committee, Rough Minutes, COL/CC/NGC/02/01/002, [n.p.], July 18, 1755.

15. LMA, Newgate Gaol Committee, Minutes, COL/CC/NGC/01/01/001, 10–12; LMA, Newgate Gaol Committee, Rough Minutes, COL/CC/NGC/02/01/002, [n.p.], July 31, 1755. Newgate's neighbors may have been exhibiting their own variation of "smellwalking" as explored by Victoria Henshaw in *Urban Smellscapes: Understanding and Designing City Smell Environments* (New York: Routledge, 2014). For historical work on urban scents and danger see Alain Corbin, *The Foul and the Fragrant: Odor and the French Social Imagination* (Cambridge: Harvard University Press, 1986), 89–160; Cockayne, *Hubbub,* 208–216; and Jonathan Reinarz, *Past Scents: Historical Perspectives on Smell* (Urbana: University of Illinois Press, 2014), especially chapters 5 and 6: "Uncommon Scents: Class and Smell" and "Mapping the Smellscape: Smell and the City," 145–175, 176–208.

16. LMA, Newgate Gaol Committee, Minutes, COL/CC/NGC/01/01/001, 20, 32; LMA, Newgate Gaol Committee, Rough Minutes, COL/CC/NCG/02/01/001, [n.p.], [n.d.], and COL/CC/NCG/03/01/001, [n.p.]; *London Evening Post,* August 30, 1755; Harold Kalman, "Newgate Prison," *Architectural History* 12 (1969): 50–61, 50; Wayne Joseph Sheehan, "The London Prison System, 1666–1795," Ph.D. diss., University of Maryland, 1975, 392–394.

17. LMA, Newgate Gaol Committee, Rough Minutes, COL/CC/NGC/02/01/001, [n.p.]; Janssen, *Letter,* 4–5.

18. 27 Geo. II cap. 17; Sheehan, "London Prison System," 387–390; *London Chronicle,* July 26–29, 1760; *Lloyd's Evening Post and British Chronicle,* July 30–August 1, 1760; *London Evening Post,* July 29–31, 1760; "Report to Comon. Council about removing the Prisoners in Ludgate to the London Workhouse," December 3, 1760. Contained in "Reports and Papers of Committees concerning the removal of prisoners from Ludgate to part of the London Workhouse, 1760–61," LMA, CLA/033/01/014.

19. 7 Geo. III, c. 37; Kalman, "Newgate Prison," 50; Sheehan, "London Prison System," 394; Evans, *Fabrication of Virtue,* 108; Tim Hitchcock and Robert

Shoemaker, *London Lives: Poverty, Crime, and the Making of a Modern City, 1690–1800* (Cambridge: Cambridge University Press, 2015), 325–326; *St. James's Chronicle or the British Evening Post*, February 16–18, 1762; *Public Advertiser*, December 2, 1763; *The Universal Museum. Or, Gentleman's and Ladies Polite Magazine of History, Politicks and Literature for 1763*, vol. 3 (London, 1764), 153; *Lloyd's Evening Post*, March 12–14, July 25–27, 1764. This last newspaper also contained as its next item the frightening report that more than four hundred people had died of an "epidemical distemper" in Naples. Invoices submitted by "The Worshipful Committee appointed by the Court of Common Council to prosecute the Petition to Parliament for Rebuilding the Gaol of Newgate" and "Hallkeepers Bill for Disbursements for the Worshipfull Committee Applying to Parliament for the removal of Newgate," in LMA, Newgate Gaol Committee, Rough Minutes COL/CC/NGC/03/01/001; Middlesex Sessions: Sessions Papers—Justices' Working Papers, April 1765. *London Lives, 1680–1800: Crime, Poverty, and Social Policy in the Metropolis*, LMSMPS505470113 (www.londonlives.org, version 1.1, June 1, 2017).

20. Evans, *Fabrication of Virtue*, 94–117. Worthy of note is that such silos are absent in the residences of the keeper and turnkeys (center, front—marked A, B, and L), suggesting that their bodily waste was not thought as dangerous.

21. Janssen, *Letter; St. James Chronicle or the British Evening Post*, February 16–18, 1762; *Public Advertiser*, December 2, 1763; *The Universal Museum. Or, Gentleman's and Ladies Polite Magazine of History, Politicks and Literature for 1763*, vol. 3 (London, 1764), 153. *Gazetteer and New Daily Advertiser*, February 20, 1767. It is notable that it was even newsworthy that a jail was *free* of jail fever. *Lloyds Evening Post*, March 12–14, 1764; *Gazetteer and London Daily Advertiser*, March 14, 1764.

22. LMA, "Committee for Rebuilding Newgate, Journal, 1767–1785," COL/CC/NGC/04/01/001, 22–25, 40, 55–59. My emphasis.

23. Kalman, "Newgate Prison," 51. Indeed, the phenomenon of polite Londoners visiting prisoners has been raised as a cogent counterpoint to my argument. Yet even when drawn to gape at famous criminals like the gentleman highwayman Paul Lewis, well-heeled men like John Boswell kept their distance. Listen to Boswell's account of remaining in an outer courtyard when he went to see Lewis in May 1763: "I stepped into a sort of court before the cells. They are surely most dismal places. There are three rows of 'em, four in a row, all above each other. They have double iron windows, and

within these, strong iron rails; and in these dark mansions are the unhappy criminals confined. I did not go in, but stood in the court." Frederick A. Pottle, *Boswell's London Journal, 1762–1763* (London: Heinemann, 1950), 250–251. Robert Shoemaker discusses such visitation in "Fear of Crime in Eighteenth-Century London," in *Understanding Emotions in Early Europe*, ed. Michael Champion and Andrew Lynch (Turnhout, Belgium: Brepols, 2015), 233–249. My thanks to him for raising this issue.

24. Daniel Peter Layard, *Directions to Prevent the contagion of Jail Distemper, commonly called the Jail-Fever* (London: James Robson, 1772), 27–46. The epidemic was first reported on September 30, and Layard dedicated his book on October 18 (n.p.). *London Chronicle*, September 29–October 1, 3–6, 1772; *General Evening Post*, October 6–8, 1772; *London Evening Post*, October 8–10, October 31–November 3, 1772; *Bingley's London Journal*, September 26–October 3, 1772, October 10–17, 17–24, 1772; *Craftsman or Say's Weekly Journal*, October 24, 1772; *Middlesex Journal or Universal Evening Post*, September 1–3, October 20–22, 22–24, 27–29, 1772; *Morning Chronicle and London Advertiser*, September 5, 30, October 14, 17, November 2, 4, 7, 1772; *Public Advertiser*, October 2, 1772; *Gazetteer and New Daily Advertiser*, October 19, 1772. On October 27 the *Middlesex Journal* reported: "The felons at the Old-Bailey have this session been tried in a dress like waggoners frocks, to prevent the communication of the goal distemper." *Middlesex Journal or Universal Evening Post*, October 27–29, 1772.

25. *London Chronicle*, October 3–6, 1772; *Middlesex Journal or Universal Evening Post*, October 13–15, 1772.

26. *Middlesex Journal or Universal Evening Post*, October 13–15, 1772; *Public Advertiser*, October 13, 1772.

27. *Proceedings of the Old Bailey*, Edward Brocket, Breaking Peace, Riot, December 9, 1772, ref. t17721209-99; *Public Advertiser*, November 16, December 19, 1772.

28. The literature on Wilkes and his supporters is vast. The key works are George Rude, *Wilkes and Liberty: A Social Study* (Oxford: Clarendon, 1962); John Brewer, *Party Ideology and Popular Politics at the Accession of George III* (Cambridge: Cambridge University Press, 1981), 163–200; Arthur Cash, *John Wilkes: The Scandalous Father of Civil Liberty* (New Haven: Yale University Press, 2006). *London Chronicle*, November 12–14, 1772; *Public Advertiser*, November 16, 1772; *Morning Chronicle and London Advertiser*, October 1772.

29. *Public Advertiser*, October 23, 1772; *Lloyd's Evening Post*, January 29–February 1, February 12–15, 1773.

30. *Middlesex Journal or Universal Evening Post,* October 8–10, 31, 1772; *Bigley's London Journal,* October 17–24, 1772; *Public Advertiser,* October 14, 1772; *Morning Chronicle and London Advertiser,* October 17, 1772; *Gazetteer and New Daily Advertiser,* October 19, 1772.

31. *Morning Chronicle and London Advertiser,* October 15, 1772.

32. *Public Advertiser,* October 14, 1772.

33. *St. James's Chronicle or the British Evening Post,* October 13–15, 1772; *Gazetteer and New Daily Advertiser,* October 6, 10, 1772; *Public Advertiser,* October 7, 14, 1772; *London Evening Post,* November 5–7, 1772.

34. Even critical histories like Ignatieff's advance versions of this picture. Michael Ignatieff, *A Just Measure of Pain: The Penitentiary in the Industrial Revolution, 1750–1850* (New York: Penguin, 1978), 47–57.

35. Porter has made the case for not seeing Howard as alone in the crusade to reform prisons, though he does not explore the earlier roots of this movement. Roy Porter, "Howard's Beginning: Prisons, Disease, Hygiene," in *The Health of Prisoners: Historical Essays, ed.* Richard Creese, W. F. Bynum, and J. Bearn (Amsterdam: Rodopi, 1995). See also Robert Alan Cooper, "Ideas and Their Execution: English Prison Reform," *Eighteenth Century Studies* 10, no. 1 (1976): 73–93.

36. Surveys include Sean McConville, *A History of English Prison Administration,* vol. 1 (London: Routledge, 1981), 78–104; Randall McGowan, "The Well-Ordered Prison: England, 1780–1865," in *The Oxford History of the Prison,* ed. Norval Morris and David J. Rothman, 71–99, 77–83; Cooper, "Ideas and Their Execution"; Sidney Webb and Beatrice Webb, *English Prisons under Local Government* (1922; rpt. Hamden, CT: Archon, 1963); Leon Radzinowicz, *The History of English Criminal Law and Its Administration,* vol. 1 (London: Stevens, 1948). For an appraisal of the theological implications of the prison reform movement see Laurie Throness, *A Protestant Purgatory: Theological Origins of the Penitentiary Act, 1779* (Burlington, VT: Ashgate, 2008).

37. Margaret DeLacy, *Prison Reform in Lancashire, 1700–1850: A Study in Local Administration* (Stanford: Stanford University Press, 1986), 94; Porter, "Howard's Beginning," 16; Philippa Hardman, "Fear of Fever and the Limits of Enlightenment: Selling Prison Reform in Late Eighteenth-Century Gloucestershire," *Cultural and Social History* 10, no. 4 (2013): 511–531. Hardman usefully situates the issue of fever at the heart of Gloucestershire reform activity. However, she presents reformers like G. O. Paul as strategically deploying fever to drum up support for reform, suggesting that the fear

was more manufactured than real. Outbreaks of fever were, in her telling, "relatively isolated incidents . . . [that] certainly never developed into the so-called 'general national calamity' referred to by Paul" (523). On this score she and I decidedly differ. Foucault has, of course, put the body at the center of his formulation of the modern prison, but I wish to draw attention to issues rather different from institutional technologies of discipline and the production of what he calls "docile bodies." Michel Foucault, *Discipline and Punish: The Birth of the Prison*, trans. Alan Sheridan (New York: Pantheon, 1977), esp. 135–169. On this theme of the body and punishment see also Randall McGowan, "The Body and Punishment in Eighteenth-Century England," *Journal of Modern History* 59, no. 4 (1987): 651–679; Paul Griffiths, "Bodies and Souls in Norwich: Punishing Petty Crimes, 1540–1700," in *Penal Practice and Culture, 1500–1900: Punishing the English*, ed. Paul Griffiths and Simon Devereaux (Hampshire: Palgrave Macmillan, 2004), 85–120; and Michael Meranze, *Laboratories of Virtue: Punishment, Revolution, and Authority in Philadelphia, 1760–1835* (Chapel Hill: University of North Carolina Press, 2012), 131–216.

38. McConville, *History of English Prison Administration*, 86. On Fothergill's importance advancing putrid theories of contagion see Margaret DeLacy, *Contagionism Catches On: Medical Ideology in Britain, 1730–1800* (New York: Palgrave Macmillan, 2016), 34–38; Thirteenth Parliament of Great Britain, Seventh Session, *A Bill for the Relief of Prisoners charged with Felony or other Crimes, who shall be acquitted, or discharged by Proclamation . . . and for more effectively securing the Health of Prisoners in Gaol during their Confinement* (London, 1774), 3; 14 George III, cap. 59; *Morning Chronicle and London Advertiser*, March 18, 1774; *Middlesex Journal and Evening Advertiser*, March 26, 1774; *St. James Chronicle or British Evening Post*, April 2, 1774; *Gazetteer and New Daily Advertiser*, April 28, 1774. Deliberations on the bill began on February 13 and lasted until it was passed the House of Commons on May 20, finally receiving royal assent on June 2. *Journal of the House of Commons, From the 26th, 1772, in the Thirtieth Year of the Reign of King George the Third, to September the 15th, 1774, In the Fourteenth Year of the Reign of King George the Third*, vol. 34 (London, 1774), 469, 486, 524, 535, 545, 563, 566, 576, 581, 591, 601, 605–606, 732, 740, 779. On prison infirmaries see Joe Sim, *Medical Power in Prisons: The Prison Medical Service in England, 1774–1989* (Milton Keynes: Open University Press, 1990), and Peter McRorie Higgins, *Medical Care in English Prisons, 1770–1850* (Bloomington, IN: Trafford, 2007).

39. Hitchcock and Shoemaker, *London Lives*, 333–334, plus their additional dataset "Old Bailey Punishment Sentences, 1690–1800," http://www.cambridge.org/gb/academic/subjects/history/british-history-after-1450/london-lives-poverty-crime-and-making-modern-city-16901800#CY030EFLDC3rSXEv.97, file name: "Punishment_statistics-1690–1800.xlsx," accessed 24 June 2017. Simon Devereaux, "The Making of the Penitentiary Act, 1775–1779," *Historical Journal* 42, no. 2 (1999): 405–433, 406; John Beattie, *Crime and the Courts in England, 1660–1800* (Oxford: Oxford University Press, 1986), 565.

40. 16 George III c. 43; Charles F. Campbell, *The Intolerable Hulks: British Shipboard Confinement, 1776–1857* (Bowie, MD: Heritage, 1994); Randall McGowan, "The Well-Ordered Prison: England, 1780–1865," in *The Oxford History of the Prison*, ed. Norval Morris and David J. Rothman, 71–99 (Oxford: Oxford University Press, 1998), 76–77, 89–92; Beattie, *Crime and the Courts*, 566–569, 573–574, 576–582, 593–597; Hitchcock and Shoemaker, *London Lives*, 334–338; *Morning Chronicle and London Advertiser*, October 29, 1772. My thanks to Simon Devereaux for this last reference.

41. Beattie, *Crime and the Courts*, 546, 558–560, 569–582; Devereaux, "Making of the Penitentiary Act," 408–413. See also Ignatieff, *A Just Measure of Pain*, 44–79; and McConville, *History of English Prison Administration*, 78–87.

42. Devereaux, "Making of the Penitentiary Act," 413–419; *Speeches of the Right Honourable Edmund Burke in the House of Commons and in Westminster Hall*, vol. 3 (London: Longman, 1816), 188.

43. Devereaux, "Making of the Penitentiary Act," 429, 431; Beattie, *Crime and the Courts*, 574, 593–594; McConville, *History of English Prison Administration*, 109; McGowan, "Well Ordered Prison," 80–81. For local studies see DeLacy, *Prison Reform in Lancashire*; Eric Stockdale, *A Study of Bedford Prison, 1660–1877* (London: Phillimore, 1977); and Philippa Hardman, "The Origins of Late Eighteenth-Century Prison Reform in England," Ph.D. thesis, University of Sheffield, 2007, 41–74.

44. LMA, Newgate Gaol Committee, Journal, 1767–1785, COL/CC/NGC/04/01/001, 324–330; Hitchcock and Shoemaker, *London Lives*, 349. On the riots see the various contributions to Ian Haywood and John Seed, eds. *The Gordon Riots: Politics, Culture, and Insurrection in Late Eighteenth-Century Britain* (Oxford: Oxford University Press, 2012), including Ian Haywood's chapter on the burning of Newgate, " 'A Metropolis in Flames and a Nation in Ruins': The Gordon Riots as Sublime Spectacle," 117–143. See also Peter Linebaugh, *The London Hanged: Crime and Civil Society in the Eighteenth Century* (London: Verso, 2003), 333–356.

45. Hitchcock and Shoemaker, *London Lives*, 338–339, 343–352, 355–357, 362–370.

46. *Proceedings of the Old Bailey*, George Morley, Perverting Justice, April 6, 1785, ref. t17850406-81; William Bateman, Returning from Transportation, December 15, 1792, ref. t17921215-18; John Purdy, Returning from Transportation, February 20, 1799, ref. t17990220-40; George Barrington, Perverting Justice, January 15, 1783, ref. t17830115-1; Charles Peat, Returning from Transportation, July 7, 1784, ref. t17840707-6; Hitchcock and Shoemaker, *London Lives*, 375.

47. Beattie, *Crime and the Courts*, 223, 596–599; *Parker's General Advertiser and Morning Intelligencer*, July 11, 1783; McGowan, "Well-Ordered Prison," 76; McConville, *History of English Prison Administration*, 109. On transportation to Australia see Robert Hughes, *The Fatal Shore: The Epic of Australia's Founding* (New York: Vintage, 1986); Alan Brooke and David Brandon, *Bound for Botany Bay: British Convict Voyages to Australia* (London: National Archives, 2005); and Simon Devereaux, "In Place of Death: Transportation, Penal Practice, and the English State, 1770–1830," in *Qualities of Mercy: Justice, Punishment, and Discretion*, ed. Carolyn Strange (Vancouver: University of British Columbia Press, 1996), 52–76, 66.

48. Tim Hitchcock, "The London Vagrancy Crisis of the 1780s," *Rural History* 24, no. 1 (2013): 59–72, esp. 62–68; Tim Hitchcock, Adam Crymble, and Louise Falcini, "Loose, Idle, and Disorderly: Vagrant Removal in Late Eighteenth-Century Middlesex," *Social History* 39, no. 4: 509–527; and Nicholas Rogers, "Policing the Poor in Eighteenth-Century London: The Vagrancy Laws and Their Administration," *Historie Sociale/Social History* 24, no. 4 (1991): 127–147.

49. Layard, *Directions to Prevent the contagion of the Jail Distemper;* James Lind, *An Essay on the Most Effectual Means of Preserving the Health of Seamen . . . Together with Observations on the Jail Distemper, and the proper Methods of preventing and stopping its Infection* (London: Wilson and Nicol, 1774); William Grant, *An Essay on the Pestilential Fever of Sydenham, commonly called the Gaol, Hospital, Ship and Camp-Fever* (London: T. Cadell, 1775); John Heysham, *An Account of the Jail Fever, or Typhus Carcerum; as it appeared in at Carlisle in the year 1781* (London: T. Cadell, 1782); Robert Robertson, *Observations on Jail, Hospital or Ship Fever* (London: J. Murray, 1783); Thomas Day, *Some Considerations on the Different Ways of Removing confined and infectious Air . . . with Remarks on the Contagion in Maidstone Gaol* (Maidstone: J. Mark, 1784); David Campbell, *Observations on the Typhus, or Low Contagious Fever*

(Lancaster: H. Walmsley, 1785); John Mason Good, *Dissertation on the Diseases of Prisons and Poor Houses* (London: C. Dilly, 1795); James Carmichael Smyth, *The Effect of Nitrous Vapour in Preventing and Destroying Contagion . . . With an Introduction Respecting the Nature of the Contagion which gives Rise to the Jail or Hospital Fever* (London, J. Johnson, 1799).

50. John Howard, *The State of the Prisons in England And Wales, with preliminary observations, and an account of some foreign prisons* (Warrington: William Eyres, 1777); Jacob Leroux, *Thoughts on the Present State of the Prisons of this Country* (London: Printed for the Author, 1780); G. O. Paul, *Considerations on the Defects of Prisons* (London: T. Cadell, 1784); Jonas Hanway, *Observations Moral and Political, Particularly Respecting the Necessity of Good Order and Religious Oeconomy in our Prisons* (London: Dodsley, 1784); Jeremy Bentham, *Panopticon; or the Inspection House* (Dublin: Thomas Byrne, 1791).

51. William Smith, *The State of the Gaols in London, Westminster, and Borough of Southwark* (London: J. Bew, 1776); G. O. Paul, *Thoughts on the Alarming Progress of the Gaol Fever* (Glocester [*sic*]: R. Raikes, 1784); David Steuart, *General Heads of a Plan for Erecting a New Prison and Bridewell in the City of Edinburgh* (Edinburgh: n.p., 1782); and Jeremiah Fitzpatrick, *An Essay on Gaol-Abuses, and on the means of redressing them: Together with the General Method of Treating Disorders to which Prisoners are most Incident* (Dublin: D. Graisberry, 1784).

52. Quoted in DeLacy, *Prison Reform in Lancashire*, 81.

53. Gary Kelly, *English Fiction of the Romantic Period, 1789–1830* (New York: Routledge, 2016), 43; Candace Ward, *Desire and Disorder: Fevers, Fictions, and Feeling in English Georgian Culture* (Lewisburg, PA: Bucknell University Press, 2007), 113, 136, 170.

6. Braving Contagion

1. Roy Porter, "Howard's Beginning: Prisons, Disease, Hygiene," in *The Health of Prisoners: Historical Essays*, ed. Richard Creese, W. F. Bynum, and J. Bearn (Amsterdam: Rodopi, 1995), 5–6. Howard has been the subject of numerous celebratory biographies. John Aikin, *A View of the Character and Public Services of the late John Howard* (London: J. Johnson, 1792); James Baldwin Brown, *Memoir of the Public and Private Life of John Howard: Philanthropist* (London: T. and G. Underwood, 1821); W. Hepworth Dixon, *John Howard and the Prison World of Europe* (London: Jackson and Walford, 1849); Leona Baumgartner, *John Howard (1726–1790): Hospital and Prison Reformer* (Baltimore: Johns Hopkins University Press, 1939); Martin Southwood, *John*

Howard, Prison Reformer: An Account of His Life and Travels (London: Independent Press, 1958); and most recently, Tessa West, *The Curious Mr. Howard, Legendary Prison Reformer* (Sherfield-on-Loddon, UK: Waterside, 2011). A counterpoint is offered by Rod Morgan, "Divine Philanthropy: John Howard Reconsidered," *History* 62, no. 106 (1977): 388–410.

2. See the contributions in Graham Mooney and Jonathan Reinarz, eds., *Permeable Walls: Historical Perspectives on Hospital and Asylum Visiting* (Amsterdam: Rodopi, 2009).

3. A third concurred, noting that what inspections did occur were usually cursory: "The Justices think the inside of my House is too close for them; they satisfy themselves with viewing the outside." Ibid., 67–68.

4. John Howard, *The State of the Prisons in England And Wales, with preliminary observations, and an account of some foreign prisons* (Warrington: William Eyres, 1777), 3, 13–14, 52, 56, 67–68, 322, 372. Also Howard, *State of the Prisons,* 3rd edition (Warrington: William Eyres, 1784), 468. Original emphasis.

5. Howard, *State of the Prisons* (1777), 149 and passim, e.g., 151, 211, 245, 257, 269.

6. Ibid., 369 and passim, e.g., 165, 182, 186–187, 213–215, 220–221, 239, 273–277, 329, 343–344, 409–412, 426, 474–475.

7. Ibid., 192, 198, 212, 217, 226, 230, 244, 270, 322, 340, 342, 354, 382, 409, 475. Also passim, e.g., 175, 186, 190, 192, 212, 276–277, 286, 334, 344, 469.

8. Ibid., 20.

9. Oxford University, Bodleian Library, MS. Eng. Misc. c. 332, fols. 22–34, 43–45, 48–49, 50–51, 53–57; Howard, *State of the Prisons* (1777), 5, 443.

10. Oxford University, Bodleian Library, MS. Eng. Misc. c. 332, fols. 58–83, 93–101, MS. Eng. Misc. e. 399; Misc. e. 400, Misc. e. 401 and Misc. e. 402; Michael Ignatieff, *A Just Measure of Pain: The Penitentiary in the Industrial Revolution, 1750–1850* (New York: Penguin, 1978), 49–52. For an attempt to situate Howard's religious beliefs within the history of prison reform see Laurie Throness, *A Protestant Purgatory: Theological Origins of the Penitentiary Act, 1779* (Burlington, VT: Ashgate, 2008) 116–117, 130–131, 141–148, 152–156, 241–247.

11. Howard, *State of the Prisons* (1777), 13, and *State of the Prisons* (1784), 467–468. West comments on Howard's penchant for the dissenting tradition of written covenants. *Curious Mr. Howard,* 107–108. Oxford, Bodleian, MS. Eng. Misc e. 400, n.p. Original emphasis, MS. Eng. Misc. e. 401, fol. 3 and MS. Eng. Misc e. 400, fols. 95–96.

12. David Gentilcore, "The Fear of Disease and the Disease of Fear," in *Fear in Early Modern Society*, ed. William Naphy and Penny Roberts (Manchester: Manchester University Press, 1997), 184–208, and Andrew Wear, "Fear, Anxiety, and the Plague in Early Modern England," in *Religion, Health, and Suffering*, ed. John R. Hinnells and Roy Porter (London: Kegan Paul, 1999), 339–363; Andrew Wear, *Knowledge and Practice in English Medicine, 1550–1680* (Cambridge: Cambridge University Press, 2000), 242, 330; Fay Bound Alberti, "Emotions in the Early Modern Medical Tradition," in *Medicine, Emotion, and Disease, 1700–1950*, ed. Fay Bound Alberti (Basingstoke: Palgrave Macmillan, 2006), 1–21; Thomas Willis, *A Plain and Easie Method for Preserving (by God's blessing) those that are well from the infection of the Plague, or any contagious distemper in city, camp, fleet, &c* (London: W. Crook, 1691), 6–7, 25; John Browne, *The Surgeons Assistant* (London: James Knapton, 1703), 58–59; Strickland Gough, *A Discourse occasion'd by the Small-Pox and Plague now reigning in Europe* (London: Joseph Penn, 1711), 10, 25–26; Phil-anthropos, *A Brief Essay on the Small-Pox and Measles, Plague, Malignant and Pestilential fevers* (London: n.p., 1721), 23; James Lind, *An Essay on the Most Effectual Means of Preserving the Health of Seamen, in the Royal Navy* (London: Wilson and Nicol, 1762), 148–150; William Cullen, *First Lines of the Practice of Physic*, vol. 1 (Edinburgh: William Creech, 1777), 26, 42, and 81; and John Alderson, *An Essay on the Nature and Origin of the Contagion of Fevers* (Hull: G. Prince, 1788), 56.

13. Aikin, *John Howard*, 3, 43; West, *Curious Mr. Howard*, xxv–xxvi, 221–226; Morgan, "Divine Philanthropy," 389, 391.

14. The standard work on eighteenth-century charity remains Donna Andrew, *Philanthropy and Police: London Charity in the Eighteenth Century* (Princeton: Princeton University Press, 1989). Sarah Lloyd's *Charity and Poverty in England, c. 1680–1820* (Manchester: Manchester University Press, 2009) is also particularly good at exploring how charity schemes captured the eighteenth-century imagination. See also James Stephen Taylor, *Jonas Hanway, Founder of the Marine Society: Charity and Policy in Eighteenth-Century Britain* (London: Scolar, 1985); Ruth McClure, *Coram's Children: The London Foundling Hospital in the Eighteenth Century* (New Haven: Yale University Press, 1981); Hugh Cunningham and Joanna Innes, eds., *Charity, Philanthropy, and Reform from the 1690s to 1850* (London: Macmillan, 1998); and Roy Porter, "The Gift Relation: Philanthropy and Provincial Hospitals in Eighteenth-Century England," in *The Hospital in History*, ed. Roy Porter and Lindsay Granshaw (London: Routledge, 1989), 149–178. On the

celebration of Coram, see Linda Colley, *Britons: Forging the Nation, 1707–1837* (New Haven: Yale University Press, 1992), 56–61.

15. Robert Alan Cooper, "Ideas and Their Execution: English Prison Reform," *Eighteenth-Century Studies* 10, no. 1 (1976): 73–93, 73; Dixon, *John Howard and the Prison World*, vii.

16. For studies that situate Howard within eighteenth-century cultures of sentimentality see G. J. Barker-Benfield, *The Culture of Sensibility: Sex and Society in Eighteenth-Century Britain* (Chicago: University of Chicago Press, 1992), 225; and Ann Jessie van Sant, *Eighteenth-Century Sensibility and the Novel* (Cambridge: Cambridge University Press, 2004), 97. On the construction of military heroes in the period see Holger Hock, *Empires of the Imagination: Politics, War, and the Arts in the British World, 1750–1850* (London: Profile, 2010); Nicholas Rogers, "Brave Wolfe: The Making of a Hero," in *A New Imperial History: Culture, Identity, and Modernity in Britain and the Empire*, ed. Kathleen Wilson (Cambridge University Press, 2004), 239–259; Alan McNairn, *Behold the Hero: General Wolfe and the Arts in the Eighteenth Century* (Montreal: McGill-Queens University Press, 1997), and Timothy Jenks, *Naval Engagements: Patriotism, Cultural Politics, and the Royal Navy, 1793–1815* (Oxford: Oxford University Press, 2006).

17. Aikin, *John Howard*, 50–51, 74, 99, 130–131. West, *Curious Mr. Howard*, 122–123. Original emphasis.

18. Aikin, *John Howard*, 91, 129–130, 186, 188, 193–194; Oxford, Bodleian Library, MS. Eng. Misc. c. 332, fols. 48–49.

19. Aikin, *John Howard*, 215–216; Colley, *Britons*, 25–30.

20. Aikin, *John Howard*, 15–19, 27–29, 35–39, 41, 232–233, 243; Lisa Forman Cody, *Birthing the Nation: Sex, Science, and the Conception of Eighteenth-Century Britons* (Oxford: Oxford University Press, 2004, 186–197).

21. Aikin, *John Howard*, 140–147; West, *Curious Mr. Howard*, 266. Leona Baumgartner, "John Howard and the Public Health Movement," *Bulletin of the History of Medicine* 5, no. 6 (1937): 489–508, 498; William Hayley, *Memoirs of the Life and Writings of William Hayley*, vol. 1 (London: Henry Colburn, 1823), 203–204; William Hayley, *Ode inscribed to John Howard* (London: J. Dodsley, 1780), 7; *Critical Review, Or, Annals of Literature* 50 (1780): 102.

22. The basis for the character is generally acknowledged, as in the entry for Inchbald in the *Oxford Dictionary of National Biography*. See also Susan Staves, *A Literary History of Women's Writing in Britain, 1660–1789* (Cambridge: Cambridge University Press, 2006), 419–426.

23. Elizabeth Inchbald, *Such Things Are: a play in five acts* (London, 1788), 20–21, 31, 48–49, 52.

24. Ibid., 55, 61, 66; Staves, *Literary History of Women's Writing*, 425–426.

25. Porter, "Howard's Beginning," 26.

26. For background on coroners' inquests in the period see especially the work of Thomas Forbes, "Crowner's Quest," *Transactions of the American Philosophical Society* 68 (1978): 1–52, and Pamela Fisher, "The Politics of Sudden Death: The Office and Role of the Coroner in England and Wales, 1726–1888," D. Phil. thesis, University of Leicester, 2007. Also, Gary I. Greenwald and Maria White Greenwald, "Medicolegal Progress in Inquests of Felonious Deaths: Westminster, 1761–1866," *Journal of Legal Medicine* 2 (1981): 193–264, and Gary I. Greenwald and Maria White Greenwald, "Coroner's Inquests, a Source of Vital Statistics: Westminster, 1761–1866," *Journal of Legal Medicine* 4 (1983): 51–86, and for the nineteenth century Ian Burney, *Bodies of Evidence: Medicine and the Politics of the English Inquest, 1830–1926* (Baltimore: Johns Hopkins University Press, 2000). On prison inquests in that period see Joe Sim and Tony Ward, "The Magistrate of the Poor? Coroners and Deaths in Custody in Nineteenth-Century England," in *Legal Medicine in History*, ed. Michael Clark and Catherine Crawford (Cambridge: Cambridge University Press, 1994), 245–267.

27. John Impey, *The Office and Duty of Coroners* (London: A. Strahan, 1800), 3; John Impey, *The Office of Sheriff: Shewing its History and Antiquity* (London: Printed for the Author, 1786), 79–80; Edward Umfreville, *Lex Coronatoria: or, the office and duty of coroners*, vol. 2 (London: R. Griffiths, 1761), 263; Anon., *Coroner's Guide: or the office and duty of the coroner* (London: Henry Lintot, 1756), 11. My emphasis.

28. Westminster Abbey Library and Muniments Room [WA], Westminster Coroner's Inquests [WCI], 1760–1799. These are now available electronically on *London Lives, 1690–1800: Crime, Poverty, and Social Policy in the Metropolis*, www.londonlives.org. For analysis of the Westminster inquests see Greenwald and White Greenwald, "Medicolegal Progress," and "Coroner's Inquests." This jail housed an average of 83.6 inmates during Howard's five inspections in the 1770s. Howard, *State of the Prisons* (1777), 193.

29. On bridewells see Joanna Innes, "Prisons for the Poor: English Bridewells, 1555–1800," in *Labour, Law, and Crime: An Historical Perspective*, ed. Francis Snyder and Douglas Hay, 42–122 (London: Tavistock, 1987); Tim Hitchcock, *Down and Out in Eighteenth-Century London* (London: Hambledon, 2004), chapter 7, 151–180; Robert Shoemaker, *Prosecution and Punishment:*

Petty Crime and the Law in London and Rural Middlesex, c. 1660–1725 (Cambridge: Cambridge University Press, 1991), chap. 7, 166–198; William Hinkle, *A History of Bridewell Prison, 1553–1700* (London: Edwin Mellen, 2006).

30. William Smith, *The State of the Gaols in London, Westminster, and Borough of Southwark* (London: J. Bew, 1776), 25–26; Howard, *State of the Prisons* (1777), 193–194. The property requirement to serve on a coroner's jury was lower than for some other juries, leading Joe Sim and Tony Ward to wonder whether by the early nineteenth century we should consider the coroner a "magistrate of the poor," presiding over a political process in which relatively common people could participate. See Sim and Ward, "Magistrate of the Poor?" Although jurors were supposed to be propertied local men, and were frequently identified in summonses as "Householders," Saunders Welch remarked in 1758 that coroners occasionally had to summon "very indifferent people, both of character and worth," because serving on coroners' juries was so unpopular. Quoted in Gregory Durston, *Whores and Highwaymen: Crime and Justice in the Eighteenth-Century Metropolis* (Hook, UK: Waterside, 2012), 284. WA, WCI, George Hancock, August 27, 1777. Professionals such as attorneys or men simply identified as "Gentlemen" also served on these juries: see for example, WA, WCI, Catherine Stanfield, March 15, 1791.

31. WA, WCI, John Arthur, April 1, 1766; Charles Price, January 25, 1786; George Pricard, June 16, 1791. The one occasion when prisoners served on the jury was WA, WCI, William Bradnock, May 5, 1770. *Proceedings of the Old Bailey*, www.oldbaileyonline.org, John Stevens, murder, April 9, 1766, ref. t17660409-67.

32. The sample group consists of 109 inquests on adults dying in Westminster outside the prison during the same period for which inquests on the Tothill Fields Bridewell survive, 1764–1799. (There were no deaths recorded in Tothill Fields from 1760 to 1763, so although inquests survive for these years, they were omitted from the control group.) To control for possible seasonal variances that might affect factors like mortality or jury participation, the control group was constructed by choosing the first three inquests on adult deaths held in January 1764, the first three in February 1765, the first three in March 1766, and so on. Since all inmates were adults, the numerous inquests on dead (usually abandoned) infants were skipped for the exercise. Juries on dead prisoners heard on average just 1.4 witnesses per inquest, while juries on adult deaths outside the prison heard 2.4 witnesses per inquest. Seventy-five

of 106 prison inquests relied on the testimony of a single deponent. Thomas
Forbes, "A Mortality Record for Coldbath Fields Prison, London, in 1795–
1829," *Bulletin of the New York Academy of Medicine* 53, no. 7 (1977): 666–670;
Sim and Ward, "Magistrate of the Poor?" 246–248; and Margaret DeLacy,
Prison Reform in Lancashire, 1700–1850: A Study in Local Administration
(Stanford: Stanford University Press, 1986), 126.

33. WA, WCI, Daniel Bradley, January 23, 1776.

34. WA, WCI, Thomas Guy, December 24, 1764; Joseph Blatchford, January 4,
1768, and William Edwards, January 4, 1774.

35. WA, WCI, John Clark, December 24, 1777. Howard published his book in
March. West, *Curious Mr. Howard*, 172.

36. WA, WCI, Mary Fokes, March 18, 1785; Mary Price, February 8, 1785;
Benjamin Higgs, March 18, 1785, and Edward Towser, July 20, 1785.

37. Work on the politics of inquests suggests how and why they might have done
so. Ian Burney and Pamela Fisher have pointed to conflict between local
magistrates and coroners, while Joe Sim and Tony Ward have suggested that
in the case of prison inquests nineteenth-century magistrates exerted pressures on the process and even packed the juries. Burney, *Bodies of Evidence*,
21–23; Fisher, "Politics of Sudden Death," 12; Sim and Ward, "Magistrate of
the Poor?" 247–248.

38. The first two of the seven inquests conducted in March on deaths in Tothill
Fields occurred on March 1 and 10. Rumors of plague at the Lock Hospital
circulated March 3–7: *Whitehall Evening Post*, March 3–5, 1785; *Morning
Chronicle and London Advertiser*, March 7, 1785; *Morning Post and Daily
Advertiser*, March 7, 1785. Tim Hitchcock and Robert Shoemaker, *London
Lives: Poverty, Crime, and the Making of a Modern City, 1690–1800*
(Cambridge: Cambridge University Press, 2015), 335–338; *Proceedings of the
Old Bailey*, April 6, 1785, trial of William Gibbons, ref. t17050406-100.

39. There were 1.65 deaths per year in the prison up to 1784, while in 1785–1799 its
mortality rate was more than two and a half times as high, fully 4.5 deaths per
year. Even omitting the anomalous epidemic year of 1785, the prison was still
the site of 3.78 deaths per year during the period 1786–1799, a mortality rate
more than double that from 1762 to 1784. Forbes found inquests at Coldbath
Fields Prison similarly vague. "Mortality Record for Coldbath Fields Prison."

40. WA, WCI, James McDaniel, January 3, 1765. Umfreville, *Lex Coronatoria*,
263.

41. WA, WCI, Jane Smith, September 12, 1783. The proximity of the Green
Coat Boy to the prison emerges in the trial about the aforementioned escape

attempt of William Stewart, when Thomas Pearce described witnessing the events from the coffeehouse. *Proceedings of the Old Bailey,* ref. t17050406-100; Thomas Forbes, "Inquests into London and Middlesex Homicides, 1675–1782," *Yale Journal of Biology and Medicine* 50, no. 2 (1977): 207–220, 208; Durston, *Whores and Highwaymen,* 285.

42. WA, WCI, William Stephens, July 11, 1793.

43. WA, WCI, Henry Young, November 8, 1786. It is notable that the formal inquest was vague, failing to follow the pattern set by almost every previous inquest held on a death in Tothill Fields, and did not list the bridewell as the locale, merely noting that the proceedings occurred "at the parish of St. Margaret's Westminster."

44. For example, WA WCI, Thomas Tushop, September 20, 1787, and Patiance Hipditch, February 23, 1788.

45. WA WCI, Andrew Farrell, August 27, 1792.

46. WA, WCI, John Patrick, April 13, 1767; Nicholas Martin, September 10, 1770; Sarah West, March 21, 1771; Ann Cole, September 23, 1773; Woman unknown, March 6, 1776; James Barkley, December 10, 1776; and Francis Bolier, September 2, 1785. Typical Westminster inquests saw jury pools smaller than twenty-four only 17.6 percent of the time, but the frequency of such small pools rose to 26.1 percent for prison inquests. Anon., *Coroner's Guide,* 12. John Langbein, "The English Criminal Trial Jury on the Eve of the French Revolution," in *The Trial Jury in England, France, Germany, 1700–1900,* ed. Antonio Padoa Schioppa, 13–39 (Berlin: Duncker and Humblot, 1987), 27.

47. WA, WCI, Elizabeth Whetston, September 1, 1766; Eleanor Fielders, September 1, 1766. (Note that this was a single jury that served on two inquests. Both women were vagrants, the second sick with fever.) Margaret Lane, February 25, 1778; Mary Jones, June 13, 1786; Henry Young, November 8, 1786; Thomas Tushop, September 20, 1787; Jane Jones, May 1, 1788; Daniel Dixon, April 7, 1790; Anonymous, April 2, 1792; and Mrs. Davis, November 24, 1798. Nonprison inquests had jury pools of twenty-six or more 17.6 percent of the time and pools of twenty-eight or more 5.88 percent of the time. Those frequencies rise in prison inquests to 34.7 percent and 19.5 percent, respectively.

48. WC, WCI, Susannah Robinson, March 1, 1785; John Ferguson, March 10, 1785; Thomas Wheeler, March 28, 1785; and Sarah Rowlinson, April 30, 1785.

49. WA, WCI, Mary Price, February 8, 1785; Susannah Robinson, March 1, 1785; John Ferguson, March 10, 1785; Thomas Bloxam, March 12, 1785; Joly de

St. Valier, March 18, 1785; Benjamin Higgins, March 18, 1785; Mary Fokes, March 18, 1785; Sarah Rowlinson, April 30, 1785; Robert Doe, June 6, 1785; Thomas Brown, June 18, 1785; William Sharp, December 12, 1785; and Elizabeth Barton, December 27, 1785.

50. Smith, *State of the Gaols in London;* G. O. Paul, *Considerations on the Defects of Prisons* (London: T. Cadell, 1784). For Ireland see Jeremiah Fitzpatrick, *An Essay on Gaol-Abuses, and on the means of redressing them: Together with the General Method of Treating Disorders to which Prisoners are most Incident* (Dublin: D. Graisberry, 1784).

51. John Howard, *An Account of the Principal Lazarettos of Europe, with various papers relative to Plague* (Warrington: William Eyres, 1789), 1; Aikin, *John Howard,* 128–129. On British maritime quarantine practices see John Booker, *Maritime Quarantine: The British Experience, c. 1650–1900* (Aldershot, UK: Ashgate, 2007), esp. 217–220 on Howard's influence.

52. Aikin, *John Howard,* 155. West mistakenly identifies him as William Jebb; *Curious Mr. Howard,* 368. John Jebb certainly came in contact with Howard, as they were both dissenters with interests in numerous late-eighteenth-century reform movements, not the least of which concerned prisons. Inspired by Howard, Jebb published his own treatise on the issue, *Thoughts on the Construction and Polity of Prisons* (Bury St. Edmunds: J. Rackham), in 1785, the same year that Howard embarked on his lazaretto tour—meaning that he, Aikin, and Howard were discussing institutions and disease just as Howard prepared for his trip. Another clue to their connection is that Howard was listed as a subscriber to Jebb's posthumously published *Works* in 1787. John Disney, *The Works, Theological, Medical, Political and Miscellaneous of John Jebb,* vol. 1 (London, 1787), xix. Jebb's most recent biographer, Anthony Page, discusses Howard's influence on Jebb, although in a general sense, failing to note that the two were in direct contact. *John Jebb and the Enlightenment Origin of British Radicalism* (London: Praeger, 2003), 163, 231–234.

53. John Aikin, *Thoughts on Hospitals* (London: Joseph Johnson, 1771), 8–10, 14–16, 20, 27–28, 32, 37–38, 41, 45–46, 50, 61–62, 87–88, 91–98; Aikin, *John Howard,* 154–156. On Aikin's medical theory see Margaret DeLacy, *Contagionism Catches On: Medical Ideology in Britain, 1730–1800* (New York: Palgrave Macmillan, 2016), 247–248. Jebb, *Thoughts on the Construction and Polity of Prisons,* 3; Howard, *Principal Lazarettos,* 32. It is also worth noting that Howard also cited Pringle directly in the first edition of *The State of the Prisons* (1777), 19.

54. Howard, *Principal Lazarettos*, 32–41.

55. Ibid., 25.

56. Howard, *State of the Prisons* (1777), 5, 13–14, and Howard, *Principal Laza-rettos*, 3, 15, 41.

57. Lind, *Health of Seamen*, 145, 345; *Morning Chronicle and London Advertiser*, October 14, 1772; *London Evening Post*, October 9–11.

58. Discussions of the medicine and advertisements for it were ubiquitous in newspapers throughout the second half of the century. For example, *London Chronicle*, January 17–20, 1767, issue 1574; *London Evening Post*, January 6–9, 1770, issue 6581; *London Chronicle*, June 7–9, 1774, issue 2730; *Gazetteer and New Daily Advertiser*, December 8, 1780, issue 16,182; *Lloyd's Evening Post*, March 27–29, 1793, issue 5580.

59. The only earlier reference I discovered in ECCO (using proximity searching to ensure catching phrases like "Vinegar of the Four Thieves") was a paper delivered to the Royal Society in 1755. Claude Nicholas Le Cat, "An Account of those malignant Fevers, that raged in Rouen, at the End of the Year 1753, and the Beginning of 1754," *Philosophical Transactions of the Royal Society* 49 (London: L. Davis and C. Reymers, 1756): 60. Search conducted on *Eighteenth Century Collections Online*, September 30, 2016. Within news-papers, only 13 of 170 references to the vinegar predate 1777, the first appearing in 1770. Virtually all were advertisements for Arnaud's medicine. Search conducted on *17th-18th-Century Burney Newspaper Collection*, September 30, 2016.

60. Anon., *The New Dispensatory* (Edinburgh: Charles Elliot, 1786), 374–375; *London Evening Post*, October 9–11, 1770; *Parker's General Advertiser and Morning Intelligencer*, August 8, 17, 1784; *Public Advertiser*, June 16, 1779; *World*, April 19, 21, 1790; *Morning Post and Daily Advertiser*, May 12, 1791; *Morning Herald*, June 30, 1791. One of the first recipes in a popular manual about cosmetics that went through eight editions between 1772 and 1784 instructed women how to concoct "An excellent Preservative Balsam against the Plague." Pierre Joseph Buc'hoz, *The Toilet of Flora* (London: W. Nicoll, 1772), 4, 254–255.

61. Elizabeth Craven, *A Journey through the Crimea to Constantinople* (London: G. G. J. and J. Robinson, 1789), 252; Stéphanie Félicité de Genlis, *Lessons of a Governess to her Pupils*, vol. 3 (London, 1792), 95–96; Anon., *An inquiry into the causes which produce, preserve, and propagate Febrile Contagious Diseases* (Newcastle: S. Hodgson, 1804), 50; *Gazetteer and New Daily Advertiser*, January 7, 1778; Joshua Lucock Wilkinson, *The Wanderer; or anecdotes and*

incidents, the results and occurrences of a ramble on foot through France, Germany and Italy, in 1791 and 1793, vol. 2 (London: J. Higham, 1798), 75; William Falconer, *Experiments and Observations in Three Parts* (London: W. Goldsmith, 1776), 99–105; *General Advertiser and Morning Intelligencer,* August 19, 1778; *Public Advertiser,* November 27, 1786; *London Chronicle,* February 26–March 1, 1785.

62. Samuel Pratt, *Family Secrets, Literary and Domestick,* vol. 3 (London: T. N. Longman, 1797), 392–393; Charles Dickens, *Barnaby Rudge; A Tale of the Riots of Eighty* (London: Chapman and Hall, 1841), 375–376.

63. Howard, *Principal Lazarettos,* 232; Peter Kennedy, *An Account of a Contagious Fever that Prevailed at Aylesbury* (Aylesbury: W. Nicholls, 1785), 43–44; Lind, *Health of Seamen,* 144–145, 344–345; Richard Mead, *A Short Discourse concerning Pestilential Contagion, and the Methods to be used to Prevent it* (London: Sam. Buckley, 1720), 52.

64. Howard, *Principal Lazarettos,* 1, 3–4, 8, 19.

65. "This plan I was also induced to adopt from a recent work of Dr. Lettsom on the Frequency and liberality of putrid and other fevers in a Poorhouse for want of Cleanliness and suffocation of Air." London, Guildhall Library [GL], MS 3226, St. Sepulchre (London Division), Minutes of the Committee for Rebuilding the Workhouse (1796–1838), 2; John Mason Good, *Dissertation on the Diseases of Prisons and Poor Houses* (London: C. Dilly, 1795), 94–95, 107, 127.

66. Lynn Hollen Lees, *The Solidarities of Strangers: The English Poor Laws and the People, 1700–1948* (Cambridge: Cambridge University Press, 2006), 33–39; GL, MS 3226, Minutes of the Committee for Rebuilding the Workhouse, 3–4. Also notable is that the architect designed the structure with separate staircases for paupers and vestrymen. Fruitful conversations with Susannah Ottaway alerted me to the importance of this design feature, which may have had similarly been intended to limit close bodily encounters between parish notables and pauper inmates.

7. Typhus Ever After

1. Charles Creighton, *A History of Epidemics in Britain,* 2 vols. (Cambridge: Cambridge University Press, 1891), 2: 123–127; James Johnstone, *Historical Dissertation Concerning the Malignant Epidemical Fever of 1756* (London: W. Johnston, 1758), 17–19.

2. Creighton, *History of Epidemics,* 2: 140–150, Hunter quoted on 134.

3. John Pickstone, *Medicine and Industrial Society: A History of Hospital Development in Manchester and Its Region, 1752–1946* (Manchester: Manchester University Press, 1985), 23–41; John V. Pickstone, "From Ferriar's Fever to Kay's Cholera: Disease and Social Structure in Cottonopolis," *History of Science* 22 (1984): 401–419, esp. 402; John V. Pickstone, "Dearth, Dirt, and Fever Epidemics: Rewriting the History of British 'Public Health,' 1780–1850," in *Epidemics and Ideas: Essays on the Historical Perception of Pestilence,* ed. Terrance Ranger and Paul Slack, 125–148 (Cambridge: Cambridge University Press, 1992); Brian Keith-Lucas, "Some Influences Affecting the Development of Sanitary Legislation in England," *Economic History Review* 6, no. 3 (1954): 290–296; E. P. Hennock, "Urban Sanitary Reform a Generation before Chadwick?" *Economic History Review* 10, no. 1 (1957): 113–120; Carla Susan Patterson, "From Fever to Digestive Disease: Approaches to the Problem of Factory Ill-Health in Britain, 1784–1833," Ph.D. diss., University of British Columbia, 1995; James Riley, *The Eighteenth-Century Campaign to Avoid Disease* (London: Macmillan, 1987); Roy Porter, "Cleaning up the Great Wen: Public Health in Eighteenth-Century London," *Medical History* 11 (1991): 61–75; Margaret Pelling, *Cholera, Fever, and English Medicine, 1825–1865* (Oxford University Press, 1978), esp. 41–46. Emphasis original.

4. William Buchan, *Domestic Medicine* (London: W. Strahan, 1772), 94–95; John Heysham, *An Account of the Jail Fever, or Typhus Carcerum; as it appeared at Carlisle in the year 1781* (London: T. Cadell, 1782), 1 and 5; Jeremiah Fitzpatrick, *An Essay on Gaol-Abuses, and on the means of redressing them: Together with the General Method of Treating Disorders to which Prisoners are most Incident* (Dublin: D. Graisberry, 1784), 8. On Buchan see Charles Rosenberg, "Medical Text and Social Context: Explaining William Buchan's *Domestic Medicine,*" in *Explaining Epidemics and Other Studies in the History of Medicine,* 32–56 (Cambridge: Cambridge University Press, 1992).

5. Fitzpatrick, *Essay on Gaol-Abuses,* 8–9; John Alderson, *An Essay on the Nature and Origin of the Contagion of Fevers* (Hull: G. Prince, 1788), 5; Heysham, *Account of the Jail Fever,* 31–34.

6. David Campbell, *Observations on the Typhus, or Low Contagious Fever* (Lancaster: H. Walmsley, 1785), 3, 6–7, 10, 15–17, 29, 31–32, 36, 39–43, 45–50, 53, 73, 75, 77, 81–82, 101, 113–114, 116, 125–126; Francis Milman, *An Enquiry into the Source from whence the Symptoms of the Scurvy and of Putrid Fevers Arise* (London: J. Dodsley, 1782), 65–66, 87, 103–104.

7. Ibid., 3, 51–53.

8. Peter Kennedy, *An Account of a Contagious Fever that Prevailed at Aylesbury* (Aylesbury: W. Nicholls, 1785), 50–51. Emphasis mine.

9. James Currie, *Medical Reports on the Effects of Water, Cold and Warm, as a Remedy in Fever, and Febrile Diseases* (Liverpool: James M'Creery, 1797), 201–211. He also conveyed, when discussing the cost of supporting of workers who lose wages when felled by fever, that his wide definition of the poor included the working poor (212). And like so many physicians, he also signaled that physiological class distinctions were medically relevant, as in his claim that symptoms and treatments, varied accordingly: "The fever that prevails among our poor is remarkably uniform; it is the pure typhus, to which cordial treatment can be applied with safety. Whereas among the higher classes, fever is often attended with inflammatory symptoms in the first instance, sometimes with pneumonic symptoms through a considerable part of the disease; and in such cases the indications of practice being contradictory, success is much less certain" (213).

10. Currie, *Medical Reports*, 202.

11. John Aitken, *Elements of the Theory and Practice of Physic and Surgery*, vol. 1 (London, 1782), 23; Robert Hooper, *A Compendious Medical Dictionary* (London: Murray and Highley, 1798), n.p.; Ephraim Chambers, *Cyclopedia: or An Universal Dictionary of Arts and Sciences*, vols. 1 and 2 (London: D. Midwinter, 1741), n.p.; *Report of the Select Committee on Contagious Fever in London: Ordered by the House of Commons to be printed, 20th May 1818*, reprinted in *Public Health in the Victorian Age*, vol. 1, ed. Ruth Hodgkinson (Westmead, UK: Gregg International, 1973), 414–415.

12. Campbell, *Observations on the Typhus*, 3; A. Meiklejohn, "Outbreak of Fever in Cotton Mills at Radcliffe, 1784," *British Journal of Industrial Medicine* 16 (1959): 68–69; A. Meiklejohn, "Industrial Health—Meeting the Challenge," *British Journal of Industrial Medicine* 16 (1959): 1–10; Charles Webster, "Two Hundredth Anniversary of the 1784 Report on Fever at Radcliffe Mill," *Society for the Social History of Medicine Bulletin* 7 (1985): 63–65; Pickstone, *Medicine and Industrial Society*, 23–39; Pickstone, "Ferriar's Fever to Kay's Cholera"; John Pickstone and S. V. H. Butler, "Politics of Medicine in Manchester, 1788–92," *Medical History* 28 (1984): 227–249; Webster, "Two Hundredth Anniversary"; Joanna Innes, "Origins of the Factory Act: The Health and Morals of Apprentices Act, 1802," in *Law, Crime, and English Society, 1660–1830*, ed. Norma Landau, 230–255 (Cambridge: Cambridge University Press, 2002).

13. *Manchester Mercury,* October 19, 1784.

14. Ibid.; Campbell, *Observations on the Typhus,* 25–27. On Bayley's various reform activities see Margaret Delacy, *Prison Reform in Lancashire, 1700–1850: A Study in Local Administration* (Stanford: Stanford University Press, 1986), 70–82; also Innes, "Origins of the Factory Act," 238.

15. Campbell, *Observations on the Typhus,* 22–23. William White clearly drew on jail fever traditions when he advertised a ventilator that could sustain health by pumping air scented with "aromatics, sulphur &c.," into "Mines, Ships, Hospitals, Prisons, Workhouses, Slave-Ships, &c." *Extracts from the Reports of the Royal Humane Society* (London, 1794), 30–32.

16. The records of the Board of Health in its early years were published as *Proceedings of the Board of Health in Manchester* (Manchester: S. Russell, 1805). The manuscript on which this treatise was based survives at University of London, Senate House Library (SHL), MS 142, Manchester Board of Health Book. *Proceedings of the Board of Health,* 33–34; Patterson, "From Fever to Digestive Disease," 9–20, 26–29, 35–36, 61–64, 81–88, 94–98, 116–120; 42 Geo. III c.73; Innes, "Origins of the Factory Act," 237–238, 247.

17. Pickstone, "Ferrier's Fever to Kay's Cholera," 402–407; Margaret DeLacy, *Contagionism Catches On: Medical Ideology in Britain, 1730–1800* (New York: Palgrave Macmillan, 2016), 207–280.

18. Pickstone, *Medicine and Industrial Society,* 24; John Ferriar, "Origin of Contagious and New Diseases," 218–248 in *Medical Histories and Reflections,* vol. 1 (Warrington: Eyres, 1792), 218–219, 222, 228–229, 235, 243–247. On the importance of putridity see 230–235. It is important to remark on the language of poisons in these passages. As we saw in Chapter 1, the concept of the poison had been an important mechanism for theorists explaining plague and plebeian diseases since at least the seventeenth century, and Ferriar here demonstrates its continued importance at the dawn of the nineteenth century. It is notable that some historians of Victorian public health mistakenly present this connection as a novel development. Michael Brown, "From Foetid Air to Filth: The Cultural Transformation of British Epidemiological Thought, 1780–1840," *Bulletin of the History of Medicine* 83, no. 2 (2008): 515–544, esp. 532–533.

19. Pickstone, *Medicine and Industrial Society,* 24; Pickstone, "Ferrier's Fever to Kay's Cholera," 404; John Ferriar, "Of the Prevention of Fever in Great Towns," in *Medical Histories and Reflections,* vol. 2 (London: Cadell and Davies, 1795), 188, 191–192, 200.

20. Ferriar, "Of the Prevention of Fever in Great Towns," 178–183, 197, and John Ferriar, "On the Conversion of Diseases," in *Medical Histories and*

Reflections, 2: 1–80. See also Ferriar's discussion of an outbreak at Ashton-under-Line in *Proceedings of the Board of Health*, 18.

21. On Haygarth see Christopher Charles Booth, *John Haygarth, FRS (1740–1827): A Physician of the Enlightenment* (Philadelphia: American Philosophical Society, 2005). On his establishment of fever wards see 63–72; DeLacy, *Contagionism Catches On*, 165–205; Kevin Siena, "Contagion, Exclusion, and the Unique Medical World of the Eighteenth-Century Workhouse," in *Medicine and the Workhouse*, ed. Jonathan Reinarz and Leonard Schwarz, 19–39 (Rochester, NY: University of Rochester Press, 2013). On the dispensary movement see Irvine Loudon, "Origins and Growth of the Dispensary Movement in England," *Bulletin of the History of Medicine* 55 (1981): 322–342; Robert Kilpatrick, " 'Living in the Light': Dispensaries, Philanthropy, and Medical Reform in Late-Eighteenth-Century England," in *The Medical Enlightenment of the Eighteenth Century*, ed. Andrew Cunningham and Roger French (Cambridge: Cambridge University Press, 1990), 254–280; Bronwyn Croxson, "The Public and Private Faces of Eighteenth-Century London Dispensary Charity," *Medical History* 41 (1997): 127–149. It is useful to note of Lettsom that the longest and most prominent chapter in his treatise on London's dispensaries for the poor was chapter 1, "Observations on fevers, with symptoms of putrescency." John Coakley Lettsom, *Medical Memoirs of the General Dispensary in London, for part of the years 1773 and 1774* (London: Edward and Charles Dilly, 1774), 1–118.

22. John Haygarth, "On the Population and Diseases of Chester, in the year 1774," *Philosophical Transactions* 68 (1778): 131–153. For example, "Another reason of greater mortality in the suburbs seems to be, that the inhabitants in general are of the lowest rank: they want most of the conveniences and comforts of life: their homes are small, close, crouded and dirty: their diet affords them very bad nourishment, and their cloaths are seldom changed or washed. These parts of the town are supplied less plentifully than the rest with water. The air they breathe at home is thus rendered noxious by respiration and putrefaction. . . . It cannot therefore, be wonderful that diseases should be produced where such poison is inspired with every breath. This noxious air is the most frequent cause of malignant fevers" (139–141).

23. John Haygarth, *A Letter to Dr. Percival, on the Prevention of Infectious Fevers* (Bath: Cruttwell, 1801), 3, 8; Haygarth, "On the Population and Diseases of Chester," 140; Booth, *John Haygarth*, 64–66.

24. SHL, MS 142, 6–11; *Proceedings of the Board of Health in Manchester*, 7–11. On the Strangers Friend Society see G. B. Hindle, *Provision for the Relief of the*

Poor in Manchester, 1754–1826 (Manchester: Chetham Society, 1975), 78–89, and Pickstone, *Medicine and Industrial Society,* 24–25.

25. SHL, MS 142, 17; *Proceedings of the Board of Health,* 81, 85, 117, 121–130, 181–186; *Manchester Mercury,* June 14, 1796. On nuisance law as it related to health in the period, see James Hanley, *Healthy Boundaries: Property, Law, and Public Health in England and Wales 1815–1872* (Rochester: University of Rochester Press, 2016), 17–38.

26. *Proceedings of the Board of Health,* 85–89.

27. Ibid., 88–90. The Russell mentioned here is Patrick Russell, a Levant Company Physician in Aleppo and expert on lazarettos, who published *A Treatise of the Plague* (London: G. G. G. and J. Robinson, 1791).

28. *Proceedings of the Board of Health,* 91–92.

29. Ibid., 96–97, 131–136.

30. Ibid., 5, 169, 195–197.

31. Ibid., 7, 11, 12, 14, 23.

32. Ibid., 67–69, 214. My emphasis.

33. Ibid., 108, 148–150, 231–237; William Clerke, *Thoughts upon the Means of Preserving the Health of the Poor, by Prevention and Suppression of Epidemic Fevers* (London: J. Johnson, 1790), 14.

34. Clerke, *Thoughts upon the Means of Preserving the Health of the Poor,* 5, 9, 12–14, 23–25; *Proceedings of the Board of Health,* 113–115; *Manchester Mercury,* July 5, 12, August 2, 16, 1796.

35. Clerke, *Thoughts upon the Means of Preserving the Health of the Poor,* 12–14, 17; John Howard, *An Account of the Principal Lazarettos of Europe, with various papers relative to Plague* (Warrington: William Eyres, 1789), 3. On the use of mustard in treatments for fever see Buchan, *Domestic Medicine,* 238–239.

36. Howard, *Principal Lazarettos,* 11, 15, 41; *Proceedings of the Board of Health,* 113–115.

37. Here is where some of DeLacy's claims in her otherwise excellent study appear to my eye slightly off base. When she argues that prior to the Manchester Board of Health "no agent of government had intervened in personal hygiene (beyond regulating the dumping of night soil in public places or neighbors' properties), or compelled residents to accept specific medical interventions, therapies or regimens," she seems to have entirely neglected the history of British plague regulations. *Contagionism Catches On,* 208. Indeed, her first volume on contagion covers the period of the great London epidemic yet curiously omits the event, devoting an entire chapter to bovine rinderpest but ignoring 1665/6. Margaret DeLacy, *The Germ of an*

Idea: Contagionism, Religion, and Society in Britain, 1660–1730 (New York: Palgrave Macmillan, 2016).

38. London, Royal Free Archive Centre, London Fever Hospital, Committee Minutes, LFH/1/C/4/1, [hereafter LFH] 1–2. Note: since I first consulted these records in 2010, they have been transferred to the LMA, where they can be found under the new shelf mark H71/LF; Robert Willan, *Reports on the Diseases of London* (London: R. Phillips, 1801), 262–263.

39. W. F. Bynum, "Hospital, Disease, and Community: The London Fever Hospital, 1801–1850," in *Healing in History*, ed. Charles Rosenberg, 97–115 (New York: Wm. Dawson and Sons, 1979).

40. LFH, 5–11, 20–21, 34–43. On the spread of these techniques see Peter Baldwin, *Contagion and the State in Europe, 1830–1930* (Cambridge: Cambridge University Press, 1999); Graham Mooney, *Intrusive Interventions: Public Health, Domestic Space, and Infectious Disease Surveillance in England, 1840–1914* (Rochester, NY: University of Rochester Press, 2015); Christopher Hamlin, *Public Health and Social Justice in the Age of Chadwick* (Cambridge: Cambridge University Press, 1998); Anthony Wohl, *Endangering Lives: Public Health in Victorian Britain* (London: Methuen, 1984); Anne Hardy, *The Epidemic Streets: Infectious Diseases and the Rise of Preventative Medicine, 1856–1900* (Oxford: Clarendon, 1993). Michael Worboys, *Spreading Germs: Disease Theories and Medical Practice in Britain, 1865–1900* (Cambridge: Cambridge University Press, 2000). On Scotland and Ireland, see John V. Pickstone, "Dearth, Dirt, and Fever Epidemics: Rewriting the History of British 'Public Health,' 1780–1850," in *Epidemics and Ideas: Essays on the Historical Perception of Pestilence*, ed. Terrance Ranger and Paul Slack, 125–148 (Cambridge: Cambridge University Press, 1992), 132. On similar measures in France see David S. Barnes, *The Great Stink of Paris and the Struggle against Filth and Germs* (Baltimore: Johns Hopkins University Press, 2006).

41. Baldwin, *Contagion and the State*, 123–243; Mooney, *Intrusive Interventions*, passim; Hamlin, *Public Health and Social Justice*. Also, Anna F. La Berge, "Edwin Chadwick and the French Connection," *Bulletin of the History of Medicine* 62 (1988): 23–41.

42. Christopher Hamlin, "Predisposing Causes and Public Health in Early Nineteenth-Century Medical Thought," *Social History of Medicine* 5, no. 1 (1992): 43–70; Michael Brown, "From Foetid Air to Filth: The Cultural Transformation of British Epidemiological Thought, 1780–1840," *Bulletin of the History of Medicine* 83, no. 2 (2008): 515–544, 518, 524–528; Roy Porter,

"Cleaning Up the Great Wen: Public Health in Eighteenth-Century London," *Medical History* 11 (1991): 61–75, 71; Pickstone, "Dearth, Dirt, and Fever," 144–145. Pelling is notable for acknowledging that Smith's views on fever were "if not wholly derivative, at least not original," and she makes a more concerted effort to explore the older roots of key concepts like putrefaction. Margaret Pelling, *Cholera, Fever, and English Medicine, 1825–1865* (Oxford University Press, 1978), 18, 136–138.

43. George Leith Roupell, *A Short Treatise on Typhus Fever* (Philadelphia: A. Waldie, 1840), 86.

44. Gabriel Andral, *Pathological Haematology: An Essay on the Blood in Disease*, trans. J. F. Meigs and Alfred Stillé (Philadelphia: Lea and Blanchard, 1844), passim, esp. 52–60, 92–106; Roupell, *Short Treatise on Typhus*, 87. My emphasis.

45. Hamlin, "Predisposing Causes," passim; Hamlin, *Public Health and Social Justice*, 106, 116–120; Thomas Southwood Smith, "Report on the Physical Causes of Sickness and Mortality to Which the Poor are Particularly Exposed," *Fourth Annual Report of the Poor Law Commissioners, Supplement, Parliamentary Papers*, 1837–1838, 28, no. 147: 83–88.

46. Smith, "Report on the Physical Causes of Sickness," 83–84, 86; Thomas Southwood Smith, *The Philosophy of Health: or An Exposition of the Physical and Mental Constitution of Man*, vol. 1 (London: Charles Knight, 1835), 355; Baldwin, *Contagion and the State*, 127–128; Pelling, *Cholera, Fever, and English Medicine*, 16–24; Hamlin, "Predisposing Causes," 64; Hamlin, *Public Health and Social Justice*, 112–118; Brown, "From Foetid Air to Filth," 538–539; Dorothy Porter, *Health, Civilization, and the State* (London: Routledge, 1999), 85–87. On disease specificity see K. Codell Carter, *The Rise of Causal Concepts of Disease: Case Histories* (Aldershot, UK: Ashgate, 2003).

47. Smith, "Report on the Physical Causes of Sickness," 84. Hamlin contends that Smith retained the concept of predisposition but "emasculated" it by shifting the emphasis to a more singular focus on the causative agent of the specific morbid poison that struck all bodies in a "lawlike manner" regardless of constitutional qualities. "Predisposing Causes," 62. I do not agree that the shift was as stark as he describes. Given Smith's claims, as well as Pelling's argument that many doctors held to constitutional theories in spite of Smith's position, and the fact that Michael Worboys and Peter Baldwin have shown that predisposition remained influential even in the age of bacteriology, it would seem that continuity rather than discontinuity may provide a more useful way of thinking about the history of this idea. Pelling, *Cholera, Fever,*

and English Medicine, 21–22, 29–30, and Worboys, *Spreading Germs*, 39–42. Baldwin, *Contagion and the State*, 186–188.

48. Thomas Southwood Smith, *Epidemics, Considered with Relation to their Common Nature, and to Climate and Civilization* (Edinburgh: Edmonston and Douglas, 1856), 10–11. Hamlin demonstrates that Smith argued against hunger—that is, an insufficient *amount* of food—as a predisposing cause, but Smith here still clearly believed that the consumption of *poor-quality* food could be a factor in generating epidemics. Moreover, he was not always consistent, even when it came to his views on hunger. Later in the same treatise he gave a canned history of epidemics in which the agricultural revolution put an end to a bygone age in which epidemics were more common because of both poor-quality (putrescent) food and pure dearth. Describing the allegedly epidemic-prone Middle Ages he asserted: "This condition of the country and this mode of life themselves constitute the most powerful causes of epidemics; and an extraordinary concurrence and concentration of these causes are manifested in the combination of the circumstances which have been enumerated, namely, in the malarious state of the greater part of the kingdom, in the confined space of the towns, in *the deficiency and putrescency* of the food, in the inadequacy of the means of protection from cold, and in the intemperance of the people. These were the true sources of the malignity and mortality of the pestilences of that age." Ibid., 35. Emphasis added.

49. Smith, "Report on the Physical Causes of Sickness," 84–85.

50. Ibid., 85; Hamlin, *Public Health and Social Justice*, 118–119.

51. Potter, a student of Benjamin Rush, was interested primarily in yellow fever. However, transatlantic exchanges make clear both that European and North American doctors followed each other's work and that ideas about typhus, yellow fever, and plague were intimately linked throughout this period. For a discussion of Rush and yellow fever, see the Conclusion. Nathaniel Potter, *Memoir on Contagion, more especially as it respects the Yellow Fever* (Baltimore: Edward J. Coale, 1818), 50–55; Thomas Southwood Smith, *A Treatise on Fever* (London: Longman, Rees, Orme, Brown and Green, 1830), 369–374.

52. Pelling, *Cholera, Fever, and English Medicine*, 20–21; Smith, *Treatise on Fever*, 361–365.

53. Christopher Hamlin, *More than Hot: A Short History of Fever* (Baltimore: Johns Hopkins University Press, 2014).

54. That is not to suggest that physiological presentations of class did not continue in the nineteenth century, an issue that I will address in the Conclusion.

Conclusion

1. Kevin Siena, "The Moral Biology of 'The Itch' in Eighteenth-Century Britain," in *A Medical History of Skin: Scratching the Surface,* ed. Jonathan Reinarz and Kevin Siena, 71–84 (London: Pickering and Chatto, 2013); Roy Porter and G. S. Rousseau, *Gout: The Patrician Malady* (New Haven: Yale University Press, 2000); Roy Porter, ed., *George Cheyne: The English Malady (1733)* (London: Routledge, 2013), xxvii–xxix. Michael MacDonald noted some time ago that seventeenth-century physicians already diagnosed polite and plebeian patients' mental disorders differently, with the former prone to melancholy and the latter prone to "mopishness." *Mystical Bedlam: Madness, Anxiety, and Healing in Seventeenth-Century England* (Cambridge: Cambridge University Press, 1981), 160–164. On the eighteenth century see R. A. Houston, "Class, Gender, and Madness in Eighteenth-Century Scotland," in *Sex and Seclusion, Class and Custody: Perspectives on Gender and Class in the History of British and Irish Psychiatry,* ed. Jonathan Andrews and Anne Digby (Amsterdam: Rodopi, 2004), 45–68; Roy Porter, "Consumption: Disease of Consumer Society?" in *Consumption and the World of Goods,* ed. John Brewer and Roy Porter (London: Routledge, 1993), 58–81.

2. Londa Schiebinger, *The Mind Has No Sex? Women in the Origins of Modern Science* (Cambridge: Harvard University Press, 1989); Thomas Laqueur, *Making Sex: Body and Gender from the Greeks to Freud* (Cambridge: Harvard University Press, 1992). The classic study of female nervous disorders is Elaine Showalter, *The Female Malady: Women, Madness, and English Culture, 1830–1980* (New York: Pantheon, 1985). See also G. J. Barker-Benfield, *The Culture of Sensibility: Sex and Society in Eighteenth-Century Britain* (Chicago: University of Chicago Press, 1992). For the most recent survey of hysteria in the eighteenth century see Sabine Arnaud, *On Hysteria: The Invention of a Medical Category between 1670 and 1820* (Chicago: University of Chicago Press, 2015). For recent explorations of other conditions see Kathleen Hardesty Doig and Felicia Berger Sturzer, eds., *Women, Gender, and Disease in Eighteenth-Century England and France* (Newcastle-upon-Tyne: Cambridge Scholars Press, 2014).

3. Siena, "Moral Biology of 'The Itch,' " 74; Jason Szabo, *Incurable and Intolerable: Chronic Disease and Slow Death in Nineteenth-Century France* (New Brunswick, NJ: Rutgers University Press, 2009), 15–57; E. H. Ackerknecht, "Diathesis: The Word and the Concept in Medical History," *Bulletin of the History of Medicine* 56 (1982): 317–325; Christopher Hamlin, "Predisposing Causes and Public Health in Early Nineteenth-Century Medical Thought,"

Social History of Medicine 5, no. 1 (1992): 43–70; Charles Rosenberg, "The Bitter Fruit: Heredity, Disease, and Social Thought," in *No Other Gods: On Science and American Social Thought* (Baltimore: Johns Hopkins University Press, 1997), 25–53, esp. 26–27 and 29–30; Staffan Müller-Wille and Hans-Jörg Rheinberger, eds., *Heredity Produced: At the Crossroads of Biology, Politics, and Culture, 1500–1870* (Cambridge: MIT Press, 2007); and Staffan Müller-Wille and Hans-Jörg Rheinberger, eds., *A Cultural History of Heredity* (Chicago: University of Chicago Press, 2012). I tend to agree with John Waller, who looks at longer continuities in ideas about heredity, " 'The Illusion of an Explanation': The Concept of Hereditary Disease, 1770–1870," *Journal of the History of Medicine and Allied Sciences* 57 (2002): 410–448; "Poor Old Ancestors: The Popularity of Medical Hereditariansim, 1770–1870," in *A Cultural History of Heredity II: 18th and 19th Centuries,* ed. Staffan Müller-Wille and Hans-Jörg Rheinberger (Berlin: Max Planck Institute, 2003), 131–144; and *Breeding: The Human History of Heredity, Race and Sex* (Oxford: Oxford University Press, 2015); Porter and Rousseau, *Gout,* 56–59, 72–74, 139–142, 154–155, 160–169; Philip K. Wilson, "Erasmus Darwin and the 'Noble' Disease (Gout): Conceptualizing Heredity and Disease in Enlightenment England," in Müller-Wille and Rheinberger, *Heredity Produced,* 133–154; Erasmus Darwin, *Zoonomia; or, the Laws of Organic Life,* vol. 1 (London: J. Johnson, 1794), 498. On Darwin and hereditary disease, see Wilson, "Erasmus Darwin and the 'Noble' Disease," and Philip K. Wilson, "Erasmus Darwin on Human Reproductive Generation: Placing Heredity within Historical and *Zoonomian* Contexts," in *The Genius of Erasmus Darwin,* ed. C. U. M. Smith and Robert Arnott (Burlington, VT: Ashgate, 2005), 113–132.

4. Roxann Wheeler, *The Complexion of Race: Categories of Difference in Eighteenth-Century British Culture* (Philadelphia: University of Pennsylvania Press), 21–28. See also Mary Floyd-Wilson, *English Ethnicity and Race in English Drama* (Cambridge: Cambridge University Press, 2006), part I; Dror Wahrman, *The Making of the Modern Self: Identity and Culture in Eighteenth-Century England* (New Haven: Yale University Press, 2005), 83–126; Clarence J. Glacken, *Traces on the Rhodian Shore: Nature and Culture in Western Thought from Ancient Times to the End of the Eighteenth Century* (Berkeley: University of California Press, 1967), 501–705. The term is "soft hereditarianism," associated with the work of Carlos López-Beltrán. See "Forging Heredity: From Metaphor to Cause, a Reification Story," *Studies in the History and Philosophy of Science* 25, no. 2 (1994): 211–235, and "Medical

Origins of Heredity," in Müller-Wille and Rheinberger, *Heredity Produced,*
105–132; Kevin Siena, "Pliable Bodies: The Moral Biology of Health and
Disease," in *A Cultural History of the Human Body in the Enlightenment,* ed.
Carole Reeves, 33–52 (Oxford: Berg, 2010); Mark Harrison, *Climates and
Constitutions: Health, Race, Environment and British Imperialism in India,
1600–1850* (Oxford: Oxford University Press, 1999); and Mark Harrison,
*Medicine in an Age of Commerce and Empire: Britain and Its Tropical Colonies,
1660–1830* (Oxford: Oxford University Press, 2010), 64–88. Harrison's argument is also important for the current discussion because he makes the case
that when beliefs in biological racism came, theories of predisposition played
a significant role. "These physiological differences manifested themselves
most clearly in the susceptibility of whites and blacks to different diseases,
and in the different course taken by those diseases in persons of the two
races." "The Tender Frame of Man: Disease, Climate, and Racial Difference
in India and the West Indies, 1760–1860," *Bulletin of the History of Medicine*
70, no. 1 (1996): 68–93, 83. See also Alan Bewell, *Romanticism and Colonial
Disease* (Baltimore: Johns Hopkins University Press, 1999), 27–65. Indeed,
Suman Seth's new study emphasizes the centrality of the putrefactive paradigm to eighteenth-century constructions of race and disease and lends
considerable support to the current argument. Unfortunately, it came out as
this book was going to press and thus cannot be engaged: *Difference and
Disease: Medicine, Race, and the Eighteenth-Century British Empire*
(Cambridge: Cambridge University Press, 2018).

5. Andrew S. Curran, *The Anatomy of Blackness: Science and Slavery in an Age of
Enlightenment* (Baltimore: Johns Hopkins University Press, 2011); Christina
Malcolmson, *Studies of Skin Color in the Early Royal Society* (Burlington, VT:
Ashgate, 2013), esp. 75–76; James Delbourgo, "The Newtonian Slave Body:
Racial Enlightenment in the Atlantic World," *Atlantic Studies* 9 (2012):
185–208; Justin E. H. Smith, *Nature, Human Nature, and Human Difference:
Race in Early Modern Philosophy* (Princeton: Princeton University Press, 2015);
Wendy Churchill, "Bodily Differences: Gender, Race, and Class in Hans
Sloane's Jamaican Medical Practice, 1687–1688," *Journal of the History of Medi-
cine and Allied Sciences* 60, no. 4 (2005): 391–444, 435; Thomas Trapham, *A
Discourse of the State of Health in the Island of Jamaica* (London, 1679), 112–122.

6. Atkins included the following among causes of the distemper in Africans:
"By their Sloth and Idleness the Blood becomes more depauperated; and
those recrementitious Humours bred from it, that Exercise would throw off
through the proper secretory Organs, are here disposed towards the weakest

Part, which in the Generality of Negroe Slaves I take to be the Brain." John Atkins, *The Navy Surgeon; or, practical system of surgery* (London: J. Hodges, 1742), 366. Atkins should not be confused with those doctors of similar names John Aikin and John Aitken, explored earlier. Norris Saakwa-Mante, "Western Medicine and Racial Constructions: Surgeon John Atkins' Theory of Polygenism and Sleepy Distemper in the 1730s," in *Race, Science, and Medicine, 1700–1960*, ed. Bernard Harris and Waltraud Ernst, 29–57 (London: Routledge, 1999).

7. Edward Long, *The History of Jamaica*, vol. 2 (London: T. Lowndes, 1774), 336, 356, 403–404, 433–436, 505–596. On Long see Howard Johnson, Introduction to Edward Long, *The History of Jamaica* (Montreal: McGill-Queens University Press, 2002), i–xxv; Wheeler, *Complexion of Race*, 209–233; Suman Seth, "Materialism, Slavery, and *The History of Jamaica*," *Isis* 105, no. 4 (2014): 764–772; Sean Quinlin, "Colonial Bodies, Hygiene, and Abolitionist Politics in Eighteenth-Century France," in *Bodies in Contact: Rethinking Colonial Encounters in World History*, ed. Tony Ballantyne and Antoinette Burton, 107–121 (Durham: Duke University Press, 2005), 113.

8. Long, *History of Jamaica*, 2: 86, 265, 412, 415, 505–506, 533; and Edward Long, *History of Jamaica*, vol. 1 (London: T. Lowndes, 1774), 318.

9. James Grainger, *An Essay on the More Common West India Diseases* (London: T. Beckett, 1764), 7–8, 15–16, 19, 21, 31, 34, 42–44, 50, 53, 55–56, 60, 62–63, 77; also James Grainger, *Essay on the More Common West India Diseases* (Edinburgh: Mundell and Longman, 1802), 29–31.

10. On yellow fever see the contributions to J. Worth Estes and Billy G. Smith, eds., *A Melancholy Sense of Devastation: The Public Response to the 1793 Philadelphia Yellow Fever Epidemic* (Canton, MA: Science History Publications, 1997); Thomas A. Apel, *Feverish Bodies, Enlightened Minds: Science and the Yellow Fever Controversy in the Early American Republic* (Stanford: Stanford University Press, 2016); J. H. Powell, *Bring Out Your Dead: The Great Plague of Yellow Fever in Philadelphia in 1793* (1949; rpt. Philadelphia: University of Pennsylvania Press, 1993). On theories of black immunity see especially Rana A. Hogarth, *Medicalizing Blackness: Making Racial Difference in the Atlantic World, 1780–1840* (Chapel Hill: University of North Carolina Press, 2017), 17–47. For a discussion that connects Philadelphia's experiences with the disease to the sorts of concerns about urban filth and hygiene explored in this book see Kathleen Brown, *Foul Bodies: Cleanliness in Early America* (New Haven: Yale University Press, 2014), 195–211.

11. Colin Chisholm, *An Essay on the Malignant Pestilential Fever Introduced into the West Indian Islands from Boullam, on the coast of Guinea, as it appeared in 1793* (London: C. Dilly, 1795), 35–36, 83–84, 94, 99–101, 130–133, 145, 220–221. Chisolm said of "negroes" that "the disease did not spread much among them, nor was it marked with the fatality which attended it when it appeared among the whites" (97). Also Harrison, *Medicine in an Age of Commerce*, 105, 111.

12. Rush's passage is oft-quoted. See for example, Mariola Espinosa, "The Question of Racial Immunity to Yellow Fever in History and Historiography," *Social Science History* 38, nos. 3–4 (2014): 437–453, 441–442, and Joanna Brooks, *American Lazarus: Religion and the Rise of African American and Native American Literatures* (Oxford: Oxford University Press, 2003), 157. Curran, *Anatomy of Blackness*, 121–127; Quinlan, "Colonial Bodies," 108–112; Winthrop Jordan, *White over Black: American Attitudes toward the Negro, 1550–1812* (Chapel Hill: University of North Carolina Press, 1968), 517–521, 528; Benjamin Rush, "Observations Intended to Favour a Supposition That the Black Color (As It Is Called) of the Negroes Is Derived from the Leprosy," *Transactions of the American Philosophical Society* 4 (1799): 289–297; and Ibram X. Kendi, *Stamped from the Beginning: The Definitive History of Racist Ideas in America* (New York: Nation Books, 2016), 128–129. Harrison similarly shows that early-nineteenth-century doctors like James Johnson attributed blackness to "permanent hereditary jaundice." Mark Harrison, "Pathology, Physiology, and Race," in *Medicine in an Age of Commerce*, 89–115, esp. 95, 98–99, 111–112.

13. The intersectional scholarship on gender and race in the Enlightenment is considerable. Sample works include Schiebinger, *The Mind Has No Sex?;* Londa Schiebinger, *Nature's Body: Gender in the Making of Modern Science* (New Brunswick, NJ: Rutgers University Press, 1995); Felicity Nussbaum, *Torrid Zones: Maternity, Sexuality, and Empire in Eighteenth-Century English Narratives* (Baltimore: Johns Hopkins University Press, 1995); Felicity Nussbaum, *The Limits of the Human: Fictions of Anomaly, Race, and Gender in the Long Eighteenth Century* (Cambridge: Cambridge University Press, 2003); Kathleen Wilson, *The Island Race: Englishness, Empire, and Gender in the Eighteenth Century* (London: Routledge, 2002); Malcolmson, *Studies of Skin Color*, 113–168; Susan Lettow, ed., *Reproduction, Race, and Gender in Philosophy and the Early Life Sciences* (Albany: SUNY Press, 2014); and for the sixteenth and seventeenth centuries Kim Hall, *Things of Darkness: Economies of Race and Gender in Early Modern England* (Ithaca, NY: Cornell University

Press, 1995). Anne McClintock, *Imperial Leather: Race, Gender, and Sexuality in the Colonial Context* (London: Routledge, 1995); Wahrman, *Making of the Modern Self,* 145–153.

14. Wheeler demonstrates the profound attention stadial thinkers devoted to levels of commercial development among different races. *Complexion of Race,* 176–233.

15. Silvia Sebestini, *The Scottish Enlightenment: Race, Gender, and the Limits of Progress* (New York: Palgrave Macmillan, 2013), offers the most comprehensive survey of stadial theory and its implications for race. See also Wheeler, *Complexion of Race,* 176–233, esp. 181–190. On four stages theory and conjectural history more generally, see Ronald Meek, *Social Science and the Ignoble Savage* (Cambridge: Cambridge University Press, 1976), 131–176, Robertson quoted on 140; Robert Wolker, "Anthropology and Conjectural History in the Enlightenment," in *Inventing Human Science: Eighteenth-Century Domains,* ed. Christopher Fox, Roy Porter, and Robert Wolker, 31–52 (Berkeley: University of California Press, 1995); and most recently Frank Palmeri, *State of Nature, Stages of Society: Enlightenment Conjectural History and Modern Social Discourse* (New York: Columbia University Press, 2016). For example, Kames presents hunger as the most powerful force driving racial advancement. Throughout his chapter "Progress Respecting Food and Population" he presents peoples in lower stages of development prompted to change because of hunger. Describing how hunting nations developed into farming ones, he writes: "Men will always be hunters, till they be forced out of that state by some overpowering cause. Hunger, the cause here assigned, is of all the most overpowering and the same cause, overcoming indolence and idleness, has introduced manufactures, commerce and variety of arts." Obviously, the similarity to discourses about the idle poor is noteworthy. Henry Home, Lord Kames, *Sketches of the History of Man* (Edinburgh: A. Strahan, 1788), 1: 98, and see more generally 85–115; also Adam Ferguson, *An Essay on the History of Civil Society* (London: T. Caddel, 1773), 18–19, and John Millar, *Observations Concerning the Distinction of Ranks in Society* (London: J. Murray, 1779), 3–5. The insight about the historicity of Enlightenment thought is usually attributed to Michel Foucault's *The Order of Things* (New York: Pantheon, 1970). For a summary of the implications of this mode of thought when applied to imperialism and race see Dorinda Outram, *The Enlightenment,* 3rd ed. (Cambridge: Cambridge University Press, 54–66, 109–111).

16. Ferguson, *Essay on the History of Civil Society,* 32, 43, 135–136, 141; Kames, *Sketches of the History of Man,* 3: 66–119. It is worth pointing out that when

Kames sought to compare Europeans to savages on the question of hygiene, he chose to highlight the declining rates of plague in Europe as evidence of the advancement of European civilization from its savage roots. This, of course, would have suggested to readers that the different levels of fever and plague between rich and poor so frequently remarked at home could serve as a key marker of a similar quasi-racial distinction between them, a distinction that his chapter on the poor would have gone a long way to support (2: 323–325). His comments on the predisposition of the wealthy to gout and other diseases in his chapter "On Luxury," and on the progress represented by Spanish calls for increased provisions of privies to protect Spaniards "habituated to dirt" against "putrescent particles of air," further demonstrate the ways in which medical debates—specifically those pertaining to class and disease—informed his thought. Moreover, when discussing workhouses he references jail fever directly: "A poor-house tends to corrupt the body no less than the mind. It is a nursery of diseases, fostered by dirtiness and crouding" (2: 118–119, 138–139, 328). Millar, *Observations Concerning the Distinction of Ranks*, 3–5. Millar repeatedly linked poverty to barbarism, as in the section entitled "The effects of poverty and barbarism, with respect to the condition of women." 17–56. Adam Smith, *An Inquiry into the Nature and Causes of The Wealth of Nations* (Dublin: Whitestone et al., 1776), 1: 286, 2: 247; Thomas Hobbes, *Leviathan, or the Matter, Form, and Power of a Common-Wealth Ecclesiastical and Civil* (London: Andrew Crooke, 1651), 62 (my emphasis); David Cannidine, *Ornamentalism: How the British Saw Their Empire* (Oxford: Oxford University Press, 2002). Meek also usefully charts the roots of eighteenth-century stadial thought about the role of property accumulation in the ideas of seventeenth-century thinkers like Grotius and, of course, Locke: *Social Science and the Ignoble Savage*, 14–23.

17. Samuel Stanhope Smith, *An Essay on the Causes of the Variety of Complexion and Figure in the Human Species* (London: John Stockdale, 1789), 15–17, 20, 49. My emphasis. It is also useful to note that he included diseases among the essential heritable characteristics of ethnic groups, claiming that a race's "figure, stature, complexion, features, diseases, and even powers of the mind, become hereditary" (91). On debates about the role of bile see Harrison, *Medicine in an Age of Commerce*, 106–107.

18. Stanhope Smith, *Essay on the Causes of the Variety of Complexion and Figure*, 27–28, 61–64, 82. Rana Hogarth notes that the same distinction between domestic and field laborers was invoked to explain the aforementioned presumptions about black immunity to yellow fever. She cites William

Wright's 1797 treatise on the diseases of the West Indies, which asserted a constitutional distinction between "house-servants" and "field Negroes," with the latter immune but the constitutions of the former rendering them more akin to whites and thus susceptible. Note that Wright here seizes on the sense of disease susceptibility acting as preexisting quality of bodies. "People of colour, and Negroes, are in a manner totally exempted from this disease, except such as are employed as house-servants, and fare the same as white people. . . . But why the yellow fever should attack some, and not others, can only be accounted for in this way,—that in order to receive or resist contagion, men's bodies and minds must be in particular state; and that field Negroes should not be liable to it is to me inexplicable. They, however, have their epidemics, from which white people are exempted." Quoted in Hogarth, *Medicalizing Blackness*, 34.

19. Stanhope Smith, *Essay on the Causes of the Variety of Complexion and Figure*, 15–17, 25–27; Brooks, *American Lazarus*, 160.

20. Stanhope Smith, *Essay on the Causes of the Variety of Complexion and Figure*, 26–27, 57, 69. He extended the point to other nations of Europe and the East. "A similar distinction takes place between the nobility and peasantry of France, of Spain, of Italy, of Germany. It is even more conspicuous in many of the eastern nations, where a wider distance exists between the highest and the lowest classes of society. The *naires* or nobles of Calicut, in the East Indies, have . . . been pronounced a different race from the populace." The former are distinguished by "manly beauty," while the "poor and laborious [are] exposed to hardships, and left, by their rank, without the spirit or the hope to better their condition, are much more deformed and diminutive in their persons, and in their complexion, much more black" (56–58). Wheeler has noted that Samuel Johnson similarly framed Scottish Highlanders' poverty as a key element of their savagery. *Complexion of Race*, 192–203. See also H. M. Hopfl, "From Savage to Scotsman: Conjectural History in the Scottish Enlightenment," *Journal of British Studies* 17, no. 2 (1978): 19–40, and Mary Poovey, *A History of the Modern Fact: Problems of Knowledge in the Sciences of Wealth and Society* (Chicago: University of Chicago Press, 1998), 249–263.

21. Stanhope Smith, *Essay on the Causes of the Variety of Complexion and Figure*, 39–40, 50–51, 56, 88–90, 95.

22. Ibid., 72–73, 75. The last passage comes from James Cook, *A Voyage to the Pacific Ocean*, vol. 3 (London: W. and A. Strahan, 1784), 126. In fact, Smith did not quote the whole passage. Cook's original claim brings us back to the

issue of disease, because he pointed not only to the superior beauty of elite Pacific Islanders but to their superior health, noting that those who he called "the lower sort" were distinguished by their susceptibility to diseases, in this case skin ailments. Cook elsewhere defines the *Erees* as "Chiefs" or "Great chiefs," whom he contrasts with "the lower class," for example, 141, 153.

23. Louis Chevalier, *Labouring Classes and Dangerous Classes of Paris in the First Half of the Nineteenth Century* (1958; New York: Howard Fertig, 1973); Gareth Stedman Jones, *Outcast London: A Study in the Relationship between the Classes in Victorian Society* (Oxford: Clarendon, 1971), 127–130; Engels quoted in George W. Stocking, *Victorian Anthropology* (London: Macmillan, 1987), 213–214; Tocqueville quoted in Asa Briggs, *Victorian Cities* (Berkeley: University of California Press, 1993), 115; Henrika Kuklick, *The Savage Within: The Social History of British Anthropology, 1885–1945* (Cambridge: Cambridge University Press, 1991), esp. chapter 3, "Civilization and Its Satisfactions," 75–118; Alastair Bonnett, "How the British Working Class Became White," *Journal of Historical Sociology* 11, no. 3 (1998): 316–340. Gertrude Himmelfarb connects such constructions of the poor directly to Chadwickian public health reforms. *The Idea of Poverty: England in the Early Industrial Age* (New York: Knopf, 1984), 323–360. Greta Jones similarly connects eugenics and Edwardian public health policies targeting the working class. *Social Hygiene in Twentieth-Century Britain* (London: Croom Helm, 1986). While Dorothy Porter responded that such connections may have been more muted, she concedes that wider popular discourses indeed applied eugenic conceptions of degeneration to the working class frequently. " 'Enemies of the Race': Biologism, Environmentalism, and Public Health in Edwardian England," *Victorian Studies* 34, no. 2 (1991): 159–178, 161–163; Judith Walkowitz, *City of Dreadful Delight: Narratives of Sexual Danger in Late Victorian London* (Chicago: University of Chicago Press, 1992), 195; John V. Pickstone, "From Ferriar's Fever to Kay's Cholera: Disease and Social Structure in Cottonopolis," *History of Science* 22 (1984): 401–419, 408, 415; Pauline Mazumdar, *Eugenics, Human Genetics, and Human Failings: The Eugenics Society, Its Sources and Its Critics in Britain* (London: Routledge, 1992); G. R. Searle, *Eugenics and Politics in Britain, 1900–1914* (Leiden: Noordhoff, 1976), esp. 50–66; and G. R. Searle, "Eugenics and Class," in *Biology, Medicine, and Society, 1840–1940,* ed. Charles Webster, 217–242 (Cambridge: Cambridge University Press, 1981).

24. Daniel Bender, " 'A Foreign Method of Working': Racial Degeneration, Gender Disorder and the Sweatshop Danger in America," in *Sweatshop*

USA: The American Sweatshop in Historical and Global Perspective, ed. Daniel E. Bender and Richard A. Greenwald, 19–36 (New York: Routledge, 2003); Daniel Bender, *Sweated Work, Weak Bodies: Anti-Sweatshop Campaigns and Languages of Labor* (New Brunswick, NJ: Rutgers University Press, 2004); and Samuel Kelton Robert Jr., *Infectious Fear: Politics, Disease, and the Health Effects of Segregation* (Chapel Hill: University of North Carolina Press, 2009), esp. chapter 2.

Index